T0093852

TELe-Health

Series Editors
Fabio Capello
North Cumbria University Hospitals
Cumberland Infirmary
Carlisle, UK

Giovanni Rinaldi
Ospedali Riuniti Marche Nord
Pesaro, Italy

Giovanna Gatti
European Institute of Oncology (IEO)
Milan, Italy

Recent advances in technology and medicine are rapidly changing the face of health care. A revolution is occurring in diagnosis and treatment thanks to the implementation of instrumentation and techniques deriving from engineering and research. In addition, a cultural conversion is taking place in which geographical and social boundaries are about to be overcome, resulting in enhanced availability and quality of care. Telemedicine has been considered a possible means of improving health care worldwide that is likely to change the way in which doctors deal with patients and diseases. While various restraints continue to limit the application of telemedicine in different settings and different areas of health, the innovations emerging from eHealth and telecare could stimulate a great leap forward for medicine, provided that some basic rules are taken into consideration and followed. In this series, diverse aspects of tele-health – preventive, promotive, and curative – will be covered by leading experts in the field with the aim of realizing the full potential of the new and exciting technological solutions at our disposal.

More information about this series at https://link.springer.com/bookseries/11892

Tanupriya Choudhury • Avita Katal
Jung-Sup Um • Ajay Rana
Marwan Al-Akaidi

Editors

Telemedicine: The Computer Transformation of Healthcare

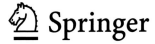 Springer

Editors
Tanupriya Choudhury
School of Computer Science
University of Petroleum and Energy
Studies (UPES)
Dehradun, Uttarakhand, India

Jung-Sup Um
Department of Geography
Kyungpook National University
College of Social Sciences
Daegu, Korea (Republic of)

Marwan Al-Akaidi
Vice President for Research and Innovation
American University in the Emirates
Dubai International Academic City, Dubai,
United Arab Emirates

Avita Katal
School of Computer Science
University of Petroleum and
Energy Studies (UPES)
Dehradun, Uttarakhand, India

Ajay Rana
Amity University
Uttar Pradesh, India

ISSN 2198-6037   ISSN 2198-6045   (electronic)
TELe-Health
ISBN 978-3-030-99456-3   ISBN 978-3-030-99457-0   (eBook)
https://doi.org/10.1007/978-3-030-99457-0

This Springer imprint is published by the registered company Springer Nature Switzerland AG
The registered company address is: Gewerbestrasse 11, 6330 Cham, Switzerland

Foreword

Telemedicine has been used to improve patient outcomes for more than 50 years. Telemedicine, a state-of-the-art concept, utilizes the advanced technologies to accommodate healthcare services in the remote areas. Initially, the tele-based healthcare services were thought to be "fortuitous future" for the medical federations and associations, but with the incoming of vivacious and apex technologies; it has become a successful reality today. Telemedicine enables advanced healthcare systems electronically which improves patient health care. This system reduces infrastructure costs and is useful in providing healthcare services at home, understaffed areas such as rural health centers, ships, trains, and airplanes.

This book provides an overview of the innovative concepts, methodologies, and frameworks that will increase the feasibility of the existing telemedicine system. With the arrival of advanced technologies, telehealth has become a new subject requiring a new understanding of IT devices and how to utilize them to fulfill health needs. The book discusses topics such as the basics of Telemedicine to help the readers understand the technology from ground up, details about the infrastructure and communication technologies to help readers in gaining deeper insights into the technology. This book also discusses the details about the use of IoT and cloud services along with the use of blockchain technology in Telemedicine. This book provides in-depth knowledge of Telemedicine with detailed information about the use of machine learning and computer vision techniques for the proper transmission of medical data keeping in mind the bandwidth of the network. This book will be a readily accessible source of information for the professionals working in the area of information technology as well as the healthcare sector.

Praveen Kumar
Amity University Tashkent
Uzbekistan

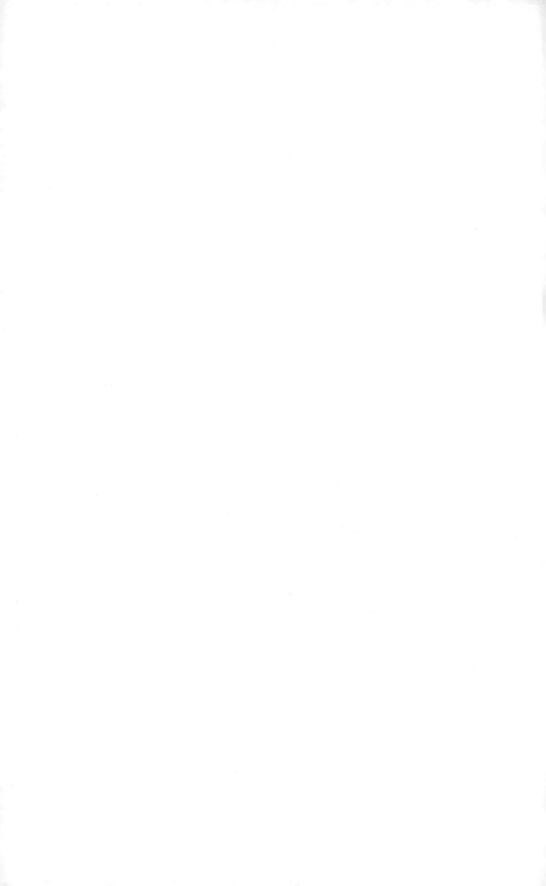

Preface I

In a world of fast growth in medical devices, clinical advances, data analytics, and information technology, there is a rising interest in engineering approaches to healthcare delivery. Recent advances in digital health technologies (e.g., electronic health records, health monitoring, and wearable devices) are not only transformative for reengineering care processes and improving healthcare outcomes such as care quality and patient safety but can also have a significant socioeconomic impact. Industry 4.0 has ushered in a new era in the manufacturing industry. In a similar way to manufacturing, healthcare delivery is on the verge of a fundamental shift into the new era of smart and connected healthcare, dubbed HealthCare 4.0. Telemedicine is the use of electronic communications and software to offer therapeutic services to patients who are unable to visit a doctor in person. Telemedicine technology is commonly used for follow-up visits, chronic disease management, medication management, specialist consultation, and a variety of other clinical services that may be given remotely via secure video and audio links. Early in the COVID-19 pandemic, telehealth utilization skyrocketed as consumers and providers looked for safe methods to access and administer care. This book gives an overview of the novel concepts, techniques, and frameworks that will improve the viability of the current telemedicine system. With the introduction of new technology and the advancement of internet access, telehealth has evolved into a new subject that necessitates a new understanding of IT devices and how to use them to meet health requirements. The book consists of 23 chapters based on telemedicine and its different use cases. Each chapter will give detailed information about telemedicine. We have divided the book into two parts, in Part I, telemedicine infrastructure and potential of blockchain have been introduced from Chapter 1 to Chapter 11. And in Part II, the methodologies and applications of telemedicine have been presented for better understanding.

Chapter 1, **"Telemedicine and Its Role in Innovating the Provision of Healthcare,"** describes telemedicine as an important tool for advancement, with the current focus on cost control strategies and meeting patient needs. It discusses tremendous opportunities and obstacles in pharmacy and other healthcare professions.

Chapter 2, **"Infrastructure and System of Telemedicine and Remote Health Monitoring,"** includes the technology developments in the field of telemedicine including the role of QoS, interoperability, and adaptability for the users. The chapter will also go over by realizing the barriers towards telemedicine. The growth towards remote health monitoring is listed through various applications along with its impact on the environment.

Chapter 3, **"Infrastructure and Systems of Telemedicine,"** discusses in detail the infrastructure of telemedicine services and remote health monitoring.

Chapter 4, **"Patient–Physician Relationship in Telemedicine,"** focusses on the communication established between physician and patient and its transformation due to digitization. The issues involved in the new communication processes allowed by telemedicine that can transform into powerful obstacles are discussed and reflections on how to keep the relevance of the patient–physician relationship alive are included.

Chapter 5, **"Smart Health Monitoring System,"** proposes a smart health monitoring system (SMS) based on machine learning techniques in order to reduce the high rate of false alarms and detect the relevant ones. It takes profits of the advantages of the k-prototypes method and an improved version of support vector machines (SVM) consisting of the real-time SVM (RTSVM).

Chapter 6, **"Machine Learning Techniques for Big Data Analytics in Healthcare: Current Scenario and Future Prospects,"** discusses various platforms that can handle healthcare data along with different algorithms based on machine learning techniques. The chapter reviews different big data lifecycle challenges like storage, processing, data sharing, security, privacy, etc. The study also presents and implements a framework for big data analytics that can be used for real-time disease prediction showcasing diabetes.

Chapter 7, **"Efficient Analysis in Healthcare Domain Using Machine Learning,"** focusses on the intelligence that is used by machine learning for the healthcare domain and providing accurate results for the prediction on the patient's condition with the healthcare dataset in python language.

Chapter 8, **"Choice of Embedded Processor for IoT-Based Teleradiology Applications and a Pilot Study on Need for Portable Teleradiology System in Rural Areas,"** focuses on investigating the need of portable embedded system for teleradiology application in rural areas and choice of appropriate processor for IoT-based teleradiology application in rural areas. The outcome of survey reveals the problems faced by rural area hospitals and scan centers for the transfer of medical images in an authenticated manner.

Chapter 9, **"Providing Efficient e-Healthcare System: Web-Based Telemedicine System,"** focuses on the importance of e-Healthcare systems and what all problems it aims to solve. It also talks about the design and working of various efficient telemedicine systems for managing diseases in detail.

Chapter 10, **"Potential of Blockchain in Telemedicine,"** provides an introduction to telemedicine and blockchain technology along with the use of blockchain technology in telemedicine. A framework for remote health monitoring integrated with blockchain is proposed. The chapter discusses various research challenges faced in the blockchain technology integration with telemedicine.

Chapter 11, **"Security and Privacy Issue in Telemedicine: Issues, Solutions, and Standards,"** presents the issues, standards, and solution for major security and privacy concern in using telemedicine systems.

Dehradun, Uttarakhand, India   Tanupriya Choudhury
Dehradun, Uttarakhand, India   Avita Katal
Daegu, Republic of Korea   Jung-Sup Um
Noida, Uttar Pradesh, India   Ajay Rana
Dubai, United Arab Emirates   Marwan Al-Akaidi

Preface II

Telemedicine can be an appealing alternative to traditional acute, chronic, and preventive treatment, and it has the potential to enhance clinical results. Telemedicine is projected to continue to shift healthcare delivery from the hospital or clinic to the home in the developed countries. Telemedicine will mostly be employed in applications that connect providers stationed at health centers, referral hospitals, and tertiary centers in the poor world or in places with insufficient infrastructure. Its future will be determined by three variables: (1) human aspects, (2) economics, and (3) technology. Technology-related behaviors influence change at the individual, corporate, and social levels. Personnel shortages and declining third-party reimbursement are major drivers of technology-enabled healthcare in the developed world, notably in home care and self-care. Prior to the advent of COVID-19, telemedicine was already being hailed as a possible game changer—a diverse sort of treatment that may make life simpler, particularly for older patients and those living in remote locations. Telemedicine allows for contact-free consultations, which eliminate the need for clinicians to endanger themselves or others. If a patient becomes unwell, a virtual appointment can give advice, test appointments, and, if necessary, a prescription. The majority of telemedicine implementations include virtual consultations; however, the technology may go beyond video conferencing to include the implementation of more tailored care solutions. Researchers are also working on ways to distribute dosages and medicine combinations that take into account individuals' genetic and biological makeup. Telemedicine is more convenient for both healthcare providers and patients. It avoids crowded waiting rooms and long waits; patients can receive care in the comfort of their own homes and visit a physical place only when necessary for testing or other procedures that need face-to-face interaction. Meanwhile, healthcare practitioners can give diagnostic and consulting services on their own time. This means they do not have to miss work because they're isolated owing to an exposure risk, for example, or because of transportation concerns. This book provides an overview of new concepts, methodologies, and frameworks that will improve the viability of today's telemedicine system. Telehealth has grown into a new issue with the advent of new technology and the growth of internet connectivity, necessitating a new understanding of IT equipment and how to use them to satisfy health requirements. The book is divided into 23 chapters that address telemedicine and its many applications. Each chapter will provide in-depth information regarding telemedicine.

Chapter 12, **"Virtual Diet Counseling as an Integral Part of Telemedicine in COVID-19 Phases,"** focusses on the awareness of proper nutrition and in-clinic diet counseling that has already proved their indispensability almost everywhere, primarily in urban areas and in COVID-19 crisis.

Chapter 13, **"Telemedicine and Healthcare Ecosystem in India: A Review, Critique and Research Agenda,"** gives conceptual footing for various modes of telemedicine in terms of its accessibility, applicability, adaptability, affordability, and accountability across geographical regions of the country. The study found that in all telemedicine as a strategy for better use and access to healthcare system has a significant role particularly in the post-pandemic times and also as a futuristic policy measure for optimal allocation of the healthcare system to underserved rural and remote areas of the country.

Chapter 14, **"Methodologies for Improving the Quality and Safety of Telehealth Systems,"** aims at overcoming the limitation of present market scenario and providing the efficient way of communication between user and doctor with the help of blockchain technology in cloud-based medical system.

Chapter 15, **"Application of Bioinformatics in Telemedicine System,"** explains various health services that can be provided remotely using bioinformatics.

Chapter 16, **"Role of Telemedicine in Children Health,"** gives detailed information about the financial impact of pediatric telemedicine and the infrastructure of telemedicine. The chapter also goes into the detail of the various applications of pediatric telemedicine and concludes with the barriers and the future of pediatric telemedicine.

Chapter 17, **"Telemedicine: The Immediate and Long-Term Functionality Contributing to Treatment and Patient Guidance,"** discusses the utilization of telemedicine and its stratification. It also discusses in detail how it is now appropriate for healthcare practitioners and patients who are self-isolating to lessen COVID-19 disease transmission.

Chapter 18, **"Web Application Based on Deep Learning for Detecting COVID-19 Using Chest X-Ray Images,"** presents a web application based on a deep learning technique to examine the X-ray image of patients.

Chapter 19, **"Telemedicine in Healthcare System: A Discussion Regarding Several Practices,"** discusses how Telehealth is rising as a successful and economical arrangement for safety measure, avoidance, and treatment to stem the spread of COVID-19. It also covers details on several practices in telemedicine.

Chapter 20, **"Telemedicine: Present, Future, and Applications,"** aims for a detailed investigation of the evolution of the concept of telemedicine in VHA and private sector and reviews the use of current telemedicine. The goals of telemedicine are to provide quality and cost-effective health services to everyone.

Chapter 21, **"Security and Privacy Issues in Telemedicine: Solutions and Standards,"** deals with healthcare data security and privacy concerns both in information systems and non-information systems fields like public health, health information, law, and medicine.

Chapter 22, **"Perception of Parents About Children's Nutritional Counseling Through Telemedicine,"** is a study conducted to understand the perceptions of parents as it relates to children's eating and exercise habits.

Chapter 23, **"Telemedicine: A Future of Healthcare Sector in India,"** is an attempt to explore telemedicine's trajectory and evolution in India; what would be telemedicine's general perception? How will this perception shape the future of telemedicine in India? Can a technology-based healthcare system be able to compensate for human presence and touch?

Dehradun, Uttarakhand, India   Tanupriya Choudhury
Dehradun, Uttarakhand, India   Avita Katal
Daegu, Republic of Korea   Jung-Sup Um
Noida, Uttar Pradesh, India   Ajay Rana
Dubai, United Arab Emirates   Marwan Al-Akaidi

Contents

Telemedicine and Its Role in Innovating the Provision of Healthcare

Shalini Yadav ⓘ, Saurav Yadav ⓘ, Vikash Chaturvedi ⓘ,
Preeti Verma ⓘ, Aishwarya Rajput ⓘ,
and Ratnesh Chaubey

1.1 Introduction

1.1.1 Telemedicine: As a Facilitator of Access and Affordability in Healthcare

Inadequate medical infrastructure and unbalanced resource sharing have become a worldwide concern as a part of the medical concerns and patients' high standards for healthcare facilities [1]. To counter this, China's governing party has introduced a modified medical policy initiative for the healthcare sector, strengthening the incorporation and use of telemedicine systems [2]. Telemedicine is a rapidly emerging service that seeks to enhance accessibility, productive, and cost-effective healthcare, notably in context of the present COVID-19 pandemic and proves to be a powerful tool for reducing patient overcrowding. Telemedicine, according to the ministry of health department, is "the use of automated intelligence and communications systems to convey and sustain patient services by allowing two-way, real-time digital engagement between the patient and a physician at a remote location." As an outcome, telemedicine has the ability to revolutionize healthcare and enhance the integrity and efficacy of healthcare dissemination while also increasing patients' access to specialized information that was antecedently inaccessible or impossible to access [3]. Despite their parallels, telehealth words should not be applied in telemedicine synonymous. Telehealth refers to "as is the distribution of medical services by healthcare practitioners over long distances by the use of the application of information technologies and networking to share accurate and correct information regarding patient evaluations, treatments, therapies, and appointments accessible"

S. Yadav · S. Yadav (✉) · V. Chaturvedi · P. Verma · R. Chaubey
Dr. M.C. Saxena College of Pharmacy, Lucknow, Uttar Pradesh, India

A. Rajput
School of Pharmaceutical Science, RGPV, Bhopal, Madhya Pradesh, India

T. Choudhury et al. (eds.), *Telemedicine: The Computer Transformation of Healthcare*, TELe-Health, https://doi.org/10.1007/978-3-030-99457-0_1

[4]. There have been reported several advantages of using telehealth technologies, particularly in non-emergency / maintenance screening and cases where treatments do not desire direct patient provider contact, such as delivering psychiatric services. Improvements of technology have greatly improved the accessibility and standard of treatment accessible online over the last few decades. Tele-pharmacy serves the same underlying intent but extends to the provision of prescription treatment. The ISRO has also seen the usability of telemedicine which, through its geosynchronous, has networked 22 specialist hospitals and 78 rural and local hospitals all around the sovereign country. This network has provided access to consultations with specialists from specialist medical institutions if there are multiple patients in remote places such as Jammu and Kashmir, Andaman Islands and Nicobar Islands, Lakshadweep Islands, and tribal regions of Central and North-east India. In the field of urban health and visionary disease, ISRO has established access for mobile telemedicine equipment units in villages [5].

Despite this, telemedicine still has to be broadly adopted owing to stringent legislative requirements and a scarcity of supportive payment systems. During the ongoing pandemic, telemedicine offers the potential to extend patient access to effective, minimal therapies, while maintaining clear distance for both healthcare providers and patients' well-being.

1.2   Background of Telemedicine [6, 7]

The use of ancient hieroglyphs and scrolls to exchange knowledge about health-related events like illnesses and diseases can be traced back to the founding of telemedicine. The telephone and the typewriter revolutionized the way patients and doctors exchanged clinical knowledge as the nineteenth century progressed. The telegraph was used during the Civil War to give reports about casualties and to request medical supplies. During the Korean and Vietnam wars, the telephone was accustomed to deploy emergency teams. The television was invented in the 1950s, and the Nebraska Psychological Institute began using videoconferencing for tele-psychiatry in 1959. A big component of telemedicine as it is known today was indeed due to the essential role played by National Aeronautics and Space Administration (NASA). Owing to that with medical attention during space flight, doctors have the ability to monitor astronauts' health status and can provide diagnostic information and medication while in space. Between 1970s and 1980s, NASA has aided the availability of telemedicine facilities in remote areas. The availability of telemedicine services to rural areas was also aided by NASA. Minnesota, New Hampshire, Maine, Alaska, Arizona, and Washington are among the states represented. The Internet revolutionized the way we utilized telemedicine systems in the 1990s. Health image exchange, such as X-rays or MRI, vital signs, ECG, and authentic audio and video interaction, has drastically enhanced due to the Internet. Telemedicine is now more popular than it has ever been, thanks to advances in smartphone and computer engineering. Both patients and caregivers can retain and view medical information with the aid of electronic medical records.

Patients may use these programs to view results, refill prescriptions, and email notes directly to their doctors. Furthermore, synchronous telemedicine, also known as face-to-face telemedicine, helps us to connect with providers in real time using live video. Both patients and caregivers can retain and view medical information with the aid of electronic medical records. Patients may use these programs to view results, refill prescriptions, and email notes directly to their doctors. Furthermore, synchronous telemedicine, also known as face-to-face telemedicine, helps us to connect with providers in real time using live video. We will also post imaging, lab results, and analysis results so that they can be interpreted at a later time.

1.3   Types of Telemedicine

Three major categories can be classified into telemedicine: shop / store and forward, remote surveillance, and immersive (in real time) facilities (summarized in Table 1.1).

Telemedicine is the use of electronic and information technologies when individuals are positioned in separate places to deliver therapeutic services. Telemedicine is one form of this, including medical imagery, video consultancies, remote medical diagnosis and assessments, teletherapy, and drug management (summarized below in Table 1.2).

Table 1.1 Three different types of telemedicine along with their elucidation [8, 9]

Types of telemedicine	Elucidation
1. Store-and-forward telemedicine	• This entails the acquisition of patient records (such as medical photographs) and then transferring the data at a suitable time for offline review to a physician or health professional • No requirement of both sides to be present simultaneously • An adequately designed medical record should be a part of this transition, ideally in electronic form • Instead of a physical inspection the "inventory and forward" procedure allows the clinician to use historical report and audio/visual material
2. Remote surveillance (self-monitoring)	• This procedure is mainly used to treat chronic disorders or certain complications such as cardiac failure, hyperglycemia disease, or asthma • These programs will provide the typical patient encounters with equal clinical benefits, provide patients with increased loyalty • It is economical
3. Immersive telemedicine	• Phone calls, Internet contact, and home visits are indeed examples of extreme encounters between patient and provider • Many tasks, such as history taking, medical examinations, psychological tests, and ophthalmology evaluations, can be performed remotely in the same way that they are in conventional face-to-face appointments • Telemedicine programs that are "clinician interactive" can be less expensive than in-person hospital appointments

Table 1.2 What is telemedicine and what isn't…? [10]

Telemedicine	Characterization
Televisits	Typical patient–provider contact, but through videoconference
Teleconsultation	With or without the involvement of the individual, a consultant in one area brings a case to a specialist in another location
Telemonitoring	Patient's signs or indications are transmitted remotely to a physician team in another area
Tele-interpretation	Radiology and other measures can be performed remotely
Not telemedicine	
Social media	There is no patient–provider interaction, because it isn't traditionally called healthcare
Remote education	There is no patient in this study; it is purely for medical education

1.4   Telemedicine Principles [11]

The Multidisciplinary Telehealth Guidelines Advisory Group has published a collection of telemedicine core principles "to protect clients accessing telemedicine services, to provide a shared ground for healthcare professions, and to offer a framework for analysis of technical requirements, clinical measure, and the need for telemedicine recommendations by professions and government agencies."

The below are the major tenets of telemedicine:

1. In telemedicine, the fundamental principles of ethical ethics must not be changed.
2. The use of telemedicine technology does not necessitate the acquisition of additional licenses.
3. Telemedicine cannot be used by healthcare personnel or practitioners to perform treatments that are not constitutionally or medically licensed.
4. There should be no weakening of technical and clinical requirements.
5. There's more a shortage of documentation, telemedicine practice recommendations should be focused on expert consensus rather than scientific proof.
6. It is relevant to acquire informed consent.
7. Clients' and clinicians' welfare must be assured.
8. Reasonable, accurate, and confidential documentation is needed.
9. The client–practitioner relationship's dignity and clinical importance must be protected.

The creation of these "interdisciplinary" telemedicine concepts did not involve pharmacy. The profession's telepharmacy rules and regulations should be derived from this series of principles.

1.4.1   Prior to Every Telemedicine Appointment, There Are a Few Things to Remember…..[12]

Until engaging in any telemedicine consultation, there are seven factors to remember.

- Context
- Identification of RMP and Patient
- Mode of Communication
- Consent
- Type of Consultation
- Patient Evaluation
- Patient Management

Context: There's no doubt that telemedicine would be appropriate in this situation. Licensed Medical Practitioners should use their professional judgment to determine if a telemedicine consultation is sufficient in a given circumstance or whether a face-to-face assessment is needed in the patient's best interests. Before embarking on any form of health instruction, therapy, or treatment, they should analyze the modes and options available and their relevance for a diagnosis.

1.5   Identification of the Registered Medical Practitioner and the Patient Is Required

- Both the patient and the RMP must be conscious of each other's identities during a telemedicine session.
- It is possible for an RMP to verify a patient's identity by using the patient's first and last names as well as the patient's age and address.
- When prescribing a prescription, the RMP must inquire the patient's age directly, and if in doubt, ask for it to be verified. It would only be allowed if the juvenile was interacting with an expert whose identity had to be validated.
- On prescriptions, websites, electronic correspondence (WhatsApp/ email, etc.) and receipts, etc., any RMP must show the identification number assigned to him by the State Medical Council/MCI.

1.6   Modes of Connectivity and Technologies Included

Telemedicine consultations may be delivered using a variety of tools. Video, audio, and text are the three major modes (chat, messaging, email, fax, etc.). Each of these technological frameworks has its own set of capabilities, disadvantages, and situations in which it may or may not be suitable for delivering a proper diagnosis (summarized below in Table 1.3).

Table 1.3 Different formats of communication: strength and weakness

Modes	Strengths	Weakness
Audio: phones, apps, etc.	• There is no need for a distinct infrastructure • It's simple and fast • Appropriate for emergency situations • Privacy is assured • Interaction in real time	• Not recommended for disorders that necessitate an examination of the epidermis, eyes, or tongue or physical touch are forms of ocular examinations • Patient identity must be more precise, since there is a higher risk of imposters impersonating the actual patient
Video: Telemedicine facility, apps, video on chat platforms, etc.	• RMP will meet with the patient and have a conversation with the caretaker • It is now easier to identify patients • An assessment of the patient is possible	• Is focused on both ends having a high-quality Internet connection; otherwise, the information sharing would be sub-optimal
Text based: Specialized chat-based telemedicine, SMS, websites, messaging systems, e.g., WhatsApp, FB, Messenger.	• Documentation and identification may be a key component of the platform • Suitable for critical situations or follow-ups, as well as second opinions if RMP has more context from other outlets • There is no need for a different infrastructure	• The doctor's or the patient's name is unknown • Text-based experiences are often devoid of verbal signals, in addition to visual and tactile contact
Asynchronous: E-mail, fax, recordings, etc.	• It's convenient and simple to record • There is no prerequisite for a particular program or download	• In the absence of real-time contact, there is no context other than the patient's specifics • Since the doctor will not get the mail right away, there may be a wait

In general, while telemedicine consultation prevents the RMP from infectious diseases, it cannot replace a physical inspection that may involve pulsation, percussion, or exultation; touch and sensation are essential.

Patient Consent: Any telemedicine appointment requires patient consent. Depending on the circumstances, permission may be implicit or explicit:

(a) The permission is implied whether the patient begins the telemedicine appointment.
(b) If the following conditions apply, an explicit medical consent is required:
  • A telemedicine consultation is started by a health nurse, an RMP, or a caregiver.

(c) Explicit agreement can take several different forms. A document, text, or audio/video message may be received by the patient. The patient may express his or her intent to the RMP over the phone or by video (e.g., "Yes, I agree to obtain consultation via telemedicine" or some other clear communication). This must be documented in the RMP's medical history.

Consultation Types: There are two primary types of meetings with patients: the first consultation and the follow-up consultation.

When a patient attempts teleconsultation for the first time and there has been no previous in-person appointment, an RMP can only have a basic knowledge of the patient. However, if the initial consultation is done by video, RMP will be able to make a much better decision and, as a result, will be able to offer much better recommendations, including supplementary prescriptions if appropriate. It's feasible to be extra cautious when treating a patient who has already been examined by the RMP in person, but it's not recommended.

1.6.1 First Consult Means

- This is the patient's first appointment with the RMP; **OR.**
- The patient has previously spoken with the RMP, but it has been over 6 months since their last meeting. **OR.**
- Previous consultations with an RMP had been for different health issues (illustrated below in Fig. 1.1).

1.6.1.1 Follow-Up Consult(s) Means

The patient continues to see the same RMP every time for the same health issue within 6 months of his or her last in-person appointment. Nonetheless,

A follow-up would not be recognized if:

- In addition, there are novel symptoms that are not part of the delivery of the same medical problem.
- RMP has little recollection of the circumstances surrounding prior care and recommendations (summarized below in Fig. 1.2).

1.7 Patient Evaluation

Before making any clinical decision, RMPs must make every attempt to obtain adequate medical knowledge about the victim condition.

- An RMP would use his or her independent conduct to collect the kind and amount of patient data (history/examination findings/investigation reports/past documents, etc.) needed to make proper clinical decisions.

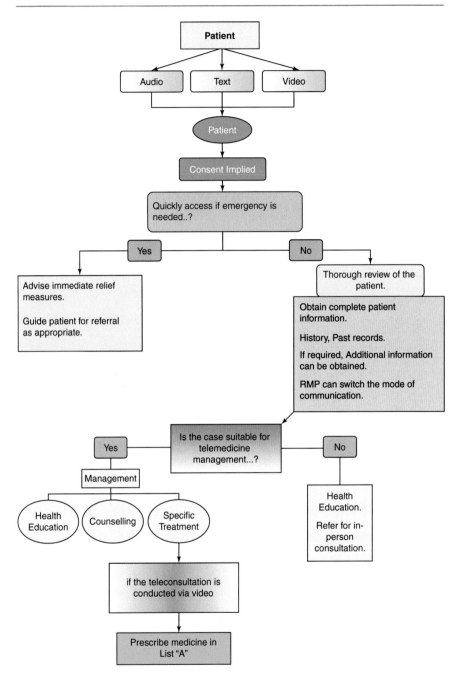

Fig. 1.1 Flowchart for teleconsultation for first consult

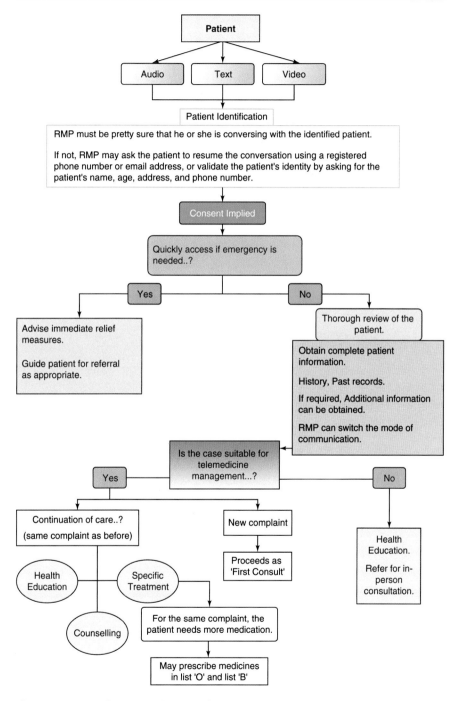

Fig. 1.2 Flowchart for teleconsultation on follow-up consult

- Telemedicine has its own range of drawbacks when it comes to doing a thorough analysis. RMP does not start until a physical assessment can be arranged with an in-person consult where a physical examination is vital evidence for consultation. Wherever possible, the RMP will make the following recommendations based on his or her professional judgment:
- Consultation through video conferencing.
- Another RMP/Health Worker examines the patient.
- In-person consultation.

1.8 Patient Management

If, depending on the form of consultation, the condition can be properly treated by telemedicine, the RMP can continue with a clinical awareness to:

- Assist in educating people about health as required in the situation; and/ or.
- Counseling in relation to a particular psychiatric disorder is given; and/ or.
- Prescribed medicine (summarized below in Table 1.4).

1.8.1 Telemedicine's Challenges and Prospects [13, 14]

Video telemedicine, the Internet, and other telecommunications technology are now being used in the delivery of healthcare, and this trend will continue. One of the most difficult tasks in today's complex, computer-driven environment is to provide recommendations to assist organizations and individuals in developing future strategies. An in-depth review of medical technology innovations by a researcher was recently performed and concluded that within five years, telemedicine-related applications are expected to be in operation. Smartphones, for example, possess the ability to combine the capabilities of a combining a mobile phone for a graphical user interface, allowing people to track telemetry patients while doing other things. These devices have the potential to improve patient safety, promote patient contact among general practitioners, and lower liability by reducing errors caused by poor

Table 1.4 Various aspects of consultation treated by telemedicine

Health education	• An RMP will provide messages about disease prevention and health promotion • An RMP will provide disease treatment and prevention instructions
Counseling	• In addition to dietary constraints, anticancer drug guidelines, hearing aid use, home physiotherapy, and other methods to relieve the underlying problem, patients are offered with practical advice
Prescribing medicines	• The RMP has the clinical discretion to prescribe medications through telemedicine consultation • In order for RMP to prescribe drugs through telemedicine, RMP must be sure that he/ she has gathered enough relevant data regarding the patient's medical state and that the prescribed meds are in the patient's best interests

handwriting. The Internet would almost certainly "conquer all," transforming the living room into a virtual experience. A critical concern is how the healthcare system can react to customer demand for instant access to doctors, goods, services, and facts.

1.8.2 Final Thoughts

Telemedicine's role in future practice is difficult to anticipate due to rapid developments in technology and healthcare. Telemedicine's popularity has grown, and it shows great promise when it comes to increase access to healthcare, encouraging patient disease treatment, and enabling in-between healthcare-visit surveillance.

References

1. AlDossary S, Martin-Khan MG, Bradford NK, Smith AC. A systematic review of the methodologies used to evaluate telemedicine service initiatives in hospital facilities. Int J Med Inform. 2017;97:171–94.
2. Kamsu-Foguem B, Tiako PF, Fotso LP, Foguem C. Modeling for effective collaboration in telemedicine. Telematics Inform. 2015;32(4):776–86.
3. Monaghesh E, Hajizadeh A. The role of telehealth during COVID-19 outbreak: a systematic review based on current evidence. BMC Public Health. 2020;20(1):1–9.
4. Fisk M, Livingstone A, Pit SW. Telehealth in the context of COVID-19: changing perspectives in Australia, the United Kingdom, and the United States. J Med Internet Res. 2020;22(6):e19264.
5. Indian Space Research Organisation (2005) ISRO Annual Report 2004–2005: space applications. Available: http://www.isro.org/rep2005/SpaceApplications.htm. Accessed 27 Dec 2015.
6. Kichloo A, Albosta M, Dettloff K, Wani F, El-Amir Z, Singh J, Aljadah M, Chakinala RC, Kanugula AK, Solanki S, Chugh S. Telemedicine, the current COVID-19 pandemic and the future: a narrative review and perspectives moving forward in the USA. Family Med Commun Health. 2020;8(3):e000530.
7. Hurst EJ. Evolutions in telemedicine: from smoke signals to mobile health solutions. J Hosp Librarianship. 2016;16(2):174–85.
8. Salehahmadi Z, Hajialiasghari F. Telemedicine in Iran: chances and challenges. World J Plastic Surg. 2013;2(1):18.
9. Gibson KL, Coulson H, Miles R, Kakekakekung C, Daniels E, O'Donnell S. Conversations on telemental health: listening to remote and rural First Nations communities. Rural Remote Health. 2011;11(2):94.
10. Serper M, Volk ML. Current and future applications of telemedicine to optimize the delivery of care in chronic liver disease. Clin Gastroenterol Hepatol. 2018;16(2):157–61.
11. Angaran DM. Telemedicine and telepharmacy: current status and future implications. Am J Health Syst Pharm. 1999;56(14):1405–26.
12. Telemedicine Practice Guidelines: Enabling Registered Medical Practitioners to Provide Healthcare Using Telemedicine. [This constitutes Appendix 5 of the Indian Medical Council (Professional Conduct, Etiquette and Ethics Regulation, 2002]; 25 March 2020.
13. Herman WA, Marlowe DE, Rudolph H. Future trends in medical device technology: results of an expert survey. Center for Devices and Radiological Health; 1998.
14. Angaran DM. Telemedicine and telepharmacy: current status and future implications. Am J Health-Syst Pharmacy. 1999;56(14):1405–26.

Infrastructure and System of Telemedicine and Remote Health Monitoring

2

Neha Mehta and Archana Chaudhary

2.1 Introduction

Telemedicine is the collaboration of multiple branches of science that allows the establishment of effective way that reduces the congestion and introduces the improvement in the utilization of medical facilities. The concept of telemedicine offers the aggregation in the medical needs and the patient's expectations. It allows the dual-channel highlighted healthcare system through the implementation of information and communication theory (ICT) and has given a great level of support in the offline traditional outpatient treatment. The important features of the telemedicine have allowed decreasing the terms of geographical variability for diagnosis and treatment. Telemedicine is being successfully practiced in many countries along with various ICT projects involved as technological resources. The telemedicine has allowed the patient access to the expertise specialist who is available at a longer distance through communication media and who is difficult to be physically available. Thus, telemedicine reduces the traveling time and the waiting time from the healthcare management system. However, the core issues including system architecture, interaction with technology, patient and also related to healthcare professional understanding are required to be timely addressed and updated. The telemedicine has served as the solution towards many barriers in the healthcare, for example, access issues, quality of care, cost of care, and depending on the locality from rural to the underserved areas. According to [1], the Institutes of Medicine has published about the telemedicine that the telemedicine is a discrete set of technologies, and is a large heterogeneous collection of related technologies, clinical

N. Mehta (✉)
Chhattisgarh Swami Vivekanand Technical University, Bhilai, Chhattisgarh, India

A. Chaudhary
Department of Biosciences & Environmental Science, Faculty of Science, SGT University, Gurugram, Haryana, India

© The Author(s), under exclusive license to Springer Nature
Switzerland AG 2022
T. Choudhury et al. (eds.), *Telemedicine: The Computer Transformation of Healthcare*, TELe-Health, https://doi.org/10.1007/978-3-030-99457-0_2

13

practices, and different organizational arrangements. But not to be confused between telehealth and telemedicine, from the University of California, Dr. T. Nesbitt has explained that there is a coordination of these both terms, that is, using the technology for the exchange of information with the perspective of providing an improvement in the patient health. However, these terms are being interchangeably used, but they are different. The term "telemedicine" often describes the direct clinical services and health information using telecommunication technology. But the advancement in the speed of communication technology along with the signal processing techniques and cloud computing has given a range of opportunities towards remote healthcare [2]. According to the authors in [3], the telemedicine may also be defined as a "technological take- away" for health services, which is being viewed as a tool towards the healthcare. In the developing countries, like India, the telemedicine tool substantially contributes towards the healthcare facilities by bridging a gap between demand, supply, and utility. The different areas which are involved in the healthcare setup have the different type of electric signals that is required to be transferred between the patient's site and the doctor's site, for example, in the radiology, the imagery is the part of medical report which is required to be transferred, a display-based physical finding of the test reports like ECG and EEG are required to be remotely displayed which may further need interactive or psychiatric examinations. Thus, with the advent of telemedicine, the usefulness of telemedicine is defined in the two different aspects when: (1) there is a physical barrier present between the patient and the physician, and (2) when there is a lack of medical information [4]. The wide range of applications of telemedicine, according to the authors in [5], includes patient care, diagnosis, administering patient care, training and research, sending and receiving of health information, educating healthcare professionals, analyzing X-rays, CT, MRI, and other radiology reports and pathology reports. The medical field is also exploded with many complexes and innovative internet-based medical sites containing enormous information about treatments, diseases, images, pathology, pharmaceuticals, and many more. This forms the part of e-health. According to ATA (American Telemedicine Association), the core word "telemedicine" is defined as the "natural evolution of healthcare of the digital world" [6], and similarly according to WHO, "telemedicine is defined as a delivery of healthcare services by the healthcare professionals using ICT for the exchange of valid information related to treatment, diagnosis and prevention, including research and evaluation and also for the continuous education of the healthcare professionals in the interest of making advancement in the health of individuals and to their communities." Telemedicine can also be defined under an umbrella, i.e., "healing at a distance."

2.2   Literature Review

Factually, the published concept of telemedicine can be traced back in early twentieth century where electrocardiograph data were transmitted over telephone wires [6]. However from the mid of nineteenth century, the use of telegraphy was deployed for the planning and providing of medical care. This usage was done in the American Civil War to order the medical needs and to communicate the casualty list. Later, advancement in the technology has allowed X-ray images to be transmitted through the communication channel. According to the researchers in [7], many areas of Europe and the USA have rapidly implemented telephone for the purpose of communication. However, the communication through radio waves has started by the end of nineteenth century. In 1920, the Seaman's Church Institute, New York, was known to be as the first organization, providing radio-based medical care among five nations till 1938. The modern telemedicine has got started in the earlier of first half of the twentieth century with ECG for the first time getting transmitted through the telephone lines. Later the electrical telegraph has given a kick start to the modern era of telemedicine. According to the review presented by the researchers in [8], the first real-time video consultation was occurred in 1959 at University of Nebraska and the feature of interactive telemedicine was used for transmitting the neurological reports. Afterwards, NASA used telemedicine services in 1985 for the earthquake occurred in Mexico City. With the increase in availability and utilization of information and communication technologies (ICT) the new potentials for healthcare services and delivery have emerged out in new forms which is presented in [9].

However, with the utilization of ICT and replacement of analog forms with digital methods in communication, [10] has raised further popularity in telehealth service. The advancement in internet facilities and web-based applications along with multimedia approach has created new possibilities in delivering healthcare services [7, 11]. If telemedicine is considered as a medical activity performed through a remote or peripheral area, it is facilitated at two fronts, one with the type of mode of communication and secondly with the end users and applicators. With the recent advancements in both directions, horizontally and vertically the applicability of telemedicine is achieving great heights and further getting popularized. Currently telemedicine is utilizing various technologies in different directions and getting customized as per the requirement of end user mentioned in [12].

2.3   General Architecture of Telemedicine: Conventional vs Modern

In the design of conventional medical check-ups, the healthcare seeker needs to be present at the clinic and complete all the formalities like front desk enquiry, registration, and further checking of vital signs like temperature, body weight, blood pressure, and many more. Then, the allotment of time slot in which the doctor or the specialist will be available for his check-up and prescription. This prescription may further include the laboratory tests, further examinations, or may be revisits. As a part of conventional health setup, as shown in Fig. 2.1, the medical records are then updated in the data resource system.

But sometimes there is a non-availability of specialists/qualified doctors/ medical equipment in the healthcare center, and thus unlikely the patients cannot avoid traveling for a long distance to get his medical examination, and sometimes

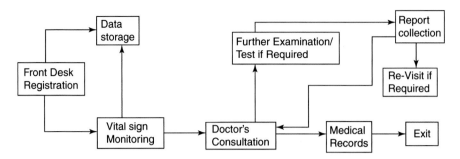

Fig. 2.1 Conventional health setup

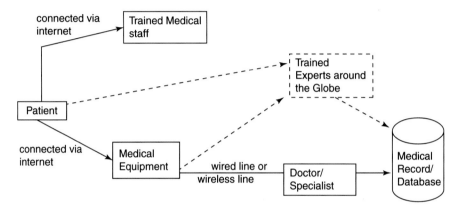

Fig. 2.2 Telehealth Setup

limited facilities or shortage of medical equipment leads the patients to wait for a long time. Thus, always a gap lies between the early and prompt medical examination; the involvement of the ICT (information and communication technology) has allowed filling this gap. ICT has allowed the healthcare facilities to be present at the doorstep through internet. The system allows the specialist to communicate with the patients through videoconferencing and the medical examinations are done with internet-enabled devices called as telehealth setup as shown in Fig. 2.2.

Telehealth allows to provide the multiple and trained expertise for the patients irrespective of the locality gaps. It is a technology driven setup, which uses a basic infrastructure and allows the communication to distant points. This technology has proved as a boon to the remote areas specifically by connecting them to the metropolitan hospitals. It has provided an opportunity to both healthcare professionals and the healthcare seekers to receive high-quality consultations and treatments along with the online pharmacy platforms. The telehealth has provided the advantage of cost saving and effort saving. From the safety point of view, the telemedicine is safer as it saves both the health workers and the patients from contagious infections.

In India, so far there are no specific guidelines nor legislations for the telemedicine practice; however, there were certain provisions under 1956, Indian Medical Council Act, Drugs and Cosmetics Act (1940), Rules (in 1945), Establishment Act (2010), IT Act (2000), and the Rules of Information and Technology (in 2011) governs the IT-based medicine.

For delivering the healthcare using telemedicine, only RMPs (Registered Medical Practitioners) are entitled to deliver the telehealth support, but the RMPs are required to upload the ethical conditions, professionals along with taking care of the limitations and in-person care of the telemedicine.

However, for carrying out the patient consultation, telemedicine needs to be connected either through any of the network topology (LAN, WAN, MAN), telephone, or may be through any of the chatting platforms like Facebook, WhatsApp, etc. or may be through data communication devices like email, fax, etc. However the applicability during the pandemics and disasters are still the challenges before telemedicine.

On the basis of different modes of communication available, the communication in telemedicine may be classified as: Audio, which is done through a simple telephone or any voice-based internet application; video, in which communication is done either through a direct telemedicine platform available with the clinicians or any video chatting applications or platforms; and Text based, which may be done with the help of general text messages or chatting platforms like WhatsApp, messengers, Google Hangout, etc. And it can also be done through asynchronous mode like Fax or emails. On the basis of interaction, the mode of telemedicine could be synchronous or asynchronous. Synchronous interaction is the mode of communication in telemedicine, in which the video or audio or text is used for the exchange of information from both the ends, i.e., for counseling, diagnosis, and/or medication. However, in the asynchronous mode of interaction, the medical reports, supplementary data, lab reports, and radiological investigation report are transmitted that can be accessed anytime as per the convenience.

2.4 Functionality of Telemedicine

There is a wide list of functionalities that are being offered by the architecture of telemedicine. According to the American Journal of Accountable care [13], the telemedicine has allowed to offer a long-term patient healthcare management along with the patient satisfaction feature. It has also happened by increasing the patient convenience by the involvement of information and communication between the patients and the practitioners through different modes like chatting, emails, messages, or videoconferencing. The different functionalities of telemedicine are:

1. Remote Monitoring.
2. (Wired or Wireless) based easy communication
3. Real-time Interaction.
4. Store-and-Forward function.

All these functionalities of the telemedicine require the basic necessity of a communication link, which is to be generated between the healthcare seekers and the professionals. For example: videoconferencing, through which the patient-related data (may be images, audio-video, data) can be transferred to a specialist using store-and-forward functionality. However, remote monitoring devices are also used to intelligently record, transmit, and acknowledge the data for interpretation, suggestion, and feedback.

The functionality of telemedicine may also be dependent upon the episode of the healthcare delivery [14], that is, pre-recorded or real time (also known as real-time healthcare delivery). In pre-recorded, the patient's data is acquired, saved in some format, and it is sent to the doctor for further interpretation. However, in real-time healthcare delivery, the interaction between the patient and the doctor is done at the site; also there is no delay of store and forward.

2.4.1 Services Interlinked

2.4.1.1 Wired/Wireless Connectivity

In order to connect the two distant persons, they are necessarily required to be connected through some media. However, this connection either is a wired connection through connection lines or the wireless connection through the internet with the good bandwidth. This connectivity necessitates the availability of some system like computer system or the mobile phone along with the back-end lines of the electricity.

Further the limitation in this service may be felt with the bi-directional communication, or the satellite connection may be facing extremely slow transfer of data. Thus, a simple communication using email (via SMTP, that is, Simple Mail Transfer Protocol) is one of the robust and most tolerant services that can be utilized.

2.4.1.2 Availability of Information

For the availability of information, the readiness of the available scientific literatures or the evidence of the clinical problems with their treatment are also required to be available, which may sometimes often be considered as a burden to treat a larger amount of research data, which is alone not sufficient and requires the evidence also. This in turn may require the translation or guidance with many of the healthcare workers along with the plenty of time.

2.4.1.3 Knowledge of Computers

Many of the healthcare workers are not happy to use computers in every minute of their life that may be due to their uncompetitiveness or the stress call to their mind. And some of them are with lack of the knowledge due to their less frequency of using computers and lack of technical training. Thus, key personnel of this field like doctors and nurses are still less familiar with most of the computer applications and are in requirement of getting the necessary basic training.

2.4.1.4 Tele-Pathology and Teleradiology

Ronald S Weinstein, in the year 1986, has coined the term called tele-pathologists, in which the pathologists render their services from a distance, where the real examination is done by examining the specimen on the glass side which is only possible through offline and later the images of the patient are electronically transmitted either through the telephone lines, satellites, or high-speed digital lines. However, there exist the chances of losing the originality of the images.

Similarly, in the teleradiology, in which the real images are already in the digital form, the images are collected, and then the process of acquisition and storage is done. Thus, there are less chances of losing the information in teleradiology as compared to tele-pathology.

2.5   Role of QoS

The services which are being offered by telemedicine often help in improving the healthcare and aid to increase the healthcare access by reducing the time and the medical costs for rural areas. By using the functions and specialties of ICT the telemedicine also offers the applications, consultations, and testing in the specialties like dermatology, neurology, general medicine, radiology, etc. In order to maintain the quality of service it should emulate a successful face-to-face interaction and effective consultation process. It is also required that the image, audio, and video transmission quality should be maintained. A need of precision can always be fulfilled through the essential quality of services maintained with respect to the critical medical environment. The ITU-T recommendation (E.800) defines that the QoS is a performance of the collective effect of services that defines the user satisfaction about the service [15]. The researchers have also defined the QoS as the network ability for providing a service with assuring its users about its service level and thus reaching to the QoE (Quality of end user Experience). However, the researchers have also produced a set of parameters that can be used in order to define the capability of the network like latency (delay), bitrate, packet rate, packet ratio, packet loss, jitter, bandwidth, delay intolerance, etc.

The telemedicine services may also be further classified as tele-consultation, tele-monitoring, telediagnosis, tele-education, and tele-data handling. The QoS requirements of these services are presented in Fig. 2.3.

The QoS is the measurement of the network performance at the network layer and the QoE is the measurement of experience on the basis of application operation, at the service layer, and the QoE is defined from the user's perspective, and thus indicating the degree of the application to meet the user needs [16]. Thus, the developmental needs of any network to reach the needs include network availability, latency, data confidentiality, and satisfying the QoS. However, the ubiquitous internet-based health services today have created a great potential to successfully implement the internet-based health services like telemedicine with often faced

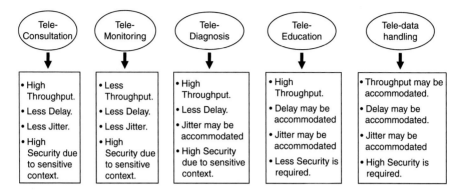

Fig. 2.3 QoS requirements of the telehealth interlinked services

challenges related to real-time transferring of multimedia, real-time storing and for-warding data, and dealing with the large amount of data.

The solutions to such challenges are sought through incorporation of signal pro-cessing techniques, signal integration and signal detection methods.

2.6   Wireless Strategies in Telemedicine

The numerous developments in the healthcare system have a series of wireless strat-egies. The wireless strategies, being used in the health services, allow the patients with diagnosis of their diseases, their treatments, and the related services inside the hospitals and outside the hospitals. To fulfill such conditions, it is required that the advanced technologies must be equipped within the healthcare units, so as to handle the queries and thirst of the patients.

According to the researchers in [17], there is a great breakthrough in 5G technol-ogy as the fifth generation offers the data transfer rate of up to 10 gbps which is between 10- and 100-fold improvement as compared to fourth generation and 4G associated LTE. However, the 5G faces a very low latency, which is less than 1 ms, and a minute response time. The wide bandwidth of 5G has produced a coverage of up to 100% with its connectivity with all the compatible devices leading to develop that ecosystem as an intelligent system, and its real-time connectivity with the mas-sive number of patients and their systems like PCs and mobile wearable devices, along with the massive medical equipment present in that health ecosystem.

In the 2020s, most of the healthcare system is dependent on the fourth-generation mobile networks but the system is facing issues with the reliability, data rate, related latency, and the bandwidth. Thus, with the advent of 5G networks most of the issues will get resolved. According to the researchers in [18], the services of 5G networks are broadly divided into three categories:

(a) Enhanced Mobile Broadband service.
(b) Ultra-reliable low latency communication.
(c) Massive Machine type communication.

The fifth-generation services provide a much enhanced quality of videoconferencing and calling for consultation along with augmented and virtual reality through enhanced mobile broadband. It provides the connectivity between medical things, technically called as IoMT, i.e., Internet of Medical Things through the service called as massive machine type communication. The 5G-based technology also supports the surveillance services through drones on the basis of ultra-reliable low latency communications. However, this technology-based architecture of the healthcare depends upon the layout of the organization in which it is going to be deployed, and there is a requirement of stable, reliable, and secure communication link. The high-speed Wi-Fi network (RF-based technology) with stability in network is preferred and is being popularly deployed in the hospitals. But the medical equipment those are prone to the electromagnetic interference have been found to be unsporting the usage of Wi-Fi networks.

2.7   Emerging Technologies in Telemedicine

The healthcare industry has always been under the stress for the delivery of internal as well as external care. The overburdening of doctors, rising demands of healthcare delivery, declining reimbursements, and the day-to-day rising risk of patients and their care takers are the reasons to enhance the advent of technologies in the healthcare sector. With the variable large-scale technology and smart technology, the healthcare industry has been able to mitigate the challenges that were being faced.

Some of the technologies which have got a huge role for shaping the broad spectrum of telemedicine are listed as follows:

2.7.1   Artificial Intelligence

The artificial intelligence has found its scope in telemedicine in various areas of telemedicine like tele-pathology, tele-psychiatry, teleradiology, tele-dermatology, etc. There are also many care-assisting apps along with the predictive methodologies that allow remote screening of the patients and thus automatically generating the prescriptions in the form of EHR (Electronic Health Record). In this way, AI-based EHR are aiding to improve the remote monitoring of the patients. Another example is artificial intelligence-based healthcare chatbots. These chatbots are gaining the huge popularity around the globe, due to their feature of making a conversation with the patients, asking their symptoms, and answering their queries along with scheduling the appointments with the healthcare specialists, if required.

2.7.2   Tele-Robots

Tele-robots are successfully running as they are making the real-time monitoring and care of the patients easier and accurate. They remotely monitor the patients and alert the clinicians in case of any adverse condition of the patient. The development of robots has also led to their applications in ICUs, wards, OTs, and many more.

2.7.3   A-V Reality

This domain includes the reality-based service like mixed reality that includes the practices of both augmented realities along with the virtual reality. This increases the accuracy in the remote diagnosis.

2.7.4   Internet of things

This technology enhances the focus of telemedicine, by making the better interaction in the healthcare network and to increase the access for in-depth data. The advantage of using IoT in telemedicine is that, it forms a closed-loop among the medical equipment and devices, then it transfers the data to the EHR (Electronic Health Record) system which helps the doctors in remote assessment and the diagnosis of the patient's disease.

2.7.5   Three-Dimensional Printing

The three-dimensional printing has got a great application in the field of tele-surgery. It allows the healthcare professionals to get the 3D contents of the scans of the patient's organs. That can be further analyzed through 3-D printed models for making error-free diagnosis of the patient's disease and further to develop the treatment plans. This 3D print technology is a great way to the prosthetists without any physical presence of the patient.

2.8   Factors Facilitating the Development of Telemedicine

Telemedicine is more compatible for those who are user friendly to technology. The adoption of telemedicine may be increased further by facilitating the development of telemedicine while considering various factors. Towards promoting and facilitating the telemedicine we need to make it more user friendly by providing training and awareness to all concerned even up to the end user. Among various factors for adopting, also exists a financial constraint which may be overcome by providing initial grants to start-up centers and make it more comfortable in the terms of financial concerns. Financial concerns may also be mitigated by using already existing infrastructure and other administrative backups to further enhance the adoption of telemedicine. However, proper digital infrastructure and organizational effort increase the acceptance of health technology on the one hand and it may otherwise become a barrier in adopting the telemedicine on the other hand. The quality of healthcare providers also affects the telemedicine outcome, and if taken into account depending upon their inputs and efforts, they may be provided with the incentives accordingly which may enhance the efficiency of physician and also promote healthy collaboration among physicians and specialist [19]. The performance of

Fig. 2.4 Factors
facilitating the use of
telemedicine

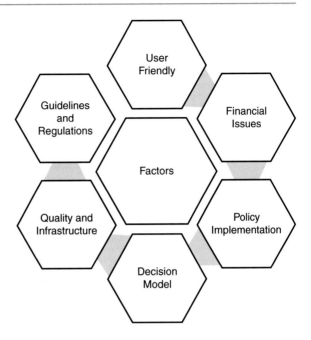

healthcare providers, service providers, and social influencers also acts as an influencing factor for the acceptance of telemedicine service which is totally concerned with the physician efficiency; therefore, physician should be considered in center before designing of setting up of a healthcare system. A concern which should be dealt at utmost is lack of clear guidelines and regulations which require further flexibility and innovation to respond to legal, technical, and political issues and challenges. There is also a need for clear ethical guidelines for cases which intentionally or unintentionally happen during telehealth services either at user end or service provider end. The policy implication if done properly helps in accessing patient support system by means of assistive technology and also plays an important factor in adopting the telemedicine [20]. Other issues may be dealt by considering proper decision model and reimbursement model so that the users do not face any issues while dealing with financial concerns. The factors which facilitate the telemedicine are shown in Fig. 2.4.

2.9   Barriers Towards Telemedicine

Telemedicine is of great benefit in terms of convenience, easy availability, and cost saving, as it is tailored to meet the patient's need and well-being along with satisfaction of both physician and healthcare receiver. However, some hidden and unidentified barriers make the patient cautious to fully adopt telemedicine as compared to interacting in physical mode. The barriers to telemedicine may be broadly classified on the basis of different grounds such as spatial, temporal, organizational, and infrastructure. There are certain basic considerations which need to be identified in a proper manner to make the telemedicine successful. And specifically, the IT barriers which include certain technical barriers are required to be identified and prompted to make it more user friendly.

Broadly, the barriers towards telemedicine are classified into two categories, i.e.:

(i) Internal Barriers.
(ii) External Barriers.

The internal barriers include patient's reluctance, which may be due to helplessness in using online platform by the patient or either due to internet accessibility or poor signals. Slow speed and inadequate knowledge of using equipment are also one of the major challenges in adopting the telemedicine. However poor body language and communication and hesitation in sharing personal details also play a major role in resisting the use of telemedicine. As patients do not feel comfortable in sharing their personal details online which may be due to their insecurity perception or may be due to the reason that patient does not feel comfortable as in case of direct conversation in physical mode to the health practitioner.

Other similar barriers include eye-to-eye contact or inability of expressing their feelings and also due to the patient's negative perception about the information of their disease or privacy may be hampered.

Thus, the communication and understanding of skills and behavior plays a major role. Sometimes, the patients feel more comfortable in face-to-face interaction for sharing and providing their information, which can even be understood by the physician easily through their body language.

Another concern for adopting telemedicine is due to its delivery and accessibility. In terms of service delivery, the related methods in telemedicine follow two different systems, that is, the gatekeeper-based system and the dual-channel-based service system. The gatekeeper system depends on only store and forward (in the form of medical images or bio-signals) for consultation as presented by researchers in [21], where the practitioner is directly in face with patient. However in the case of remote patient monitoring, the physician monitors the patient by using wearable devices or digital videos through online platforms to monitor the parameters and thus providing prescription to the patient. In dual-channel service system, both abovementioned techniques are included in real-time mode where the physician interacts through videoconferencing to the patient in real-time monitoring. There is more complexity in the later scenario as this service needs Tally-specialist or local telehealth center so that they can act as a bridge between patient at the remote area and the physician or consultant at the other end.

However, the external barriers include problems related to the outsourcing services. The telemedicine involves outsourcing for consultation, financial planning, and information technology to decrease the congestion in hospitals and thus improves the utilization of medical services by excluding financial constraints. The external barriers which are related to outsourcing services include slow internet speed, poor network signal, difficulty in operating the system, lack of organizational support in case of public health subcenters, and even some home obstructions while consulting the physician which may be due to interference of other members at home. The lack of standards and guidelines for regulating the telemedicine practices or ethical guidelines including the nature and extent of the doctor-patient relationship is also the part of external barriers. Another outmost barrier is the cyber-attack which influences the overall data of healthcare provider as well as patient in a single run. The detailed classification of barriers towards telemedicine is shown in Fig. 2.5.

Healthcare providers need to be associated with IT vendors and the communication from them needs to be improved as private security and confidential in today's scenario. Technologies are emerging for providing good faith telehealth services to patients but still some lacuna is there in safekeeping issues due to legal and other cyber concerns. The cyber issue is a major concern in the application of telemedicine. Secondly, switching from one platform of telemedicine to the other for better service and feasibility may also pose a problem for the service providers in keeping the records at a common platform with full confidentiality. However, there has been a limited research towards the adoption and successful implementation of these modalities of healthcare services in the form of telemedicine.

Another barrier is being faced due to the up-gradation of the technology and there is a lack of technical knowledge at both the ends, that is, at the patient level and the physician level. As the physician and patient compares the telehealth services, a multiple new developments and new online platforms are coming at a faster pace, which seems to be more lucrative and easily accessible so it also creates havoc at the users end. The study of sufficient literatures, related research studies and their comparison is a task of unending patience. It also creates dilemma in using the

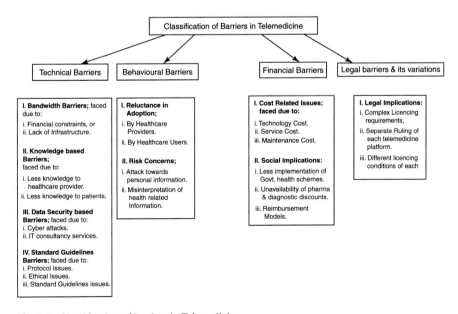

Fig. 2.5 Classification of barriers in Telemedicine

telemedicine. Thus, the group of healthcare managers, clinicians, healthcare practitioners, and other telemedicine proponents are required to be addressed for the uncertainties connected with using different telemedicine platforms and for the key adopter groups about the major uncertainties that is being faced by the physician's center on quality of medical care, quality of health services, and complexity issues. Additionally, there are many legal uncertainties which are being faced by the physicians. For patients, the key towards adoption of the uncertainties includes coordinating with the new way of interacting with healthcare providers and the concern over security, confidentiality, and privacy. However, the administrators may also face the concern over cost-effectiveness, money reimbursements, and other legally connected procedures. Finally, payers are also required to ensure that endorsement of telemedicine procedures may actually result in low healthcare service costs and to increase the penetration of telemedicine in the existing healthcare system along with the addressing of necessary issues. It is also due to lack of standards and guidelines which help in regulating the telemedicine practices or ethical guidelines effecting the nature and extent of the doctor-patient relationship.

The telemedicine has paved roads to produce improved health outcomes by providing access to health services at doorstep even at remote areas and for those who are not willing to come to the health center. Telemedicine has not only reduced the travel time but also releases financial burden not only for patients or healthcare seekers but also to the physicians and healthcare providers (administrator and other stack holders). There is a perceived assumption that telemedicine is more vulnerable towards security, confidentiality, and privacy, so it needs to be facilitated for addressing these concerns which might be due to lack of technology advancements and effectiveness. Patients usually face issues related to adjustment to the technology; however physicians are more concerned towards legal uncertainties, quality of service, and other complexities including software technologies. These technical barriers need to be dealt with proper care and utmost so that the successful rate for implementing telemedicine may be achieved.

2.10   Application in Remote Health Monitoring

Application of telemedicine in remote health monitoring is becoming boon for the patient especially where geographical distance acts as a major barrier. The geographical distance between healthcare providers and healthcare uses becomes a barrier if not projected properly. Therefore, it should be reflected in such a way that geographical distance instead of being a barrier becomes boon for quality assurance of health services as it incorporates all specialists at a single platform. Getting health facilities through telemedicine at doorstep is gaining popularity and becoming game changer in health sector. They are proving better in terms of access to healthcare facilities as a person or a patient sitting in a remote area gets advice facilities from a specialist by sitting at its own place. It is highly acceptable in case of heart patients and accidental and casualty cases, where the integration of various specialists makes better health decisions for the patient and improves the quality of care. It also allows the patients, physicians, and other healthcare providers to consult each other especially if they get stuck in a dilemma or need super-specialist advice without increasing competitiveness among stakeholders. It provides peace of mind not only to physicians but also to the patients as they get into communication with their health providers and thus improving the overall support system. The education and knowledge regarding new advancements in medicine and feedback from different researches for a case helps in strengthening the medical system. It is also applicable in providing and continuing medical education in order to promote the physician's knowledge who otherwise faces difficulties while practicing in physical mode due to time constraints. Telemedicine is proving boon for dementia patients, diabetic patients, hypertension cases, and also in clinical trials as it is providing in depth to providers. Cancer patients having high mortality rate are also relying on telemedicine as lots of advancement in techniques and diagnosis is taking place every day which needs to be updated along with the advanced technology to cope up with new emerging cases.

2.11 Conclusion

The expanding use of new health technologies is endorsing the development of more and more customized telemedicine platform. With the latest advancement in broad band spectrum, access to healthcare services, collaborative work between teams of healthcare providers and users has made a remarkable change in the improving efficiency of the telemedicine. Telemedicine has opened new horizons by facilitating collaboration among medical healthcare providers and users. The shift from conventional health setup to telehealth setup is inevitable with the application and integration of new technologies for information exchange, broadening access, cost-effective, customized and improved convenience to healthcare system.

However the challenges remain opened and needs to be dealt to implement it efficiently and effectively.

References

1. Jane L, Wilson LS. Telehealth trends and the challenge for infrastructure. Telemed e-Health. 2013;19(10):772–9.
2. Raza M, Le MH, Aslam N, Le CH, Le NT, Le TL. Telehealth technology: potentials, challenges and research directions for developing countries. In: IFMBE Proceedings, vol. XX. Singapore: Springer; 2016. p. 233–6.
3. Sood SP, Bhatia JS. Development of telemedicine technology in India: "Sanjeevni"—an integrated telemedicine application. J Postgrad Med. 2005;51(4):308–11.
4. Perednia DP, Allen A. Telemedicine technology and clinical applications. JAMA. 1995;273(6):483–8.
5. Senbekov M, Saliev T, Bukeyeva Z, Almabayeva A, Zhanaliyeva M, Aitenova N, Toishibekov Y, Fakhradiyev I. The Recent progress and applications of digital technologies in healthcare: a review. Hindawi Int J Telemed Appl. 2020;2020:8830200. https://doi.org/10.1155/2020/8830200.

6. Breen GM, Matusitz J. An evolutionary examination of telemedicine: a health and computer-mediated communication perspective. Soc Work Public Health. 2010;25(1):59–71.
7. Craig J, Patterson V. Introduction to the practice of telemedicine. J Telemed Telecare. 2005;11:3–9.
8. Chellaiyan VG, Nirupama AY, Taneja N. Telemedicine in India: where do we stand? J Family Med Prim Care. 2019;8(6):1872–6.
9. Shirzadfar H, Lotfi F. The evolution and transformation of telemedicine. Int J Biosen Bioelectron. 2017;3(4):303–6. https://doi.org/10.15406/ijbsbe.2017.03.00070.
10. Merrell RC. Changing the medical world order with technological advances: the future has only begun. Stud Health Technol Inform. 2004;104:25–9.
11. Currell R, et al. Telemedicine versus face to face patient care: effects on professional practice and health care outcomes. Cochrane Database Syst Rev. 2000;(2):CD002098. https://doi.org/10.1002/14651858.CD002098.
12. Burg G, editor. Telemedicine and teledermatology. Curr Probl Dermatol Basel, Karger. 2003;32:6–11. https://doi.org/10.1159/000067346.
13. Alvandi M. Telemedicine and its role in revolutionizing healthcare delivery. Am J Account Care. 2017;5(1):e1–5.
14. Le EW. télécardiogramme [The telecardiogram]. Arch Int Physiol. 1906;4:132–64.
15. Malindi P. QoS. In: Telemedicine. Telemedicine techniques and applications; 2014. p. 119–38. Book chapter.
16. Díez IT, Alonso SG, Hamrioui S, Coronado ML, Cruz EM. Systematic review about QoS and QoE in telemedicine and eHealth services and applications. J Med Syst. 2018;42:182.
17. Li D. 5G and intelligence medicine—how the next generation of wireless technology will reconstruct healthcare? Precision Clin Med. 2019;2(4):205–8.
18. Janjua MB, Duranay AE, Arslan H. Role of wireless communication in healthcare system to cater disaster situations under 6G vision. Front Commun Netw. 2020;1:1–10.
19. Menachemi N, Burke DE, Ayers DJ. Factors affecting the adoption of telemedicine—a multiple adopter perspective. J Med Syst. 2004;28(6):617–32.
20. Nebeker C, Torous J, Ellis RJB. Building the case for actionable ethics in digital health research supported by artificial intelligence. BMC Med. 2019;17(1):137.
21. Wang X, Zhang Z, Zhao J, Shi Y. Impact of telemedicine on healthcare service system considering patients' choice. Hindawi Discr Dynam Nat Soc. 2019;2019:7642176. 1–16

Infrastrucuture and Systems of Telemedicine

Abhineet Anand ⓘ, Naresh Kumar Trivedi ⓘ,
Vinay Gautam ⓘ, and M. Arvindhan ⓘ

3.1 Introduction

In order to prepare for this projected rise, telehealth systems should be scalable to absorb a growing quantity of data and technological components. The aim of the article is to identify the qualities that contribute to the success of a telehealth infrastructure programme. Health companies need to evaluate and build a programme that contains six critical elements of a successful telehealth infrastructure—including IT infrastructure, software, hardware, IoT, scalable design, and patient and data protection [1].

Telemedicine was discovered at the beginning of the twentieth century. This was one of the first documented occurrences of electrocardiographic data being transferred to a clinic around one kilometre away over telecommunications cables from a physiological laboratory in the early twentieth century.

One of the first instances published in the early twentieth century was that electrocardiographic data was transferred to a clinic about one mile away by telephone wires from one physiology lab. In 1964, they built a telemedicine link to provide healthcare services at a milestone of 112 miles from the campus of Norfolk State Hospital [2].

Telemedicine was also woven into many programmes supported and carried out by the US government with a much wider scope. For example, the STARPAHC space technology initiative (STARPAHC) enables the US government to provide

A. Anand (✉) · N. K. Trivedi · V. Gautam
Chitkara University Institute of Engineering and Technology, Chitkara University,
Rajpura, Punjab, India
e-mail: abhineet.anand@chitkara.edu.in; nareshk.trivedi@chitkara.edu.in;
vinay.gautam@dituniversity.edu.in

M. Arvindhan
Galgotias University, Greater Noida, Uttar Pradesh, India

Native Americans living on a remote Tohono O'odham reserve in Arizona, USA, with healthcare through the connection of patients in mobile support units in remote areas with doctors in Sells and Phoenix hospitals in Arizona, USA, and the telecommunications system was found to take a lead in crisis management, involving about 500,000 homeless people, during the 1985 earthquake in Mexico City and then again in 1988 after the Soviet Armenia earthquake, when estimated deaths exceeded 50,000. Thus, the age of global telemedicine collaboration began [3].

Telemedicine found its function in disaster management as well, with the telemedicine services first being employed by NASA after the Mexico City earthquake in 1985 and again in 1988 when the Soviet Armenia Earthquake, with an estimated 50,000 homeless victims, was affected. The age of worldwide telemedicine cooperation for a greater humanitarian goal began thus [4].

It is essential to first comprehend five causes leading to the emergence of this telehealth infrastructure. These are among the challenges of expanding care for the elderly in the US: changing rules, chronic illnesses, receptiveness of patients and suppliers, and financial restrictions. Understanding how new and existing telehealth systems can help organisations prepare for an increase in telehealth services [1].

Population changes in the United States are the initial driving force of telehealth expansion. According to the CDC, by 2030, 71 million people will be reached, or almost 20% of the population, compared with just 12% in 2000 in the US and more than 65 in the United States. This increase is particularly apparent among those aged 80 and older, from 9.3 million in 2000 to 19.5 million in 2030. Those organisations will have to reconsider how they give care as a result of this transformation. They employ technology to augment and enhance productivity and treatment to satisfy this rising requirement [5].

As more healthcare companies use telehealth programmes, it is more vital than ever to ensure that all telehealth IT infrastructure needs are satisfied. Dropped connections, security risks, and unsatisfied clinicians and patients will be experienced by organisations that do not adequately maintain their telehealth network. When contemplating telehealth, the first thing businesses should do is develop a plan that takes into account both current and future expectations. The network must be scalable, and upgrades must be done in a realistic timeframe that takes into account budget and available resources. Telehealth is a common tool used by rural hospitals to treat patients who are unable to visit their doctors on a regular basis [6]. Because rural places frequently have fewer connections than urban regions, telehealth infrastructure is essential for their support. Telehealth programmes, according to the ONC, must include:

- Broadband internet access is required for the transmission of audio and video data. Rural businesses may have trouble connecting to or securing inexpensive, dependable broadband connection.
- Imaging technologies or peripherals: These gadgets are the backbone of telehealth, allowing healthcare providers to see and hear patients from afar. Heart and lung sounds can be transmitted to remote providers using digital stethoscopes, for example.

- **Technical support staff**: Members of the technical support team can assist with questions about telehealth programmes.
- **Staff training:** Telehealth technology requires staff training, which can take some time. Organisations should think about whether modifications to process are necessary and train accordingly.

Telehealth is about ensuring consistent connections regardless of the clinician's or patient's location. According to Children's Mercy Hospital in Kansas City, any telemedicine programme will fail due to unreliable connectivity [7].

Organisations must address how professionals and patients connect to the network safely from a distance. Entities must also be aware of the strength of the connection in order to enable video streaming and other data-intensive telemedicine requirements. To compensate for the lack of coverage, organisations must put up telemedicine systems that may use whichever signal is the strongest and most dependable in the region. This may necessitate multiple contracts with several cellular or wireless carriers in various places, which can be particularly complicated for big healthcare companies. According to a recent Research and Markets analysis, the telehealth industry is estimated to reach almost 64 million by 2022 as more healthcare companies use telehealth services. Telemedicine use is growing due to a rising population, more people living with chronic diseases, and a need for individuals to consult with professionals who aren't in their region. According to the different research papers and reports, telehealth aids interoperability efforts by providing a conduit for diverse healthcare professionals to communicate on the same platform [8].

3.2 Projects for Early Telemedicine

Telemedicine has existed since the 1960s, and many of the challenges previously widely acknowledged by today's suppliers, academics and regulators (e.g. Bashshur [9]; Bashshur et al. [10]; Bashshur and Lovett [11]; Park and Bashshur [12]), have been discussed [13]. In offering a historic perspective on telemedicine for readers, Bashshur's and his colleagues' work from the 1970s are of special use. The early telemedicine projects were demonstration programmes backed by different government entities. Many of these projects were aimed to explore the ability to diagnose and treat people in remote regions via interactive telecommunications. Nearly no projects have been autonomous, and a large majority of them have been reduced by the reduction in financing. The only longstanding programme in North America is Memorial University of Newfoundland (House and Roberts 1977; House and Keough 1992) [14–16].

The first telemedicine initiative, financed by the National Institute for Mental Health, was linked to Norfolk State Hospital and the University of Nebraska School of Medicine [17–20]. Funded in 1967 by the US Public Health Service, Boston Logan's Airport and Massachusetts General Hospital established an interactive network [21]. In both city and rural areas the programmes for prisons, nursing homes and other sites were established in the early 1970s (Armstrong et al. 1975) [13, 22].

Advanced healthcare was one such endeavour applied to rural Papago (STARPAHC) [3]. The NASA, equipped with the Lockheed, supported STARPAHC and carried out the Papago Indian Reservation in Arizona, with assistance of the Indian Health Service. STARPAHC used telecommunications technology developed by NASA in concert with transportable Health Units to monitor the physiological functions of astronauts in space [23, 24]. Research has demonstrated that current technologies can be utilised to provide rural healthcare [13, 25].

The project received mixed ratings among STARPAHC providers. They enjoyed the improved availability to some treatments, but they considered the equipment to be expensive, unreliable, and sometimes unneeded for patient diagnosis and care [26]. Justice and Decker [27] determined that "no consistent variations in quality of treatment delivered by the locations equipped with telemedicine systems and manned by community health medics as compared to the other clinics staffed by physicians within the same health system" in their report on the study [26].

The first crucial step in establishing a network that can serve the connectivity and security requirements of telehealth is to start with a strong and realistic strategy. Reaching out to telehealth suppliers and working with them when planning infrastructure changes can help firms develop a stable network with no gaps after a strategy has been formed. Clinicians can no longer rely on WiFi or a single cellular carrier to exchange the information they need to treat and connect with patients since they are no longer trustworthy or secure. Telemedicine organisations must have a scalable IT infrastructure to enable telehealth [28].

3.3   Chronic Illness

Health professionals and their patients are still worried about the treatment of chronic diseases. The instances of chronic disease persisting 3 months or more are cancer, type 2 diabetes and chronic cardiac illness. Studies have shown that over 40% of the US' population—or 133 million individuals—is chronically affected. The amount is projected to reach 157 million by the end of the decade [4, 14].

In fact, over half of everyone has a chronic disease and over a third of people have many chronic conditions. A total of seven diseases with an annual economic impact of 1.3 trillion dollars include cancer, diabetes, hypertension, stroke, heart disease, lung disease and mental illness.

As a result, medical practitioners are looking for ways of reducing the price of chronic disease treatment without losing quality of service. Therapy, including remote monitoring of patients, can assist to reduce the cost of chronic disease treatment. Doctors and professionals may use living video and audio, mobile devices and other intelligent digital technology to treat the health of a patient remotely, reducing the necessity for personal consultations. Find out more about the benefits of telemedicine in chronic illness management [29].

3.3.1 Enhance Access to Specialist Care

There is a shortage of access to healthcare for many patients across the country, as most people in the world reside in rural regions. They can travel long miles to a medical doctor or specialist in rural areas, both of whom are uncommon. It is difficult to go long distances to a doctor to patients with chronic diseases. They could have restricted mobility or long periods of time with trouble sitting still. Chronic patients are also subject to specialty care in order to deal with their symptoms, which in some areas of the nation may be hard to come by, making it harder for them to see their doctor often [30].

Patients, including experts, can communicate from their own homes via telemedicine with care specialists. In this way, access to specialised therapy is improved while the expense of treatment is decreased or even eliminated through cuts or eliminations in travel costs. Patients who don't regularly see their healthcare providers may get sicker. However, telemedicine may simplify the therapy required by the patients [31].

3.3.2 Monitor Changes in Patient Lifestyle

In addition to medications and other therapy, patients with chronic illness may have to modify their lifestyles if they wish to improve their condition. Nutritional changes, cessation of smoking and greater exercise are all possible. However, if some patients are left on their own devices, they might struggle to stay to this kind of treatment regimens and aggravate their sickness.

But if a patient's state can be remotely monitored by healthcare practitioners, they can find out whether the patient meets the needs for therapy. If a patient overflows and does not get enough exercise, he or she can stroll on the Bluetooth scale to monitor how their weight altered. Doctors may use mobile devices and live video and audio to remind patients to take medicine, to eat well and to be active [32].

3.3.3 Real-Time Triage of New Symptoms

Sometimes a new symptom may occur in patients with chronic illnesses. This might be an indicator of a failing health or the start of a new chronic illness. Some people can wait until their health gets worse, particularly if they need to travel large distances for an individual session before visiting their healthcare practitioners.

However, patients may visit their healthcare provider promptly via telemedicine on a new symptom, as it occurs in real time. If the disease is significant, the doctor will either propose a modification in therapy or encourage you to attend a local emergency room. That guarantees that the patient be taken care of promptly rather than ignore the symptoms together [33].

3.3.4   Reduce Readmissions in Hospitals

81% of all hospital admissions are chronic disease patients, making them one of the most expensive treatment areas. However, if physicians and specialists can monitor a patient's health from distance, they can help the patient manage his treatment scheme and reduce the chance of being hospitalised again. This reduces care costs for both patients and caregivers. Telemedicine may be used by doctors to ensure patients follow certain lifestyle changes and respond to prescription requests and quickly assess new symptoms to minimise hospital readmission rates [34].

UPMC Health Plan, which serves 3.4 million Pennsylvanians, noticed a reduction in the number of congestive heart failure patients admitted to observation units after instituting a telemedicine service. Medicare enrollees who took part in the study were 71% less likely than non-participants to require a stay in an observation unit.

Telemedicine can help patients manage chronic diseases better by keeping them in touch with their doctors, minimising the likelihood of treatment lapses and hospital readmissions. Many patients will have difficulty consulting with a healthcare physician if these digital tools are not available. Visit in Touch Health to learn more about the advantages of telemedicine in chronic disease management [35].

3.4   Policy Change Required for Telemedicine in Context with Present Scenario

The third factor for the increase in telehealth is a shift in the laws of regulation. More than 150 pieces of legislation on telehealth have been submitted during the past 5 years. As a result of these policy developments, the compensation for telehealth and digital healthcare improves.

As of late 2018, 50 countries have reimbursed live video under Medicaid fees for services, a payment structure focused on care rather than on quality of treatment, according to the Center Government of India Connected Health Policy. Only 11 countries pay for storage, involving the collection and electronic transmission of clinical information to a second site for examination [29].

The lack of money has been recognised as the main obstacle to telehealth implementation; any reimbursement policy adjustments will increase adoption rates and fuel. The new virtual inspection plan of the Medicare & Medicaid Services Centers may indicate a change in policy on telehealth [36].

3.4.1   Telemedicine in India

Since the nation is so huge and highly inhabited, telemedicine plays an important role, especially as medical facilities are concentrated more in cities than in rural India which make the majority of the people accessible and accessible to remote locations.

A pilot project in Telemedicine in 2001 marked a modest start in telemedicine for the Indian Space Research Organization (ISRO) which connected Chennai's Apollo Hospital with the rural Apollo Hospital in the hamlet of Aragondia, Andhra Pradesh 5 district in Chittoor. All contributed to the development of telecom services in India by ISRO, the Department of Information Technology, the Ministère des Affaires Etrangères, the Ministry for Hygiene and Family Welfare, as well as state administrations. It has 45 remote and rural hospitals and 15 specialised hospitals and has connected them to it [37].

Telemedicine, in fact, is one of the most successful fields in India, in which the private sector has taken over the administration of public health and participated actively. Narayana Hrudyalaya, the Asia Heart Foundation, the Amrita Medical Science Institute and the Aravind Eye Care are some of the private-sector Indian enterprises in telemedicine. Telemedicine is the responsibility of the Indian Ministry of Health and Family Welfare and the Department of Information Technology [38].

Telescope medicine in India has been extended to traditional medicines, such as the National Rural AYUSH Telemedicine Network, using telecommunications to advocate for the public the advantages of traditional medicines.

Before 2020, telemedicine had few concerns due to the absence of standards and the resulting unpredictability. The High Courts of Bombay rejected two doctors who had been engaged in the care of the dead patient in the cases of Deepa Sanjeev Pawaskar and Anr. vs State of Maharashtra, and the spouse filed a criminal complaint against the physicians charging them with criminal negligence, which they filed. In this case, telecoms were also employed as a way of consulting. Because telemedicine consultations are not covered by law in India, medical organisations have requested on multiple times the Indian Medical Council and the government to establish explicit telemedicine regulations [39].

Due to the broad COVID-19 pandemic, which afflicted nations throughout the world, obstacles have been identified to provide healthcare services for the needy—in particular, because individuals over the world are ordering social distance and high risk of COVID-19 contracts. Telecommunications should be regulated and promoted in order to consult patients with other problems and seek medical advice in a timely manner, and RMPs should also be assisted in effective patient management and consultation as and when requested—without the patient having to go to the hospital or to the clinic [40].

The national lock-out process can help both patients and doctors minimise the spread of COVID-19, which is extremely infectious and reduce the risk of the exposure of vulnerable patients and healthcare personnel to the virus.

3.4.2 Guidelines Telemedicine Practices and Policies

The Ministry of Health and Family Welfare, the Government of India, issued on 25 March 2020 telemedicine practise guidelines, prepared in collaboration with NITI Aayog in response to the country's crisis and the need to enforce social distancing and eliminate unnecessary movement of patients into clinics and hospitals.

As described in the "Background" section of the above-mentioned guidelines, these guidelines are intended to provide practical advice to doctors so that they can use Telemedicine as part of their regular practise and to provide a sound course for effective and secure medical care based on the latest information [29].

3.5   Telemedicine Patient and Provider Receptivity

The acceptance of telemedicine by patients and providers is the next factor driving the growth of telehealth services. More than three-quarters of customers (77%) want to use telehealth services, and more than 65% want to utilise telehealth to manage their chronic conditions.

This favourable attitude of telehealth services persists after they have used these platforms. Sixty-seven percent of patients who used telehealth services said it improved their medical care satisfaction [28].

Implementing telehealth technologies is considered as critical for healthcare executives by providers. Telehealth services were ranked as a high priority by 58% of healthcare executives. Eighty-six percent of healthcare executives who have not yet implemented telemedicine feel it is a medium to high priority for them.

Many types of patients benefit from telehealth, particularly those who require frequent office visits and follow-ups. Consider how much simpler it would be for those who live in rural places, the elderly, and chronically sick patients to meet with their doctors in person without the burden of typical consultations. Patients often feel good about continuing to use telehealth after they understand how it works [41].

3.6   Budget Constraint

Finally, because there is a disparity between the demand for telehealth services and the services now offered and the available budget, finances are critical to the spread of telehealth.

Investments in telehealth programmes are minimal, with the majority of healthcare companies polled having annual expenditures of less than $ 250,000. Budgets are likely to climb in general next year, with more than half of CEOs anticipating increases of up to 25% [42].

Only 14% of healthcare executives who identified the need for telehealth services claimed they possessed such skills. This discrepancy indicates the telehealth industry's continued expansion [4].

3.7   Design of Telemedicine Workflow

The need to improve information and provide medical treatment to a large number of geographically distributed agents is one of the key drivers for the use of ICT in both public and commercial healthcare companies. Telemedicine has been proved in clinical tests to be safe and cost-effective when compared to hospital therapy, particularly for patients with chronic conditions. Furthermore, it is vital to note that the implementation of telemedicine services must overcome a number of challenges, including patient acceptability, accessibility concerns, technological expenses, patient physical and psychological limitations, and acceptability and availability of medical personnel. Despite all of the challenges and setbacks, telemedicine principles have been viewed as having a lot of promise in terms of supporting healthcare, particularly for patients with neurological illnesses. Because the majority of these patients are in their later years, it is critical to create concepts, systems, and equipment that can be used by older people and tailored to their specific requirements and limits [3].

3.7.1   Centre and Representative Telemedicine

Medical experts are essential to any healthcare industry's success. The present situation's biggest issue is a scarcity of healthcare professionals. During the current COVID-19 epidemic, the risk of contracting (SARS-CoV-2) has increased significantly, placing health professionals at risk of serious disease. With a limited number of doctors and a large number of infected patients, providing effective treatment and advice to individual patients became difficult. To enable effective workplace management and promote a culture of trust within the workplace, clear approaches for supporting and effectively handling the pandemic scenario are essential. These management techniques should be centred on risk classification, appropriate clinical supervision, low-threshold access to diagnostics, and decision-making on patient management. Hence the healthcare worker could be used for monitoring the patients at home with mild and manageable symptoms. The basic parameters (Temperature, SpO_2, Pulse rate) could be monitored by the healthcare worker and record patient's day-to-day health records. The healthcare professional should update the patients' health conditions to the nearby health centres. The health record of the patients then could be easily and regularly analysed by the medical officer. The medical officer will prescribe proper medication based on the health condition of the patient and may also suggest any further medical tests to be performed. The workflow has been discussed in Fig. 3.1. The suggestions and prescriptions are then shared with the healthcare professional and then they can communicate the information and the prescription with the patients. This will help to overcome the situation of overcrowding at hospital and further disease spreading.

3.7.2   Direct Telemedicine

Since the advent of the pandemic coronavirus (COVID-19) outbreak in 2019, social isolation and quarantining have become routine practices. Because the aforementioned control procedures are universally accepted, regular doctor visits are demotivated. Yet, some individuals' physiological critical needs continue to require

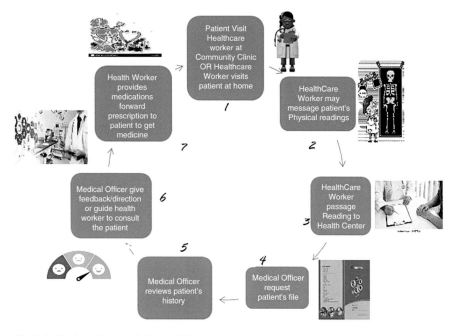

Fig. 3.1 Design of telemedicine workflow

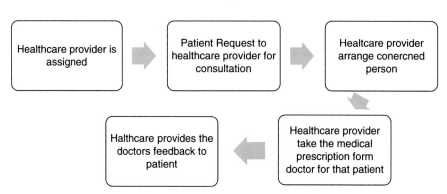

Fig. 3.2 Follow in direct telemedicine

periodic monitoring in order to ensure a healthy lifestyle. To overcome the current drawbacks associated with the direct hospital visit, with the advancement of smart home automation and hospital services, direct communication and physician visits are now considered optional. To accomplish this, a healthcare professional home medical support system is suggested for monitoring patients' health condition and obtaining prescriptions from doctors while they remain at home, which can be easily understood by taking the following into consideration (Fig. 3.2). Additionally, doctors can diagnose patients' diseases using data acquired remotely from the patient. The healthcare professional becomes the facilitator to support and provide health-related queries and suggestions given by the medical adviser.

3.8   Future Demands and Prospect

The future of the m-health sector is bright and full of prospects, with the increased demand for mobile healthcare consultations. The worldwide m-health industry is predicted to increase at a CAGR of 29.1% from USD 34.28 billion in 2018 to USD 293.29 billion by the end of 2026, according to Fortune Business Insights (2019–2026). Connected medical equipment, mobile services, and applications all fall under the umbrella of m-health. While linked medical devices and applications enable patients with chronic conditions to self-monitor, services such as tailored patient engagement, remote diagnostics, and remote monitoring are gaining great feedback.

With the use of mobile health technology, an increasing number of individuals are realising their potential to enhance healthcare services dramatically, even in the most resource-constrained and distant settings. Despite the fact that m-health is still in its early stages, it is already on the verge of revolutionising the healthcare system. This is due to a number of major advantages technology provides, including greater access and cost to healthcare services, the capacity to track and cure illnesses, and actionable public health information.

Furthermore, hospitals have started to use healthcare data systems to better patient care coordination, reach more patients, and triage them more swiftly. Furthermore, the application of AI in diagnostic processes, information flow, patient data management, and imaging has completely changed how healthcare is seen and delivered. Furthermore, linked medical devices are being utilised to monitor numerous health factors at home, allowing patients to have convenient access to healthcare and reducing the need for hospital visits. Remote patient monitoring helps care professionals to decide if hospital visits are essential by providing secure and quick information transfers.

References

1. P. Matlani, N. D. Londhe, A cloud computing based telemedicine service. In: 2013 IEEE Point-of-Care Healthcare Technologies (PHT), 2013, pp. 326–330.
2. Sharma N, Anand A, Husain A. Cloud based healthcare services for telemedicine practices using internet of things. J Crit Rev. 2020;7(14):2605–11.
3. Freiburger G, Holcomb M, Piper D. The STARPAHC collection: part of an archive of the history of telemedicine. J Telemed Telecare. 2007;13(5):221–3. https://doi.org/10.1258/135763307781458949.
4. C. O. Rolim, F. L. Koch, C. B. Westphall, J. Werner, A. Fracalossi, G. S. Salvador, A cloud computing solution for patient's data collection in health care institutions. In: 2010 Second International Conference on eHealth, Telemedicine, and Social Medicine, 2010, pp. 95–99.
5. Wurm EMT, Hofmann-Wellenhof R, Wurm R, Soyer HP. Telemedicine and teledermatology: Past, present and future. J der Dtsch Dermatologischen Gesellschaft = J Ger Soc Dermatol JDDG. 2008;6(2):106–12. https://doi.org/10.1111/j.1610-0387.2007.06440.x.
6. Wang Ping, Wang Jin-gang, Shi Xiao-bo, He Wei, The research of telemedicine system based on embedded computer. In: 2005 IEEE Engineering in Medicine and Biology 27th Annual Conference, 2005, pp. 114–117.

7. Portnoy J, Waller M, Elliott T. Telemedicine in the Era of COVID-19. J Allergy Clin Immunol Pract. 2020;8(5):1489–91. https://doi.org/10.1016/j.jaip.2020.03.008.
8. A. Jebrane, N. Meddah, A. Toumanari, M. Bousseta, New real time cloud telemedicine using digital signature algorithm on elliptic curves. In: Advanced information technology, services and systems, 2018, pp. 324–332.
9. Bashshur R. A Proposed Model for Evaluating Telemedicine. In: Parker L, Olgren C, editors. Teleconferencing and interactive medicine. Madison, WI: University of Wisconsin; 1980.
10. Bashshur RL, Armstrong PA, Youssef ZI. Telemedicine: Explorations in the use of telecommunications in health care. Springfield, IL: Charles C. Thomas; 1975.
11. Bashshur R, Lovett J. Assessment of telemedicine: Results of the initial experience. Aviat Space Environ Med. 1977;48:65–70.
12. Park B, Bashshur R. Some implications of telemedicine. J Commun. 1975;25:161–6. https://doi.org/10.1111/j.1460-2466.1975.tb00619.x.
13. Bashshur R, Doarn CR, Frenk JM, Kvedar JC, Woolliscroft JO. Telemedicine and the COVID-19 Pandemic, lessons for the future. Telemed e-Health. 2020;26(5):571–3. https://doi.org/10.1089/tmj.2020.29040.rb.
14. House M, et al. Into Africa: the telemedicine links between Canada, Kenya and Uganda. C Can Med Assoc J = J l'Assoc Med Can. 1987;136(4):398–400.
15. House AM, Keough EM. *Distance health systems—Collaboration brings success: The past, present, and future of telemedicine in Newfoundland*. Paper presented at Conference on Information Technology in Community Health; Victoria, BC.. October 1992.
16. House AM, Roberts JM. Telemedicine in Canada. Can Med Assoc J. 1977;117:386–8.
17. Benschoter R. Multipurpose television. Ann N Y Acad Sci. 1967;142:471–8.
18. Menolascino FJ, Osborne RG. Psychiatric television consultation for the mentally retarded. Am J Psychiatry. 1970;127:157–62.
19. Wittson CL, Affleck DC, Johnson V. Two-way television group therapy. Ment Hosp. 1961;12:22–3.
20. Wittson CL, Benschoter R. Two-way television: helping the medical center reach out. Am J Psychiatry. 1972;129:136–9.
21. Dwyer TF. Telepsychiatry: Psychiatric consultation by interactive television. Am J Psychiatry. 1973;130:865–9.
22. Armstrong PA, Youssef ZI, Bashshur RL. Telemedicine in the United States: A summary of operational programs. In: Bashshur RL, Armstrong PA, Youssef ZI, editors. Telemedicine: Explorations in the use of telecommunications in health care. Springfield, IL: Charles C. Thomas; 1975.
23. Lovett JE, Bashshur RL. Telemedicine in the USA: An overview. Telecommun Policy\ 1979 Mar;:3–14.
24. Pool SL, Stonsifer JC, Belasco N. Application of telemedicine systems in future manned space flight. Paper presented at Second Telemedicine Workshop; Tucson, AZ. December 1975
25. Bashshur R. Technology serves the people: The story of a co-operative telemedicine project by NASA, The Indian Health Service, and the Papago People. Tucson, AZ: The Indian Health Service; 1979.
26. Fuchs M. Provider attitudes toward STARPAHC: a telemedicine project on the Papago reservation. Med Care. 1979;17(1):59–68. https://doi.org/10.1097/00005650-197901000-00005.
27. Justice JW, Decker PG. Telemedicine in a rural health delivery system. Adv Biomed Eng. 1979;7:101–71.
28. C. Kugean, S. M. Krishnan, O. Chutatape, S. Swaminathan, N. Srinivasan, P. Wang, Design of a mobile telemedicine system with wireless LAN. In: Asia-Pacific Conference on Circuits and Systems, vol. 1, 2002, pp. 313–316.
29. Silfwerbrand E, Verma S, Sjökvist C, Stålsby Lundborg C, Sharma M. Diagnose-specific antibiotic prescribing patterns at otorhinolaryngology inpatient departments of two private sector healthcare facilities in Central India: a five-year observational study. Int J Environ Res Public Health. 2019;16(21) https://doi.org/10.3390/ijerph16214074.
30. Aldwairi M, Alwahedi A. Detecting fake news in social media networks. Procedia Comput Sci. 2018;141:215–22. https://doi.org/10.1016/j.procs.2018.10.171.

31. Shi X, Luo X, Shang M, Gu L. Long-term performance of collaborative filtering based recommenders in temporally evolving systems. Neurocomputing. 2017;267:635–43. https://doi.org/10.1016/j.neucom.2017.06.026.
32. Júnior JG, de Sales JP, Moreira MM, Pinheiro WR, Lima CKT, Neto MLR. A crisis within the crisis: the mental health situation of refugees in the world during the 2019 coronavirus (2019-nCoV) outbreak. Psychiatry Res. 2020;288:113000. https://doi.org/10.1016/j.psychres.2020.113000.
33. Sarkar K, Khajanchi S, Nieto JJ. Modeling and forecasting the COVID-19 pandemic in India. Chaos Solitons Fract. 2020;139:110049. https://doi.org/10.1016/j.chaos.2020.110049.
34. Sharma K, Anand A. Determination of COVID-19 relief centers by using Facebook Json data and providing information analysis. Int Res J Eng Technol (IRJET). 2020;7(4):2525–8.
35. Eisma MC, Boelen PA, Lenferink LIM. Prolonged grief disorder following the Coronavirus (COVID-19) pandemic. Psychiatry Res. 2020;288:113031. https://doi.org/10.1016/j.psychres.2020.113031.
36. Jin Z, Chen Y. Telemedicine in the cloud era: prospects and challenges. IEEE Pervasive Comput. 2015;14(1):54–61.
37. Iyengar KP, Jain VK, Vaish A, Vaishya R, Maini L, Lal H. Post COVID-19: planning strategies to resume orthopaedic surgery—challenges and considerations. J Clin Orthop Trauma. 2020;11:S291–5. https://doi.org/10.1016/j.jcot.2020.04.028.
38. Manupati VK, Ramkumar M, Baba V, Agarwal A. Selection of the best healthcare waste disposal techniques during and post COVID-19 pandemic era. J Clean Prod. 2021;281:125175. https://doi.org/10.1016/j.jclepro.2020.125175.
39. Deep G, Sidhu J, Mohana R. Role of Indian IT laws in smart healthcare devices in the intensive care unit in India. In: 2020 Sixth International Conference on Parallel, Distributed and Grid Computing (PDGC); 2020. p. 1–5. https://doi.org/10.1109/PDGC50313.2020.9315763.
40. Palasamudram D, Avinash S. ICT Solution for Managing Electronic Health Record in India. In: 2012 Third International Conference on Services in Emerging Markets; 2012. p. 65–74. https://doi.org/10.1109/ICSEM.2012.17.
41. Luthra S, Mangla SK. Evaluating challenges to Industry 4.0 initiatives for supply chain sustainability in emerging economies. Process Saf Environ Prot. 2018;117:168–79. https://doi.org/10.1016/j.psep.2018.04.018.
42. Fortney JC, Maciejewski ML, Tripathi SP, Deen TL, Pyne JM. A budget impact analysis of telemedicine-based collaborative care for depression. Med CareMed Care. 2011;49(9):872–80. Available: http://www.jstor.org/stable/23053673

Patient–Physician Relationship in Telemedicine

4

Aniello Leonardo Caracciolo, Maria Michela Marino, and Gennaro Caracciolo

4.1 Introduction

The COVID-19 pandemic has given a formidable push to the spread of telemedicine and as often happens in major critical events; this will mean that many things will change in the future. Hospitals and physicians' offices even before the pandemic were not perceived as safe places. *"Hospitals are dangerous places"* [1], but also in Italy, as in much of the Western world, between 5% and 8% of hospitalized patients contracted healthcare-associated infections (HAI) even before the COVID-19 pandemic, while 10–15% of hospitalized patients report damage due to hospitalization. Telemedicine, therefore, is no longer a simple option, but has become—and will increasingly be—an essential component of health services. Patient satisfaction also increased. A survey conducted by OnePoll, commissioned by DocASAP, examined, between 29 and 30 June 2020, a representative sample of 1000 adults who, in the United States, had a telemedicine experience. 92% of respondents said they were satisfied and, to define the experience, they used terms such as "easy" (45%), "efficient" (38%), and "convenient" (30%). The physician consulted in telemedicine has also numerous advantages. He can operate teleconsultation from his studio or home, has the ability to program the teleconsultation or answer an urgent call without moving, can consult a database or an electronic medical record in real time, can

A. L. Caracciolo (✉)
Integrated Telemedicine Services, Head of Department Neurosurgery, "Sant'Anna e San Sebastiano" Hospital, Caserta, Italy

M. M. Marino
Department of Precision Medicine, University of Campania "Luigi Vanvitelli", Naples, Italy
e-mail: mariamichela.marino@unicampania.it

G. Caracciolo
Studio Forensis, Caserta, Italy
e-mail: info@studioforensis.com

T. Choudhury et al. (eds.), *Telemedicine: The Computer Transformation of Healthcare*, TELe-Health, https://doi.org/10.1007/978-3-030-99457-0_4

simultaneously order diagnostic tests and all with the maximum contractual flexibility.

Telemedicine is in the daily future of the patient–physician relationship and, therefore, it must be studied in an organic way in its effects on the very relationship. It is not a commercial. The importance of studying and ensuring this ancient relationship between people is further evidenced by the need felt by the General Assembly of the World Medical Association (WMA) to adopt the *"Cordoba Declaration on the patient–physician relationship"* in October 2020.

A universal meaning is attributed to the patient–physician relationship, in which the deep motivations have remained unchanged in human history, but which has undergone a significant evolution within the social dynamics in which it evolved.

4.2 Evolution of the Patient–Physician Relationship in History

A person suffering from severe discomfort looks for another person who can alleviate that discomfort. A sick person seeks a healer. At the beginning of time, the healer was a figure cloaked in sacredness. He invoked the gods and nature to overcome the disease. Traces of primitive medical practices have already been found in the Neolithic villages discovered in Pakistan [2].

The history of the patient–physician relationship constantly accompanies the history of man and social relationships: it is not identified only with the history of medicine, but involves communication, technological development, great scientific discoveries, social organization, economics, and the history of human thought itself. The first elements of medical decision-making appear in the Egyptian papyri: examination, diagnosis, treatment, and prognosis [3]. Plato (428–348 BC) and Aristotle (384–322 BC) developed deductive reasoning, analyzing the concept of cause and effect until they considered as superior the knowledge based on proof. For Plato, the best medicine is obtained if, beyond the scientific aspects of the cure, physician and patient are placed in the context of a personal relationship. Aristotle's writings influenced both Western and Islamic culture, those ideas were inspired by Hippocrates (460–370 BC), Erofilo (335–280 BC), and Galen (129–201 BC) [4]. Hippocrates is emblematic not only for Western medicine, for which he is still a reference of professional ethics through the declaration of his ancient oath but has strongly influenced the evolution of the patient–physician relationship also in other cultures and over the centuries.

> *Into whatsoever houses I enter, I will enter to help the sick, and I will abstain from all intentional wrong-doing and harm, especially from abusing the bodies of man or woman, bond or free. And whatsoever I shall see or hear during my profession, as well as outside my profession in my intercourse with men, if it be what should not be published abroad, I will never divulge, holding such things to be holy secrets.*—Hippocratic Oath.

The Hippocratic Oath already contains the concept of confidentiality and protection of privacy, as well as that of respect for the dignity of the patient, in addition to the main declaration of its mission which is to help the sick. Hippocrates values the dialogue between physician and patient. *"If a slave doctor hears you, he will reproach you: 'But in this way you make your patient a doctor!' Just so he will have to tell you if you are a good doctor"* [5].

In a world not yet globalized, knowledge had fewer opportunities for comparison and longer exchange times.

Language and communication, also from the point of view of evolutionary theories, increasingly became a conscious tool in the relationship between people. The relationship between physician and patient perceived the effects of an increasingly complex professional and social organization in a social and environmental context that required a new alliance between physician and patient, strengthening mutual physical and moral support, which would bear fruit in the twentieth century.

In 1947 the World Medical Association (WMA) was born, an international and independent confederation that today represents 115 national medical associations from all over the world. In 1949 the WMA published the first draft of the International Code of Medical Ethics, which inherits the Hippocratic conception and extends it to include, among other things, the principle of autonomy of the patient and of health as a collective good. The Declaration on Ethical Principles for Medical Research Involving Human Subjects will follow in 1964, where, among other things, it is reiterated that the physician must always act in the best interest of the patient when he provides his professional work. The physician must protect life, health, dignity, integrity, the right to self-determination, privacy, and confidentiality of personal information. Furthermore, explicit reference is made to informed consent, the clarity and completeness of the information and the voluntary nature of consent. In 1981 the World Medical Association (WMA) proclaimed the Declaration on the Rights of the Patient, which recognizes the patient's rights in 11 points and reaffirms *"While a physician should always act according to his/her conscience, and always in the best interests of the patient, equal effort must be made to guarantee patient autonomy and justice."*

In 2019, the era of 5G, the fifth-generation mobile network, began. It is a new global wireless standard. 5G enables a new type of network designed to virtually connect people, machines, objects, and devices. 5G is designed to deliver data rates up to 20 Gbps and to support a 100× increase in traffic capacity and network efficiency, with a 10× decrease in end-to-end latency and increased reliability. It will have a big impact on every sector, especially on remote healthcare. The full economic impact of 5G around the world is likely to be realized over the next decade, contributing to the enhancement and development of virtual reality (VR), internet of things (IoT), and artificial intelligence (AI).

In 2020 the World Medical Association (WMA) proclaimed the Declaration on Patient–Physician Relationship, which reaffirms *"The patient-physician relationship is the fundamental core of medical practice. It has a universal scope and aims at improving a person's health and wellbeing."* The development of telemedicine will have to follow this path.

4.3 Definition of Health and Telemedicine

4.3.1 Health

The World Health Organization defines health as follows: *"Health is a state of complete physical, mental and social well-being and not merely the absence of disease or infirmity."*

This definition has many merits, but it no longer appears responsive to reality, as it ends up, in the current world social context, to be a sort of collective aspiration—a utopia—where the idea of health coincides with that of happiness, in an environment devoid of political, social, ethical, and economic threats, not only epidemiological, biological, or physical. Health is limited to a lucky and impromptu event, never present in the life of the majority of men and women. Even within its limits of universality and practice, this definition remains a mantra [6]. Human health arises from the interplay of basic biological processes, environmental exposures, social structures, and behaviors. The definition of health is not just a theoretical exercise. Such a definition is preparatory to any discourse in the health sector, especially in the evaluation and application of new technologies and innovation. The implications of such a definition are many: political choices, application of innovations, research strategies, organization of services, therapeutic choices, and social impact [7].

Among the many possible definitions of the concept of health, the implementation of telemedicine promotes its own: it can be broadly generalized not only to medical sciences, but also to social ones.

As will be seen better later, in telemedicine the object of medical practice is the individual in his holistic complexity, and the main applications concern the monitoring of the elderly and the chronically ill, which, in the most developed countries, constitute the largest part of the population.

With these premises, health could be defined as a condition of dynamic, measurable equilibrium between the disease (or its absence) and the symptoms, which allows the complex of capabilities we have to provide for our needs, according to our objectives and aspirations. Out of any cultural prejudice, this is a condition that is more widely achievable in the most diverse social, political, and environmental conditions, regardless of age. However, it requires some changes in the approach to the disease by both the physician and the patient himself and involves the social and family organizations, to achieve the management and economic conditions that allow you to maintain the best state of health for as long as possible.

4.3.2 Telemedicine

The history of communication in medicine is probably as old as medicine itself. A thousand different definitions (e-Health, m-Health, digital health, remote assistance, etc.) were born out of the need to define the transformation and evolution of medical management approaches in the face of the changes and new opportunities made possible by technology *Information and Communication Technology* (ICT). Telemedicine is the interrelation between players in the health system (patients, physicians, nurses, caregivers, stakeholders) through online digital tools, free from the constraints of space and time. Telemedicine is, therefore, the medicine possible through digital structures on the net. When at the beginning of the century I began to be interested in telemedicine, I shared the emotion of being able to glimpse the future of medical art, but the problems presented themselves soon: certainty of reporting, sending of complex images, compressibility and rendering of files, network coverage, cost of technology, transmission costs, low digital literacy, skepticism of policy makers, resistance to innovation or, on the contrary, excessive expectations and so on.

The COVID-19 pandemic, as often happens in times of crisis, has reminded us that with telemedicine we have an extra weapon against diseases, a weapon that we need to understand better and to perfect [8].

Telemedicine has gone through a surprising evolution in the last decade, along with an increase in the number of companies dealing with telemedicine. The size of the global telemedicine market was valued at $ 24.9 billion in 2016 and is expected to reach $ 113.1 billion by 2025. The implications of telemedicine must therefore be deepened and studied in all their aspects, being aware that innovation without strategy leads to bad practices [9].

4.4   Actuality of the Patient–Physician Relationship

The first therapy that the physician administers to the patient is the physician himself, he is himself. This ensures that the patient–physician relationship is the basis of the success of any therapy. For centuries Medicine has been considered an Art, an exaltation of inventive talent and expressive capacity, because it does not consider the sole and profound scientific knowledge and is expressed through experience, intuition, empathy, and judgment, qualities closer to art than to science. Medical art reassures the patient, who will collaborate more and better in their own care. The meeting between the healer and the patient has remained the main means by which medicine achieves its objectives. Medicine deals with the fundamental aspects of the human condition: birth, life, physical and psychological integrity, fragility, and end of life. These are universal and unavoidable issues for the human being, for which patients seek help from the physician. Regardless of advances in science or changes in politics, these aspects of the human condition will always be present.

Medicine achieves the goal of helping patients not only by treating the disease, but in many other ways: first of all, by listening when patients need to communicate their fears and anxieties, by talking to them and treating them with respect and dignity, relieving physical pain and psychological suffering, restoring the ability that the disease has taken away from them to be free and independent. All of this takes place in the context of a patient–physician relationship [10]. The patient–physician relationship takes place within a social and health system, which requires organization, structural, economic and technological resources, updating, research, good practices and cannot ignore the physical and social environment (e.g., the presence of caregivers is important in the care of the chronic). "The availability of good medical care tends to vary inversely with the need for it in the population served" is the so-called inverse care law [11].

If healthcare becomes a commodity and it is distributed as such, the rich will get more and the poor will get little or nothing. Bringing back the principles of equity and social justice is the task of public health.

Society gives an economic value to human life: for example, the entire population cannot be all subjected to screening, but the population considered most at risk must be selected. Many lives could have been spared with broad screenings, but the number of deaths due to the lack of it is considered ethically acceptable. After months into the COVID-19 pandemic, many people got tired of the restrictions and the effects on the economy, starting to tolerate a certain amount of daily deaths and trying to come back to old social habits even if the pandemic persisted. Public health must guarantee physician and patient. Physicians are not heroes, they are health professionals, and the patient is not simplistically a victim of fate. When in 2020 the World Medical Association (WMA) published the Declaration on Patient–Physician Relationship, it restored primacy of the physician's against biotechnology, while still recognizing the autonomy and self-determination of the patient.

The Declaration on Patient–Physician Relationship was the moment of synthesis of a debate on the relevance of the patient–physician relationship, accentuated in the last decade of the last century due to a greater request for autonomy—on the part of patients that generated real conflicts within the decision-making process—sometimes resulting in legal initiatives against physicians. Conflicts that were at the origin of the so-called defensive medicine, a sort of degeneration of the patient–physician relationship, which involves the loss of empathy and the detachment on the part of the physician who, worried about the possible legal consequences of the procedures adopted towards the patient, limits his action to a purely technical activity.

Particularly significant for such a synthesis were the works of Mark Siegler [12] and Ezekiel and Linda Emanuel [13]. The increase in the average age and life expectancy of the population, consequent to the improvement of medical care and living conditions in general, has led to a surge in public health expenditure, which has forced States to exercise control of the patient–physician relationship, limiting the autonomy of both.

With public health management, the patient–physician relationship is contextualized. More than the good of the patient, the good of the community is sought in a perspective of rationalization of resources (not only economic) and social equity, which however remains difficult to reach, as demonstrated by the highly asymmetrical world management of the COVID-19 pandemic. After the Second World War, the patient's awareness and his desire for autonomy within the patient–physician relationship increased. The concept of informed consent is affirmed, for which the patient, in addition to claiming the correctness and completeness of the information, seeks in the physician more than anything else a technical and scientific aid to his decisions. It is the era of autonomy. The third era is that of bureaucracy. The state intervenes on the patient–physician relationship, compressing their mutual rights and duties within the strategies that concern the well-being of the community. While in the first two previous epochs the patient's well-being was the predominant concern of physicians, in the age of bureaucracy the patient's needs must be confronted with the needs of society and with the resources available. Decision-making is no longer exclusively in the hands of physicians and patients. The patient–physician relationship is subject to the strategies of administrators and bureaucrats. This change has also led to very positive effects such as the spread of preventive medicine and the search for greater social justice. The social evolution of the patient–physician relationship is an unstoppable process, but it must not cancel itself out in a universalistic perspective that ignores the rights acquired by the individual. A society would be created that, in the name of utopia, destroys the good things we have achieved in millennia of medical history: thinking of being able to limit the patient–physician relationship to the mutual link between the institutionalized expectations of the patient and those of the physician is potentially dangerous (Fig. 4.1).

A therapy with little chance of success is seen by society as an ethical negative value, but in reality, it is an economic negative value. The other side of the coin of the apparently broader definition of health that the WHO gives is that the concept of quality of life prevails over the very concept of the right to live. It is in fact an economical choice that our society makes more acceptable by transforming it into an ethical choice. The question is how the standard of quality of life will change in the future and consequently who will be allowed to continue living?

Another tool for standardizing choices and clinical orientation is undoubtedly the large-scale application of the guidelines. These are typically based on physiological parameters that do not necessarily include the wishes, values, or preferences

Fig. 4.1 The bureaucracy compress mutual rights and duties of the patient–physician relationship within the strategies that concern the well-being of the community

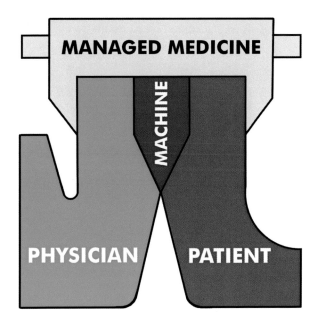

of patients or physicians. What may be right for a group may not be acceptable to individuals within the group. The guidelines, which are useful for formulating shared and evidence-based therapeutic strategies, can, however, limit the freedom and discretion of both patients and physicians and therefore substantially change the patient–physician relationship. In humans it often raises conflicts of conscience, but what about computers? If we completely rely on choices dictated by algorithms (AI) there is a risk that public management bureaucrat could insert into intelligent health management. A shared responsibility among all would be little perceived as a personal choice and would be more tolerable. Will the sick elderly or the chronic patient or the disabled person still be in the standard of living accepted by society if their cost becomes unsustainable? The good use of technology can resolve economic and ethical conflicts in decision-making. Misuse can alienate us from ethical choices. Patient autonomy has also been the subject of a long debate. Obviously, the patient's autonomy is not called into question. The debate focuses on how the physician confronts his patient's self-determination. In the paternalistic model physicians act as the patient's guardians; they know what is best for the patient and do it. This behavior is nowadays admitted almost exclusively in emergency cases, when obtaining the patient's informed consent could require times and methods that can irreversibly damage the patient himself.

In the information model, the patient considers the physician as a scientific technical tool. The physician is detached. This is generally what happens when there is only an occasional interaction between physician and patient, as in the depersonalized relationship with a super specialist. In the interpretative model, the physician takes on the role of a consultant, in addition to offering his technical knowledge, he answers the patient's questions based on his own health values. In the end, the decision is entirely up to the patient.

In the deliberative model, physician and patient assume equal dignity. The final choice will be shared and based on the comparison of the values carried by the patient with the respective values suggested by the physician. Here the conception of the patient's autonomy is identified with moral self-development. The physician is a caring friend, who spends a lot of time communicating with his patient, to clarify and articulate the values underlying the decisions to be made (Table 4.1).

Table 4.1 Benefits of the patient–physician relationship

Improvement of the health and well-being of the person
Relief of suffering
Lower frequency of diagnostic errors
Faster differential diagnostics
Reduction of unnecessary diagnostic tests
Greater adherence to therapy
Reduction of unnecessary interventions
Less use of personal and collective structural and economic resources
Support in the elaboration of decision-making processes, motivation
Respect for individual freedoms and decision-making autonomy
Reduction of inequalities and greater social justice
Diffusion of lifestyles that promote personal and collective health and well-being

Table 4.2 Degeneration of the patient–physician relationship

Medicalization of daily life
Utopia of the perfect human being and the creation of unattainable health standards
Economic estimate of human life
Exclusively reductionist approach (superspeciality)
Prejudices about science, treatment, culture, race, sex, etc.
Scientism (attributing to the sciences the ability to satisfy all human needs)
Pervasive use of the technique (AI, ML, big data, media, social, etc.)
Defensive Medicine
Depersonalization of the relationship
Creation of diseases without a nosological framework
Inverse care law
Interpret the different as pathological
Conflict of interest
Excessive bureaucracy

The physician becomes a health promoter. It is considered the optimal relationship, within which a shared decision-making process—built around mutual participation and respect—takes place.

The sick man is not a machine to be repaired, but physicians cannot be the simple executors of the patient's will, just as they cannot consider their duties resolved only towards the ideology of scientific evidence, efficiency, or profit. A good relationship with the patient is still today the main motivation of a physician in his work. In a Medscape [14] survey of a sample of about 20,000 physicians, 90% said they love their job despite the excessive bureaucratization and increasing legal problems. The gratitude of the patients, their satisfaction, and the awareness of working for the common good gratify almost 80% of physicians overall (Table 4.2).

Diagnosis is a multidisciplinary process that requires knowledge of the patient's physical state, through observation, knowledge of his clinical history and pathology, and almost always requires the support of multimodal examinations and adequate or specialized knowledge. The success of the therapy requires the patients' adherence and their motivation. Improving the bond with the patient improves the chances of therapeutic success, in favor of the quality of life and the duration of life in good health, understood as a dynamic condition, which allows the complex skills that people have to provide for their needs, according to their goals and aspirations. The patient–physician healing relationship will never be abandoned because it serves the universal needs of both patients and physicians.

4.5   Be a Good Physician

The first draft of the International Code of Medical Ethics produced by the World Medical Association (WMA) is from 1949, the last is from 2006, a sign of the need to constantly adapt medical ethics to the changes of the time. In the Declaration of Cordoba on Patient–Physician Relationship of 2020 the same WMA defines in the preamble that *"The patient–physician relationship is part of a human relationship model that dates back to the origins of medicine. It represents a privileged bond between a patient and a physician based on trust. ".*

The influences of Western traditions are evident—In God We Trust—but they manage to synthesize a universal sentiment well. Trust is a feeling that is built over time and generates security and tranquility. Obviously, there is no single way to be a good physician and this concept expresses different priorities depending on the point of view. Empathy places us into intimate contact with patients, compassion allows us not to be completely dragged into their torment, allowing us to help them in the best possible way. Empathy is our ability to recognize and understand the emotional state of our patients, in an immediate way, creating a strong bond with them, which helps them to overcome the stress of knowing the state of the disease and its evolution. Compassion is the sign of our willingness and propensity to come to the aid of those who are unhappy, approaching with respect and pity a human condition marked by pain and detachment.

There is nothing worse for a physician than being indifferent to the patient's expectations and pain. Empathy and compassion are indispensable in moments of greatest stress in the patient–physician relationship, such as in the case of an inauspicious diagnosis and at the end of life. The patients have the right to know their own condition and prognosis, but the physician must be able to use adequate communication and give access to all necessary support, overcoming, if necessary, even his own beliefs.

The physician's decision-making process generates a clinical judgment that is formed by collecting the patients' history, looking and touching them for a physical examination, prescribing diagnostic tests, proceeding with information review and differential diagnosis, making a therapeutic program, and formulating a prognosis. All this cannot happen without adapting to the characteristics of the individual patient and, above all, listening to them and communicating in a clear, complete, simple, and respectful way, but also motivating them to pursue the purposes of the treatment.

Today it is evident that technical success stems from a scientific culture through a predominantly qualitative evaluation. The evolution of this integration has given rise to today's precision medicine.

The physician must ensure the reduction of risks related to the procedures, the confidentiality and safety of patients. Confidentiality and security are elements of the quality of the medical act. These are ancient concepts, that of confidentiality, as we mentioned earlier, already appears in the Hippocratic oath. The concept of safety is contained in the *"Primum non nocere, secundum cavere, tertium sanare"* (first do not harm, secondly act safely and carefully, and finally promote healing), attributed to Scribonius Largus (48 AD). Measures and procedures must be proportionate. The physician must not subject the patient to unnecessary or potentially more harmful than beneficial investigations or therapies. The lack of safety can be due to errors of the individual (physician, patient, health workers, caregivers, etc.), procedure errors (not suitable for the complexity of the pathology, the characteristics of the patient or inflexible), and system errors (lack of organization, difficult access to services, lack of control and verification). In such a context the guidelines help to protect the patient from inappropriate practices and defend caregivers and stakeholders from accusations of negligence, but the physician will have to follow them critically, adapting them to the complexity of the disease condition.

The cognitive abilities of a physician play an important role, equal to that of his human abilities. Scientific and technological knowledge need intuition, that is the recognition of experiential patterns that repeat themselves, of analysis, in the examination of every single data, and finally of synthesis, to produce an effective action. The physician must have investigative skills, when analyzing the patient's medical, social, and family history, deductive skills, essential in differential diagnostic processes, and constructive self-criticism, for a constant verification of decision-making processes. It must be flexible enough, because often the best clinical choice is based more on compromise than on rigor, due to the complexity of the factors to be considered in formulating therapeutic choices. The good physicians still have another characteristic that distinguishes them: moral integrity, considered as intellectual honesty towards his patient, absence of conflict of interest, sense of responsibility, ethics of human and professional behavior. It is a quality that has a practical value because it predisposes to the resolution of the conflicts. It concerns, for example, the ability to recognize the need to change the care plan or facilitate the patient's access to better care systems and, if necessary, to more experienced colleagues. The ineffectiveness of the public system can cause moral anguish, anger, anxiety, frustration, fatigue, and dissatisfaction at work. The dehumanization of the patient–physician relationship, the excessive bureaucratization, the reduction of resources, the excess of workloads, the reduction of turnover, the less availability of time for oneself and for others, the weight of responsibilities and the effects medico-legal, the conflict between private and professional life, the lack of institutional support and social policies are at the origin of a widespread malaise among physicians. Chronic stress in the workplace causes burnout, a psycho-physical collapse that involves a feeling of lack of energy and lack of self-realization, which charges the most critical aspects of the medical profession with heavily negative meanings to the point of making them intolerable. Over time, it can lead to depression, substance abuse, the risk of suicide, and abandonment of the job. In the United States of America, it is estimated that 300–400 physicians commit suicide each year, at a rate more than double that of the general population [15], and it has been calculated that burnout creates a national cost of $ 4.6 billion per year [16]. Empathy, so important in the patient–physician relationship, can become a very heavy burden in the event of professional error, which does not spare the most competent and educated physician, causing the so-called Second Victim Syndrome [17]. Error is possible in all human behaviors. For a physician it involves a sense of inadequacy, shame, humiliation, fear of professional reputation, and a loss of self-confidence. If a path of reconciliation and constructive critical elaboration is not possible, if defensive medicine prevails, decision-making capacity will be compromised with the risk of making even more mistakes. Social, managerial, and economic support and protection policies are therefore necessary to create a positive and motivating environment, so that physicians find the best conditions in their work to treat the well-being of their patients, improving their resilience capacity, overcoming challenges and criticality by acquiring new energy (Table 4.3).

Table 4.3 Characteristics of the good physician

Human qualities:
• Patient
• Available and attentive
• Deserves trust
• Possesses empathy
• Show compassion
• Sense of responsibility
• Deductive and synthetic skills
• Critical sense and resilience
Technical qualities:
• Takes care of the patient's well-being, through prevention, diagnosis, and treatment
• Knows medical science and practice by integrating the principles of evidence with their own wealth of experience
• Knows the patient
• Studies and updates with diligence
• Guarantees the safety of procedures
• Communicates clearly and knows how to be understood
• Dedicates the necessary time to listening to the patient
• Guarantees confidentiality and professional secrecy
• Shares the management of the decision-making process and guides it
• Respects the patient's autonomy and supports it
• Motivates the patient to pursue the goals of treatment without false therapeutic goals
• Knows the mechanisms of health and social interaction
Ethical qualities:
• Moral integrity
• Inspired by the ethical principles that govern the patient–physician relationship
• Abstains from any action that could generate a conflict of interest
• No prejudices towards patients
• Respects the patient's privacy
• Abstains from defensive medicine practices
• Promotes equity of access to care and social justice
• Defends human dignity and the rights of the citizen
• Problem-solver

4.6 Be a Good Patient

With traditional medicine, the figure of the physician has decisively prevailed in the relationship between physician and patient. The recognition of the patient's autonomy has transformed the patient–physician relationship into an equal relationship, where the patients share the decision-making processes concerning their health condition, assuming an active and proactive role; it therefore makes sense to reflect that the patient is also required to be a *"good patient"* like the physician a *"good physician."* Obviously, there is no bad patient in an ethical sense, but only in terms of collaboration and adherence to therapeutic purposes [18, 19].

The collaborative and deliberative nature of the patient–physician relationship requires that the latter and, more generally, their family unit and caregivers participate in the decision-making and operational processes of care. The effectiveness of care and patient satisfaction with the course of treatment also depend on fulfilling certain patient responsibilities.

Generally, the patient chooses the physician, but this is not always possible, as in cases of clinical emergencies. Patients must not be prejudiced against the physician (race, sex, etc.), but they must know that they cannot ask the physician for anything they want. Like the patient, the physician is also the bearer of ethical interests and beliefs, which in daily practice are measured, however, with the main objective of pursuing the patient's health and well-being. The patient cannot force the physicians to act against their own ethical and religious beliefs.

Today the patient is often already informed about the presumed conditions of their disease through media and social networks. But the internet is also a producer of fake news, which can negatively influence the approach between physician and patient right from the start. A conflicting relationship with the physician always has negative effects on the therapeutic result [20]. The patient should refrain from showing feelings of contrast and challenge during treatment.

The good patients actively and personally participate in the search for the most suitable physician for them in terms of competence and attitudes and from the first meeting establish an open and sincere communication on their needs. They are honest with the physician and provide clear and comprehensive information on past illnesses, hospitalizations, medications, and other health-related issues.

They pay attention to the physician's instructions and, if they are not clear, ask for further information and explanations. If they foresee that there will be problems following the prescribed treatment, they inform the physician. They promptly communicate adherence to therapy, any unwanted or side effects, compliance with initial expectations, the perceived effectiveness of the therapy and do not interrupt, modify or abandon a therapy without having communicated and discussed it with the physician.

They value the empathic capacity and technical competence of their physician, at the same time they acknowledge that—within a shared decision-making process—some objectives and therapeutic strategies may change. Physician and patient sign an alliance pact, in which they have equal dignity, with mutual respect.

The patients are aware that, in addition to the treatment procedures established by their physician, their own health and well-being depend on many other factors such as their lifestyle, the adaptation of their family and social environment or the relationship with the sanitary institutions. They evaluate this impact on their life and discuss this with their physician if necessary. Commitment is also hard work, and the success of a therapy can include discomfort and lifestyle changes.

Finally, physicians cannot ignore their professional role and the patient must therefore adapt in a reasonable way to the needs of the other patients, of the physician and of the healthcare personnel involved in the treatment. Therefore, patients accept the organizational and managerial changes that involve the professional life of their physician and are aware that it is necessary to prepare sufficient economic and temporal resources for the completion of the treatment. Relationships of a different nature, friends or affective, must not alter the correct clinical judgment and adherence to therapy (Table 4.4).

Table 4.4 Characteristics of the good patient

• Chooses the physician carefully as often as possible
• Shares the decision-making processes concerning health in an active and proactive way
• Is not prejudiced against the physician (race, sex, etc.)
• Establishes an open and sincere communication
• Evaluates the impact of lifestyles, family and relational environment on his or her health
• Values the empathic capacity and technical competence of his or her physician
• Has respect for the physician as a man/woman and as a professional
• Is attentive to the physician's instructions
• promptly reports undesirable effects of therapy
• Does not interrupt or change therapy without informing the physician
• Does not ask for treatments or certificates contrary to clinical evidence or the physician's conscience
• Avoids a conflictual relationship with the physician during treatment
• Does not allow friends or affective relationships to alter the correct clinical judgment and adherence to therapy

4.7 The Pillars of the Patient–Physician Relationship

Exploring in detail the historical and functional components of the patient–physician relationship, as it has been done so far, could make us lose sight of those foundations without which the relationship itself loses its value, transforming into the simplest relationship between the provider of a service and its user. The patients are not just "customers": they need much more than the attention that a buyer deserves. Delicate issues such as death and therapeutic failure are also part of the report. These issues must be managed within the patient–physician relationship, even beyond any possible profile of fault. We have seen how social policies have become increasingly invasive, driven by laws of economics more than from the expression of the most basic human rights. There are, therefore, some elements that cannot be removed from the dynamics of the patient–physician relationship without distorting it. The first essential foundation of the patient–physician relationship is what brings the healer and the patient together: the need for a cure. The patient's health and well-being are therefore the first pillar of the patient–physician relationship. It is a universal and perennial value.

Whenever a patient is able to choose a physician, they look for one who is prepared and knows his profession well, but also his "Art." This allows the physician to be able to grasp not only the signs and symptoms of the disease, but also the conditions of social life, hygiene, the environment, exposure to physical and chemical agents, diet, frequency of physical exercise, family pathologies, the degree of education, emotional deficiencies, and the conditions of physical or psychological violence in which the patient is immersed.

Physicians with moral integrity and all those human characteristics that make them empathetic and compassionate and who observe an ethics of behavior are in tune with their patient and obtain better therapeutic results. Respect the patient and have no prejudices. Lifestyles, personal values, cultural traditions, religious beliefs, scientific and technological beliefs, political or racial affiliation, and gender identity do not influence the shared decision-making process. Moral integrity and the alliance pact always impose confidentiality, except when it represents a danger to the patient or hides abuse and violence or has effects on the health of others. The entire patient–physician relationship is based on mutual trust. Sometimes it precedes the meeting between physician and patient, more often it must be built and nurtured during the treatment relationship. When this mutual trust fails it is better to interrupt the relationship, not only for the risk of having an ineffective therapy, but also to avoid the risk of conflicts. Communication is a value in itself. It is able to nourish and make the patient–physician relationship stronger and more effective, if it is respectful of mutual sensitivities. It is always necessary to guarantee the favorable environmental and temporal conditions for the interview. Keeps mutual attention and the bond of responsibility alive. Understanding does not necessarily involve sharing, which is why it is essential to have informed and voluntary informed consent.

Sharing decision-making processes, within a deliberative relationship, is an evolution and a real social achievement for the patient–physician relationship. This parity is also expressed in manifestations of reciprocity which, outside the critical conditions of the emergency, go as far as the possibility that the patient rejects the physician and, conversely, that the physician rejects the patient (conscientious objection).

Adherence to therapy is a guarantee of success because it plays a key role in the treatment of any type of disease. Its importance is often overlooked. Failure to adhere to therapy may be due to various causes ranging from the patient's negligence to the fatigue of respecting a therapy that changes lifestyle too much, to the difficulties of practicing it in complex family and social contexts, or due to poor communication and lack of trust within the patient–physician relationship.

The absence of conflicts during treatment is a practical principle as well as an ethical one and has value for both the physician and the patient. The physician therefore refrains from any initiative that could even be interpreted as a conflict of interest, while the patient avoids taking any conflicting action during treatment (Table 4.5).

4.8   What Changes with Digitization

We perceive from the world a continuous flow of information. In communications, digital information has many advantages such as the ability to be compressed, fragmented, reconstructed, and, finally, almost completely recovered even after a strong distortion. Above all it is fast and cheap, ecologically sustainable. Technically adaptable to the most diverse needs. These features have made it increasingly accessible, becoming an indispensable tool for innovation, to promote knowledge and culture, capable of radically transforming playful activity and creating the world of social media.

Today we can communicate with computers and computers communicate with each other. Our TV is smart and a car can travel alone without a driver. Robotic aids

Table 4.5 Pillars of the patient–physician relationship

The cure
Knowledge
The ethics of behavior
Confidence
Communication
Sharing of decision-making processes
Adherence to therapy
Absence of conflicts

already exist for some disabilities. Part of our reality seems to spring directly from the world of Isaac Asimov, the man of the three laws of robotics [21]. A visionary man who read the signs of the future like Jules Verne or Leonardo da Vinci before him.

The digital world has been characterized from the outset by extreme freedom and a strong drive towards universality. The free flow of information has been a huge step forward, but it also brings with it many contradictions. In 2017 there was the first annual meeting of the United Nations World Data Forum. The UNIDO (United Nations Industrial Development Organization) and JRC (Joint Research Center) Agencies of the European Commission have become partners of the World Ethical Data Forum, which defines *"Digital ethics is the field of study concerned with the way technology is shaping and will shape our political, social, and moral existence."*

The leading international organizations take the need to ethically regulate the digital world and the explosion of artificial intelligence very seriously. Many expectations and fears that were once only present in science fiction films have become realities [22] with which we know we must measure ourselves today and in the immediate future in a world that lives in a global village [23]. When Bill Gates talked about the risks of a pandemic in 2015, not many people took it seriously, but COVID-19 has become a tragic planetary reality after only 5 years. The big topics of the discussion concern the excessive pervasiveness of the digital world, digital oligopolies, the political and economic use of big data, persuasion techniques, the influence of platforms and the network on privacy and on sensitive health-related data protection, the ease with which fake news can be spread.

Laws and guidelines are difficult to enforce in a system that by its nature pursues the free exchange of information and data. It is difficult to impose bans or safeguard clauses, difficult to create insurmountable barriers to privacy, because there will always be those who will be able to circumvent them. The solution is in the daily effort to keep a constant update to ensure that someone's freedom does not turn into oppression for someone else. Progressively, all the activities that can be digitized will become such, so it is necessary to spread a general awareness of maturity on the digital world, which requires constant implementation. It is necessary to spread a basic culture, partially present among the "digital natives," which allows them to take advantage of the main systems for accessing data, exchanging information, archiving and scheduling activities. Digitization reduces human errors but amplifies the effects of a single error.

For international investors, the development of digitization and the structural resources that allow it (network, mobile, platforms, etc.) are an indispensable motivation, for which they will tend to invest less and less in digitally underdeveloped countries.

4.9   What Changes with Telemedicine in the Patient–Physician Relationship

4.9.1   The Mediator

Telemedicine introduces a new element in the patient–physician relationship: the mediator, or the machine factor. When in 1905 Willem Einthoven carried out the transmission of heart sounds from a hospital to his laboratory using the telephone [24], he unwittingly introduced not only an innovative technical instrument, but a real mediator between the physician and the patient.

A "machine" can be defined as a set of physical and organizational elements that make up a single aggregate, which multiplies the energy applied, to perform predetermined actions saving time and resources. Machines are very present in diagnostics and therapy, where they function as tools available to the clinic, unlike what happens in telemedicine where the "machine" is interposed between two people so that each can reach their goal with the greatest advantage and lower costs, a definition that corresponds to that of a real broker (Fig. 4.2).

Without this mediation, telemedicine does not exist as a support for diagnosis, treatment, and prevention, but is only a communication system, still important, but with a more limited socio-health impact.

This concept of mediation exercised by telemedicine in the patient–physician relationship is even more valid as network systems, hardware, the Internet of things (IoT), and, above all, the support of artificial intelligence (AI) evolve. The reduction

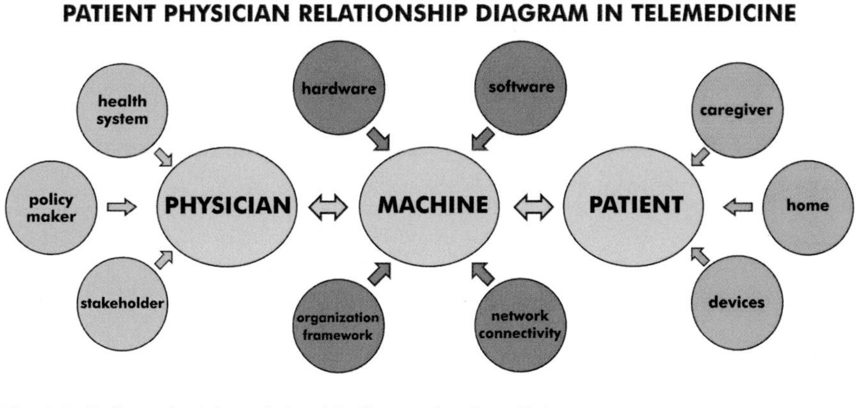

Fig. 4.2 Patient–physician relationship diagram in telemedicine

of transmission costs and the creation of less bulky devices allow us to think of telemedicine as the cornerstone of a new global health system. The decrease in data transmission costs, the increase in the capacity and speed of the networks, and the IT advances that make it possible to process large amounts of data in a short time even on mobile devices have made telemedicine more accessible and widespread, creating a general improved healthcare. Telemedicine has changed the way health-care professionals work with each other, has changed the way they provide care, and has led to new forms of engagement and relationships with patients and communities. Digitization and communication science are part of the medical baggage of this century.

The presence of a mediator, due to its nature of promoting new connections, multiplies the number of actors who contribute to therapeutic success, strengthens the role of caregivers, from whom—in addition to their willingness to support care—is also required adequate training that allows them to make full use of the new technological tools available to them.

In this new physician/machine/patient relationship, the mediator will play an increasingly important role in contributing to the decision-making process. The management of the treatment will always be a burden on the physician, who will now be able to benefit from the complementarity of judgment that the further development of artificial intelligence (AI) will be able to provide. Therapeutic success will always be characterized by uncertainty, disparity of interpretation, complexity of elaboration and organization; for this reason the role of the physician cannot be replaced by an App.

People perceive changes differently. Some feel oppressed by the eye of the "big brother" and are obsessed with the threat of privacy, others consider telemedicine to be a tool that prevents the physician's leadership as responsible for clinical management, still others are overwhelmed by the concern of medical implications: legal and by the effects on the working relationships between health personnel and on the workloads themselves [25]. On the contrary, others are attracted by the possibility of having a continuous feedback from their patients; they are satisfied by the possibility of a continuous and fast flow of information, by the possibility of having a real-time comparison with other colleagues, and of being less bound to the determinism of time and space [26]. Patients, caregivers, stakeholders, and policy makers share in different ways the fear of being excluded from decision-making processes and of the fact that these may become automatic and inflexible, not integrated into the socio-health system of their country. These fears, however, will not prevent the progress of telemedicine, due to the enormous advantages it brings.

4.9.2 The Communication

Clear, correct, and simple communication has always been essential to positively feed the patient–physician relationship. Telemedicine allows communication between physician and patient regardless of the identity of space and time. The two interlocutors may be in two adjacent rooms or on two different continents. The exchange of information can be synchronous, i.e., fully interactive, or asynchronous, i.e., offline, when the data can be analyzed at a later time than when it is generated, as occurs in accessing databases [27].

It enormously increases the amount of information we have access to, even if it is not always good quality information. All information, in fact, can be translated into digital, from data and numerical values, to text, images, diagnostic findings; but also, speech, with voice recognition and transcription, up to physical location (GPS) and the use of implantable sensors and ingestible cameras. Telemedicine, allowing more complex levels of communication, allows the intervention of multiple actors both simultaneously with teleconsultation and in the monitoring phases, with different levels of responsibility and even hierarchical when entire teams or second opinions intervene [28]. The actors involved (specialists, trusted physicians, nurses, caregivers, social workers) must be sufficiently familiar not only with the digital environment, but also with the communication methods implemented by all the other actors, to avoid giving inconsistent information, but above all to avoid conflicting and potentially harmful diagnostic and therapeutic actions [29]. A spokesperson of the team can be useful to avoid the inevitable discrepancies in a communication where people with different cultures and characters intervene. The patient must be helped in the decision-making process without being confused or manipulated. In the patient–physician relationship, communication takes place through different channels. First of all in a physical way, through the contact between the physician and the patient's body, as required by classical semeiotics, but also through the canons of verbal communication, through the non-verbal communication of mimicry, gaze, gestures and postures, finally, through para-verbal communication, such as tone and volume of the voice or speed and rhythm of language [30].

Current telemedicine does not yet allow a physical relationship between physician and patient, but it certainly allows us to satisfy the four dimensions of the interpersonal communication model proposed by Friedemann Schulz von Thun [31], which consist in the content of the communication, in the quality of the relationship between the two interlocutors, in the self-disclosure that accompanies the communication, and in the appeal that each of the two interlocutors addresses to the other party. Communication through digital tools has drastically reduced the perception of non-verbal communication at its onset, for which some paralinguistic elements have developed that help to understand intentions in ambiguous contexts such as emoji [32]. Emojis can represent not only facial expressions, abstract concepts, emotions, and feelings, but also animals, plants, activities, gestures, body parts, and objects. Emojis have both emotional and semantic functions, overcoming the limits of the lack of a universal verbal language. Some researchers believe that the use of emojis is generally consistent across all platforms, can help users convey feelings and understand the meaning of a text, can play the role of non-verbal cues to help understand the general meaning of messages, improve the performance of computer hardware and software, and they can also help in monitoring emotions. At least 5 billion emojis are used on Facebook every day. The knowledge of the dynamics of communication is fundamental to feed the patient–physician relationship in telemedicine: it will make the experience more and more comparable to the face-to-face relationship, but above all it will further improve the management of chronic patients, with whom the physician has already had a history face-to-face relationship, which can be updated periodically with remote communication techniques [33]. It is useful to guarantee the flow of communication, without sudden interruptions of both a dialogical and technical nature, to contextualize it, to create favorable environmental conditions for the interview, to share the meaning of the words and to recognize early potential crisis conditions, such as failure to adhere to therapy, interruption of care, discomfort, signs of violence or conflict, to properly manage adverse events and error. Informed consent to the use of telemedicine must have the same prerequisites used in traditional medical practice [34].

Telemedicine favors teamwork not only with healthcare personnel or staff connected to the healthcare world, but above all with caregivers and the patient himself. The exchange of information generally does not recognize a prevalence of genesis, but all actors must strive to recognize fake news, reduce mistrust, and avoid the risk of information loss. To avoid the hypertrophic fragmentation of information, which becomes misleading by not having the frequency of physical contact, it is necessary to develop a holistic approach. Patents are not a disease or a sick organ, they are the complexity of interactions and perceptions, which often go beyond their illness and involve their personal history, family, social relationships, living conditions, and environment. These interrelationships must be the subject of the systematic attention of the physician in telemedicine; they must be actively sought and investigated, because they are unlikely to emerge spontaneously in the absence of physical contact.

4.9.3 The Physician and Telemedicine

During the COVID-19 pandemic, both physicians and patients have increased the use of telemedicine, driven by the possibility of being able to exchange information without being physically in proximity.

Telemedicine still has objective limitations to the physical examination, but once awareness of the advantages and limitations is achieved, the experience is satisfactory for both the physician and the patient. Telemedicine leads to similar results in providing face-to-face care in the management of chronic patients such as heart failure, hypertension, and diabetes. Consultant time has become the most expensive element of patient–physician interaction. Many physicians have experienced that telemedicine optimizes the interaction time with patients, having a continuous flow of information, allowing a quick consultation and the evaluation of the follow-up, facilitating a team approach [35]. During the pandemic, processes using telemedicine to improve the care system were introduced, without adequate preparation, but when innovation increases production pressure, additional stress is generated in operators, and this can be a factor of quality decay. Physicians have experienced that they can be the object of judgment on social media, that bad communication can irremediably compromise the fiduciary relationship, and that they have the responsibility not to depersonalize the relationship with the patient.

4.9.4   The Patient and Telemedicine

The home becomes the first place of care, in many cases it is no longer necessary to undergo diagnosis and treatment within a hospital environment perceived as foreign if not hostile, where the sense of helplessness and abandonment increase. The possibility of involvement of the family unit and caregivers increases. Patients are more aware of their own autonomy, have access to the vast world of the internet, so they are well prepared on how to represent their condition and require adequate responses, availability and empathy from the physician. The patient has access to a wide range of information, which is not always correct, in which, on the contrary, strong prejudices can take root, which prevent adherence to the recommended therapy. The success of the therapy may not correspond to the satisfaction of the patients, who live in a world of globalized information, which increases their expectations, sometimes putting the patient themselves in competition with the updating of the physician's theoretical knowledge. Patients generally say they are satisfied with their relationship with the doctor (80%), but in fact only 1/3 of patients who experience unsatisfactory service complain about it on the Internet through social media [36].

Most of the complaints concern the limited time for medical consultation and the intolerance of physicians. Less frequently, patients complain of the therapeutic effect obtained, poor treatment schemes, incorrect information, and disrespect. The physicians' behaviors are definitely influenced by the healthcare organization and the work environment, but bad reviews damage their image even before the structure in which they work can increase the level of patients' dissatisfaction with them and can influence their self-esteem of the physicians themselves, who will more easily resort to defensive medicine in their future work.

4.9.5   The Role of the Machine

We have already spoken extensively about the role of the machine as a mediator in telemedicine, but it is right here to remember (and it does not seem pleonastic to the reader) that in order for there to be a patient–physician relationship there must be a physician and a patient. It would be very dangerous for the patient to believe that the role of the physician can be replaced by a machine or software.

Telemedicine produces complex data, called Big Data. This large amount of data can be used by machine learning (ML) techniques, which make it possible to learn and predict based on passive observations. The development of artificial intelligence (AI) allows the machine to actively interact with the environment to learn and take actions that maximize its chances of successfully achieving the objectives that have been previously loaded [37]. A medicine is born based on what is not yet evident to the individual physician but can become evident with the use of big data and deep learning techniques which are able to consider and process much more information about the probabilistic relationships between diseases and symptoms. The conditions exist for effective predictive and preventive medicine long before the onset of symptoms and for chronic and worsening pathologies this constitutes a considerable advantage in the prevention of exacerbation phases.

Such a large amount of data requires better forms of archiving, greater transparency, and better levels of access control. The goal is to make these data anonymous, but open to medical research. AI technology could perform trend analysis in order to better understand the relationship between different predictors that can help medical researchers improve public health [38]. The progress of robotics, able to offer concrete support to the therapeutic action—which can also take place at a considerable distance from the operator's seat—has undoubted advantages in procedures that do not require the physical presence of the physician, improving production efficiency and reactivity. For now, the development of robotics is burdened by the long times required by the procedures, but, as has happened in industrial applications, it is already able to generate in operators the fear of being soon obsolete and of losing their role and control, because the use of AI favors decentralization and the winner is the author of good ideas, instead of the top of the organization, increasing the risk of losing your job in the event of poor performance.

4.9.6   Potential Conflicts

Digitalization in the healthcare sector brings opportunities and risks. These consist mainly of patient confidentiality and sensitive data. The vulnerability of data relating to integrity and availability can lead to financial losses and damage to the health of data subjects.

After the scandal of 2018, in which a company that analyzes Big Data, Cambridge Analytica, allegedly used the personal data of 87 million users of the social network for the purpose of political propaganda, the correct management of big data came to the attention of the public opinion. In truth, the European Union had already adopted a regulation in 2016 [39]. On March 7, 2020, the National Information Security Standardization Technical Committee of China published the Technical Specifications for Personal Information Security GB/T 35273–2020 with the basic principles for the security of personal information, as well as a guide to the collection and storage of personal data. There are still no homogeneous international rules, capable of harmonizing regulations on consent, purpose constraint, data transfer, rights of interested parties, procedural provisions, technical and organizational measures. In many countries, issues of transparency, official oversight, analysis, and research processing often remain unresolved. The problem is that apparently incompatible needs must be reconciled. It would be useful, for example, for an intangible trace to remain in a third-party archive of all the transmissions that took place between physician and patient, always being able to trace both the traceability of the physician's prescriptions and the correct execution by the patient. The protection of the two protagonists of the contractual relationship exposes both to the violation of privacy and can come into conflict with professional law. To begin with, you need to be sure of the identity of the interlocutor (this applies to both the physician and the patient). The management of clinical errors or adherence to therapy requires transparency, awareness, and adjustment times. It is necessary to know how to manage the expectations of the patients and their families, but also the expectations of the physicians.

Pursuing patients empowerment allows you to develop a growth process in the patients, which allows then to take care of themselves and actively collaborate in the decision-making processes that concern them, but this changes the routine of the patient–physician relationship and, if not well managed, it can break the relationship of trust, for which a *"joint empowerment"* is more useful, which allows a better balance of the patient–physician relationship [40, 41]. The physician must be attentive to the apparently inconspicuous signs of disincentivization to therapy or its adherence, of distrust in the means of communication used, of unavailability for further control if not face to face. The medical act must be agreed and authorized for all the connected phases and again for the new phases, you cannot have access to therapies without the validation of the physician, who must have access to the images and not just to the reporting. Each communication must be recorded and, if possible, scheduled. Many feared that telemedicine could have conflicting effects on the patient–physician relationship, errors due to negligence, lack of standards, and reimbursement of expenses [42]. However, there is still no articulated case law of litigation in telemedicine [43], because:

(1) It is still too little practiced.
(2) It is used for chronic patients rather than acute ones.
(3) Almost only services with a low risk of negligence are accessible.
(4) Generally new or potentially dangerous drugs are not prescribed in therapy, but the therapy already practiced is modulated.
(5) A visit in person is always recommended if the teleconsultation coverage is not sufficient.
(6) Many services cannot be used directly by the patient, but are carried out through the further mediation of another healthcare professional or a caregiver.
(7) Access to a new control on teleconsultation is simplified compared to the times of a face-to-face visit.

4.9.7 Health Policies and Social Justice

The application of telemedicine changes the entire system within which the patient–physician relationship is developed, because the organization, access and distribution of resources, both economic and technological, the methods of updating, research changes; it involves new good practices and manages to have effects on the same physical and social environment. It lowers system costs and improves the quality of the service provided, improves patient satisfaction, the socio-family environment and health professionals. The most common chronic diseases take advantage of this [44, 45].

According to the World Health Organization (Dec.2020), the top three causes of death in the world are ischemic heart disease (16%), stroke (11%), and chronic obstructive pulmonary disease (6%), all together accounting for 1/3 of dead in the world. All pathologies susceptible to improvement through remote monitoring in telemedicine [46].

Telemedicine has important effects on prevention in its various forms. In the case of primary prevention, when the disease does not yet exist, but the risk factors already exist, telemedicine is useful in orienting lifestyles, such as promoting a correct diet and physical activity, refraining from cigarettes, drugs, and alcohol abuse. It can promote specific protection through the spread of vaccination practices [47]. In secondary prevention, when the disease is present in an initial presymptomatic phase, it has proved to be very useful in screening activities, in particular for cardiovascular diseases and tumors [48].The remote biometric monitoring of multiple essential parameters, particularly widespread during a pandemic, to prevent the progression of the disease towards disability or premature death, has shown all its effectiveness in tertiary prevention [49].

Telemedicine also makes its positive effects felt in quaternary prevention, managing to prevent the excess of unnecessary or potentially harmful medicalization, which risks worsening the quality of life beyond the outcome on the disease. The physician defends the patient from the physician himself [50, 51].

Having as a privileged field of action health education and the dissemination of correct lifestyles, telemedicine can also play an important role in primordial prevention, as in the case of childhood obesity and exposure of the mother to conditions, such as obesity and hypertension in pregnancy, which are at the origin of cardio-metabolic risk in children and adults [52, 53]. Telemedicine makes it possible to create a network between home, territory, and hospital, capable of integrating different functions from remote monitoring to consultation and psychological and social assistance. Healthcare resources are more easily available, accessible, and more convenient for everyone, so the effort of policy makers must be to make telemedicine available and easy to access, reviewing the organization of the health network according to more current approaches, capable of exploiting full technological innovation. The absence of valid public health policy strategies discourages investment in the private sector.

One of the most widespread organizational schemes in telemedicine is the hub-and-spoke one, which for the provision of services is based on a conventional and hierarchical positioning structure. It is a centralized hub, which acts as a point of contact and education for several spoke sites, an organization that lends itself to the implementation of AI, which includes areas of shared responsibility (Fig. 4.3).

It is therefore possible to pursue the goal of greater equity in access to care in the absence of mobility and healthcare facilities for diagnosis and treatment, reducing differences due to class, culture, organization, and geography of the territory. Traceability and interconnection can reduce the bureaucracy that today weighs on the patient–physician relationship. Access to extensive updated databases allows qualitative and quantitative economic studies on the effectiveness and efficiency of the services offered to the population.

For these reasons, the spread of telemedicine is important both for developing countries, where access to care is physically less widespread in the area, and for countries of the post-industrial era, where the number of elderly and chronically in need of support. In all cases, telemedicine contributes to improving the quality of life. The introduction of telemedicine can free the patient–physician relationship

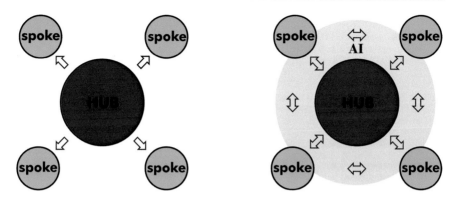

Fig. 4.3 The organization framework hub-and-spoke in telemedicine is an organization that lends itself to the implementation of artificial intelligence, which includes areas of shared responsibility

from any political and economic conditioning, or it can make it even more constrained: as always, it depends on the use that people make of it.

The physician and the patient tend to conform their behavior to the standards proposed by international globalization and any shift from the standard must be justified (economics of public and private services, planned economic investments, insurance, etc.). The spread of telemedicine opens up new fields of application which in turn become part of everyday life and modify the system. The COVID-19 pandemic has exposed structural and organizational barriers. Telemedicine has been essential for the resilience of the global health system, has allowed complex procedures to be implemented even outside hospitals in pre-critical or chronic high-care stages, and has shown the potential to act as the "safety net" of our public health response [54, 55].

4.10 The Pillars of the Patient–Physician Relationship Added by Telemedicine

Population aging is a global phenomenon, in every country of the world the number and percentage of elderly people is increasing. The number of people over the age of 65 (according to WHO 703 million in 2019) is projected to double globally to 1.5 billion in 2050, by then one in six people in the world will be elderly.

In much of the world, life expectancy and quality of life over 65 are improving, but the aging of the population will increase the financial pressure on support systems for old age and the chronicity that is often linked to it. Chronic diseases are the leading cause of death and disability worldwide, responsible for 59% of deaths and 46% of the global disease burden. Social protection programs must now be established to prevent poverty, reduce inequality, and promote social inclusion among older people. Addressing the costs of a fairer and more sustainable health system will be the biggest challenge [56]. The difficulties of an elderly person with a chronic illness and his/her family members are mostly related to lack of autonomy, fragility, and loneliness. The main difficulties for this segment of the population are travel, isolation, and economic difficulties. It is the population at greatest risk for therapeutic adherence. A phenomenon that, according to the Organization for Economic Co-operation and Development (OECD 2018), affects about half of the population receiving prescriptions, leading to serious health complications, premature deaths, and greater use of health services. Poor adherence is estimated to lead to around 200,000 premature deaths in Europe each year, at a cost of € 125 billion. In the United States, an estimated $105 billion are spent annually in avoidable hospitalizations, emergency care, and outpatient visits due to non-adherence to therapy. The reasons behind these low rates of adherence to drugs for chronic diseases are all within a patient–physician relationship that manifests poor awareness of the actors, wrong goals, little motivation, and a reductionist approach that deprives the patient of his or her personal value. The development and diffusion of telemedicine, due to the characteristics we have outlined, plays a fundamental role, adding three new pillars to the dynamics of the patient–physician relationship: proactive medicine, integrated care pathways, and computational support. Telemedicine ceases to be an impromptu process and becomes the code of a complex activity, prolonged over time with continuity and competence, which has the citizen-patient and many intermediate providers as the only final user, connected in a telematic network, but above all organizational and partner-integrated sanitary.

4.10.1 Proactive Medicine

Parity in the patient–physician relationship goes beyond mere adherence to shared therapy to transform patients into health workers themselves, in their own interest. Patient empowerment allows the development of a growth process in the patient, which actively supports self-care and collaborates in the decision-making processes that affect him or her. Patient empowerment has been associated with positive clinical outcomes for health: improved disease management, effectiveness of health services, improved health status, and drug adherence. In this regard, we have seen how a balanced view of *"joint empowerment"* is more advantageous when patients' beliefs about their abilities and control of their health coexist with their recognition of the physician's role in managing the disease. The term *"proactive"* is borrowed from the lexicon of company management. A management action is *"proactive"* when it takes charge, launches new initiatives, generates constructive changes, and leads in an expected direction, aimed at changing things for the better. All healthcare personnel are called upon to support patient self-care and ensure from triage to planning and carrying out the follow-up [57]. It has proved useful to distinguish the decision-making process of chronic patients from acute ones. The Chronic Care Model (CCM) is a medical care model for patients with chronic diseases, updated since the 1990s [58], which proposes the proactive model to promote the improvement of the conditions of the chronically ill, creating paths dedicated to diseases such as heart failure, diabetes, hypertension, and chronic obstructive pulmonary disease, which absorb a large amount of resources from the health system. The model consists of six components: (1) health system and organizational support to promote safe and high quality care; (2) clinical information systems to organize patient and population data; (3) delivery system design to ensure the provision of effective and efficient clinical care and self-management support; (4) decision support for clinical care consistent with scientific evidence and patient preferences; (5) self-management support to empower and prepare patients to manage their own health and healthcare; and (6) community resources to meet patient needs. Telemedicine strengthens proactive medicine, improves its efficiency and effectiveness, and makes it a new pillar of the patient–physician relationship.

4.10.2 Integrated Care Pathways

The integrated care pathways are a useful tool to promote the patient–physician relationship towards an effective clinical practice, capable of obtaining better results with the same available resources. They are the evolution of the guidelines which, as it is well known, represented an important progress towards the realization of an evidence medicine, but are not able to correctly represent the complexity of decision-making processes in routine clinical practice [59]. The integrated care pathways involve various service providers, not only theoretical experts, but above all those who have direct responsibility for the implementation of patient care, considered in its peculiar individuality and complexity. Each specialty involved participates in the decision-making process by integrating with the others. Everyone works together with the patient, who is directly involved in the design and development of integrated care, forming a multifunctional team, committed to providing answers quickly [60]. Many service providers work closely together regardless of the context and location of the patient. Operators in general practitioning, hospital medicine, social care, mental health services and other providers share the focus on individual cases, coordinating a wide variety of separate interventions and sharing information. Pathway design seeks to identify predictable actions that most commonly represent best practice for most patients and include suggestions for them at the appropriate time along the path to ascertain whether all the necessary has been done and results match predictions. The patient journey is individual, and an important part of the purpose of the journey documents is to acquire information about variations, which provide useful information to improve clinical practice. It also allows physicians to evaluate the effectiveness of the application of the guidelines and collect evidence of efficacy when randomized studies are impractical or not justified. It takes a long time to get validated results, according to Shaw and Levenson [61] no less than 2 years. Such a high level of integration cannot ignore the use of ICT and therefore constitutes a new pillar of the patient–physician relationship produced by telemedicine.

4.10.3 Computational Support

We have seen how telemedicine has contributed in a decisive way to giving an equal role to the two players in the patient–physician relationship, making the physician more "accessible" and less distant, both culturally and physically, and favoring the active role of the patient in taking care of self.

Computational support influences communication, allows access to data and the exchange of information in real time, can support decision-making, self-assessment of the state of health and preventive medicine in its various articulations, has a role increasingly important also in carrying out real medical and surgical actions at a distance. It makes available, if necessary, technological tools that help the patients in everyday life, to manage their health simply through devices that have become familiar: such as computers, smartphones, tablets, and smartwatches, wherever the patients are, at home, at work, or on vacation. The computer role has grown so much that it has become a real mediator in the patient–physician relationship.

4.11 Limits of the Machine Mediator

The actors can see and hear each other, but they cannot touch each other. Therefore, the face-to-face physical examination must always be considered feasible, because not all the physical signs of the disease may be evident without contact, furthermore the physical signs may be the only proof of the disease and may change over time. Lack of physical contact can lead patients and caregivers to ask for new remote contacts even if it is not necessary. It is easier to voluntarily interrupt communication, it is easier to lie. Digital divide and poor digital literacy of the actors can negatively affect the effectiveness of decision-making processes through telemedicine. To make up for the poor digital literacy of the actors or even just one of them, it is necessary to prepare a training course or to resort to auxiliary technical support. A potentially symmetrical filter for access to information can be created between physician and patient. External filters can intervene that can hide substantial information or, on the contrary, flood with redundant information that can cause serious errors of assessment during the decision-making process. Signs and symptoms can be underestimated or ignored even in the presence of standardized evaluation models. Injury can fuel patient distrust or heighten the concerns of healthcare professionals, negatively affecting their clinical skills. It can increase misunderstanding and make communication ineffective. It can generate in healthcare professionals the fear of conflicts and legal disputes or of a lack of remuneration for the service. Computer skills and access to digital services and the network can decisively influence the use of the services themselves, making the experience inadequate or even misleading. If complicated devices are used, there is a need for a trained health worker to support the patient at the place of care, so it is important that there is a planning of interventions, as in the case of chronicity, even if telemedicine has proved its usefulness, even in urgency, as in the case of teletriage [62]. For the telemedicine experience to be productive, all actors need to form a close-knit team with the patient, which ensures the smooth and consistent transition of care within a cohesive whole such as between hospital, home, and territory. The greater the number of steps to which the information is forced or the number of channels available, the higher the possibility of a breach of privacy. The value of the context may not be evident or not visible or simply not perceived. It may have been manipulated or concealed. It is influenced by the social environment and the health system: language difference, gender discrimination, discomfort with professional hierarchies, poverty, resource constraints, and staff motivation. The hub-and-spoke structure is the most widespread organization for the provision of telemedicine services, characterized by a conventional and hierarchical positioning. It is a centralized hub, serving as a point of contact and education for several spoke sites that provide assistance. This facility is particularly suitable for building and integrating telemedicine networks, but it can slow decision-making, depress innovation, and make communication between the various spoke sites difficult. For the physician, the responsibilities and the pressure on the expectations of the patient, family, society, and the entire productive and economic structure to which he belongs increase. Physicians must adapt to changes in the patient–physician relationship without losing their healer heritage. If they don't master the tools to control stress, they are doomed to burnout (Fig. 4.4).

Given the symptoms, the network system can be used to calculate (ML, AI) the probabilistic relationships between symptoms and diseases, for now with results still to be evaluated, but we are only at the beginning. The implementation of such

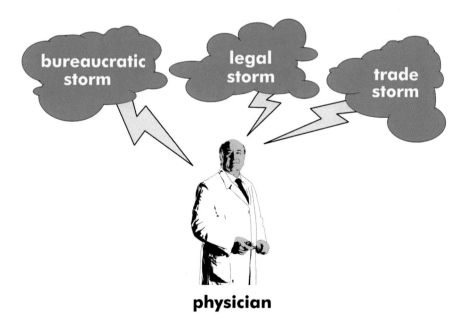

Fig. 4.4 For the physician, the responsibilities and the pressure increase. If Physicians don't master the tools to control stress, they are doomed to burnout

systems is an indispensable support to the decision-making process, but the cultural prejudices of those who design the systems can reduce the effectiveness of telemedicine, perhaps favoring the public good without considering the well-being of the individual patient. Many centers advertise robotic surgery, which has a lot of appeal even if—currently—the costs are excessive, it needs a long learning curve, the duration of the procedures is often double the normal and still lacks the surgical "touch." The degeneration of the machine effect could create a system that favors profit rather than social justice and equality in the face of care. The patient may feel that they can do without the physician to solve their health problems.

4.12   Advantages of Telemedicine in the Patient–Physician Relationship (When Everything Works)

Being in the next room or on the other side of the world is irrelevant. Physical distance is no longer a problem between physician and patient. Consultation with the physician is quick and easy. The physician knows the state of health of the patient deprived of memory distortions, he/she can easily reassess his/her condition and follow up on his/her follow-up. All actors have immediate access to data, images, and procedures. Visual contact between physician and patient is always possible and can give access to a virtual space that favors mutual knowledge [63]. Similar results can be obtained to providing face-to-face care in the management of chronic patients such as heart failure, hypertension, and diabetes. Continuous remote monitoring of these patients can prevent acute manifestations, hospitalization, and disease progression. The possibility of frequent feedback can be exploited, for example, in enhancing the peanut effect. Understanding and knowledge improve the outcome of a therapy, but, as we have already pointed out, what is decisive is the motivation. We are generally more likely to accept small risks of gains or losses, if they are close in time, especially if our life is at stake. The physician has a better chance of promoting good behaviors, such as greater therapeutic adherence, with small short-term incentives, because the motivation is linked to the perception of personal or shared advantages rather than to the perception of potential harm, which, on the contrary, it can prevent action, appearing as an ineluctable destiny [64].

Telemedicine can intercept risky behaviors early, using communication systems that have entered the daily use of large sections of the population such as mobile phones and the world of social media. You can intervene on the environment and circumstances, so that accepted behavior patterns are more likely to lead to better results and promote health.

The same provider can take care of many patients simultaneously in a short time with great effectiveness and accuracy, thanks to the possibility of resorting to health video surveillance or asynchronous evaluations, i.e., subsequent to the generation of information. The organization can be strengthened through the creation of multi-parameter pre-critical alarm systems. In this way we obtain the best rationalization of resources and an efficiency of the assistance system, focusing on supporting the physical network of integrated services and supporting the continuous flow of information between the various specialists, hospital, treating physician, home, social services, and territory. Patients reduce waiting times for appointments and follow-up visits. They can be treated at home, staying longer in the environment that is familiar to them. During the COVID-19 pandemic, telemedicine reduced social isolation. Telemedicine decreases the discomfort and anxiety of those forced to travel long distances to receive services. Hospitalization times are reduced, and it is possible to keep the decision-making process active and frequent during discharge.

The physician can respond quickly to the request for intervention. Diagnostics and therapeutic changes can be timely and appropriate. Critical stages can be prevented conveniently with remote monitoring. Hospital access is reduced and the use of the emergency room, which can take advantage of teletriage, is reduced [65]. Healthcare professionals have faster access to specialist second opinions, interact in real time to ensure the best continuity of care and share information, going back, when necessary, to the source at the first place of care. The advantages of telemedicine are increasingly attractive to many patients, thus fueling a new market. Telemedicine is able to meet the patient's expectations and makes the support of caregivers more effective, who may be involved in the evolution of the decision-making process. It is an advanced training tool, virtual reality and augmented reality can improve the training of all actors and their ability to collaborate. The whole society benefits from it, having a more efficient and less costly health system available. Preventive medicine has enormous advantages, from the spread of vaccination and screening to the containment of the expense of excess medicalization. It influences the economic planning of services. Socio-economic barriers are reduced, and the spread of services increases, with great impact effects both on the urban fabric and in extraurban or particularly disadvantaged areas. Research has the possibility of a wider and more timely sharing of information, of observational studies and randomized clinical trials on large numbers, multiplying the comparison between treatment options. The adoption of electronic medical records allows greater use of predictive statistical models useful in clinical practice and able to support, but not replace, the physician's clinical judgment, also using reminder systems that simplify monitoring and compliance with guidelines. During the pandemic, telemedicine has allowed acceptable levels of social interaction, which otherwise would have been completely impossible in some cases, facilitating protection from infections and allowing continuity and domiciliation of care.

The possibility of having computerized checklists, of having multi-parameter alarm systems, of recording and tracking any access or modification of the decision-making process, reduces the error, allows to recognize the evolution and the contributing causes. The errors inherent in the transition from a hospital to a territorial system decrease, without resorting to punitive attitudes, which usually worsen the overall quality of each subsequent decision-making process.

Telemedicine can reduce the interference of technocrats and bureaucracy on the patient–physician relationship.

4.13   Disadvantages (Even If Everything Works) and Risks of Telemedicine for the Patient–Physician Relationship

In telemedicine there is no physical contact, patients cannot be touched, it is only possible to see and hear them, the reading of body language is limited. There are objective limitations to the physical examination: physical distance is a problem. Teleconsultation could be limited to monitoring patients whose diagnosis has already been made during a face-to-face medical examination.

It can alter the perception of the context, underestimate or overestimate the social and environmental conditions that determine and influence many pathologies. In the absence of controls, there may be the introduction of incorrect data within a chain of processed events, disrupting the connection elements, making it almost impossible to reconstruct the correct chain of events.

The lack of adequate clinical support, which allows to make correct decisions in applying computerized checklists, perhaps for insufficient information on the patient's organs and systems in the case of new drug therapies, and automatisms without control stages can be due to medical error.

The ease of access to the patient–physician report can lead to an overabundance of information, often useless and redundant or inconsistent, coming from different specialists and operators, which can negatively affect the decision-making process and mislead it. The possibility that many healthcare professionals and caregivers themselves can interact on the decision-making process makes it possible for erroneous or manipulative mediation. Patients experience anxiety and discomfort from excessive exposure to information relating to their state of health, their continuous evaluation and overexposure to judgment parameters.

The repetitiveness of some actions can lower the attention threshold or lead to the use of shortcuts that expose you to registration errors. The intervention of a mechanical mediator can distance the physician and patient from one another, dehumanizing their relationship, removing the value of care, and reducing the psychological reward factors that normally feed the patient–physician relationship. Integrating and coordinating communications about tests, consultations, clinical signs, and symptoms can also be difficult. Too many interchangeable and unnecessary professional figures can prevent the establishment of a privileged trust relationship based on the patient's free choice. Information, by its nature, tends to deteriorate in each subsequent step. The transmission of information through digital tools requires a learning curve that depends very much on the culture shared by all the actors and cannot ignore their motivations, availability, learning skills and access to training channels. The habitual use of computational support can lead to the weakening of experiential medical skills, resulting in less flexibility and adaptability of judgment and, therefore, less ability to deal with the unexpected. If the economic approach prevails, communication times are reduced, monitoring is fully automated, and procedures and guidelines are applied uncritically. Insurance coverage influences decision-making processes. Computer jargon that is difficult for most patients to understand is frequently used. Telemedicine may require physicians to be able to manage complex technologies (online prescriptions, sophisticated devices, electronic medical records, robots for remote interventions, etc.) that require specific qualifications generally not required by conventional medicine. Fears of inadequacy can hinder the physician's adherence to telemedicine techniques, as well as the risk of exposing himself/herself to an additional burden of study, work, and responsibility. Patient empowerment uses self-assessment of the health condition, which if not placed within a shared assessment system can be misleading and encourage the use of *"do-it-yourself"* medicine, deeming the physician's judgment unnecessary. Self-assessment turns into self-diagnosis, which can lead to distortions of the patient–physician relationship, lack of adherence to therapy, misunderstandings, misdiagnoses, and conflicts. On the other hand, if technology prevails, while the patients think they can do without the physician, the physicians, in a certain sense, do without the patient, so they are forced to analyze only the available data, without investigating sufficiently the patient and context. The excess of bureaucracy, excessive workloads, multiplication of responsibilities, the use of rigid protocols, and the intrusiveness of health policies on the autonomy of the physician decrease the quantity and quality of the time that he/she is willing or able to allocate to the patient. On the other hand, the lower frequency of face-to-face relationships with the physician can root in the patient the idea of a lack of empathic involvement of the physician, this can reduce the fiduciary relationship and originate conflicts which also influence the decision-making process of the physician care.

The demand for higher quality services is increasing, not always available in each healthcare system, which may not be able to respond to the demand induced by telemedicine. Success is determined by the effectiveness and efficiency of all the nodes of the system: physician, patient, caregiver, stakeholder, machine, software, network connectivity, devices, system integration, competence of operators, and management policy of the health system. For failure, it is enough that the coordination of data integration is insufficient. Telemedicine is perceived as an element of quality of care; if the technology is insufficient, the treatment is also perceived as inadequate [66].

Therefore, a preliminary assessment of the ease of use of the software-hardware-devices system, the attitude of healthcare professionals, the costs of storing and protecting data, and the possibility of accessing the network is essential [67].

One of the characteristics of telemedicine is that it can be cross-border. There is still no shared standard at a global level to regulate free telemedicine activity between different countries, probably also due to the difficulty of reconciling the aspects of the health service with those of the information service [68]. There is a lack of ethical and *leges artis* rules specifically applicable to telemedicine, which would be particularly useful for a program to support third world health systems, but also for the development of second opinion exchanges in the most advanced countries and should not ignore the regulation of informed consent and privacy protection methods.

4.14   Conclusions

Telemedicine improves the quality of life. It improves the health conditions of peoples, helping to make access to care more equitable and the use of social and economic resources more rational.

For telemedicine, the principles applicable to the study of complex systems apply, taking up the holistic approach compared to the reductionist one, which for many years has prevailed in medical research and, therefore, also in the patient–physician relationship. In the reductionist approach, the analysis of the disease, understood as organ or apparatus failure, is simpler and cheaper and has allowed us great progress in the knowledge of biological mechanisms and the pathogenesis of diseases, paving the way for more effective therapies. But man is himself a complex system that is born, lives (sometimes getting sick), and dies within complex systems, which interfere with each other. Obviously, it is not a question of returning to the holistic approach of the ancestors, science and mysticism have been separated for centuries, today's challenge is to investigate all the effects and interactions that occur in a perturbed system, contributing to the realization of our target. In human history it has often been necessary to look back to go further. Telemedicine can help us in our approach to such a complex system of interactions, even if not all the effects of innovation are predictable and appear clearly to us, because they will not simply correspond to the sum of the categories we have analyzed.

The next few years will give us the answer to the questions that our reflections require us to ask, in order to continue to keep the debate on the relevance of the patient–physician relationship alive:

Will technology ever exceed the accuracy of a face-to-face visit?

Will the "machine" mediator also become an actor in the patient–physician relationship?

Will a global standard of care be achieved?

We are probably facing an era of ubiquitous computerization of daily life, but the relationship between the healer and those who ask for his or her work will remain the relationship of two people who need each other. Although the speed of spread of telemedicine depends a lot on political decision-makers, the COVID-19 pandemic has once again shown that when innovations are useful, they also have a strength of their own that guarantees their affirmation [69–72]. Political decision-makers remain responsible for intercepting the changes produced by the evolution of technology and preparing adequate legislation.

We are facing a process that has just begun, but which already announces better prevention and therapy of diseases, but also a coherent predictivity of pathological development, capable of offering more and more a personalized perspective of treatment.

Acknowledgments The authors are grateful to Annapaola Ambrosio and Paolo Caracciolo for their contributions.

References

1. Smith R. The NHS: possibilities for the endgame. Think more about reducing expectations. BMJ. 1999;318(7178):209–10. https://doi.org/10.1136/bmj.318.7178.209.
2. Coppa A, Bondioli L, Cucina A, Frayer DW, Jarrige C, Jarrige J-F, Quivron G, Rossi M, Vidale M, Macchiarelli R. Palaeontology: early Neolithic tradition of dentistry. Nature. 2006;440(7085):755–6. https://doi.org/10.1038/440755a.
3. Smith Edwin Papyrus: Egyptian medical book—Encyclopaedia Britannica, retrieved 21 December 2016.
4. Magner Lois N. A history of medicine. Taylor & Francis Group, 2005.
5. Werner Jaeger. Die Formung des griechischen Menschen – Paideia, 1934.
6. Leonardi F. The definition of health: towards new perspectives. Int J Health Serv. 2018;48(4):735–48. https://doi.org/10.1177/0020731418782653. Epub 2018 Jun 14
7. Koplan JP, Christopher Bond T, Merson MH, Srinath Reddy K, Rodriguez MH, Sewankambo NK, Wasserheit JN. Consortium of Universities for Global Health Executive Board—towards a common definition of global health. Lancet. 2009;373(9679):1993–5. https://doi.org/10.1016/S0140-6736(09)60332-9. Epub 2009 Jun 1
8. Agarwal N, Jain P, Pathak R, Gupta R. Telemedicine in India: a tool for transforming health care in the era of COVID-19 pandemic. RevJ Educ Health Promot. 2020;9:190. https://doi.org/10.4103/jehp.jehp_472_20. eCollection 2020
9. World Health Organization (WHO). Telemedicine opportunities and developments in Member States, 2009.
10. Chaet D, Clearfield R, Sabin JE, Skimming K, Council on Ethical and Judicial Affairs American Medical Association. Ethical practice in telehealth and telemedicine. Rev J Gen Intern Med. 2017;32(10):1136–40. https://doi.org/10.1007/s11606-017-4082-2. Epub 2017 Jun 26
11. Tudor Hart J. The inverse care law. Lancet. 1971;297:405–12. https://doi.org/10.1016/S0140-6736(71)92410-X.
12. Siegler M. The future of the doctor-patient relationship in a world of managed care. Med Secoli. 1998;10(1):41–56.
13. Emanuel EJ, Emanuel LL. Four models of the physician-patient relationship affiliations expand. JAMA. 1992;267(16):2221–6.
14. Medscape Physician Compensation Report 2019.
15. Farmer, Blake (2018) When doctors struggle with suicide, their profession often fails them. NPR. Retrieved December 5, 2019
16. Han S, Shanafelt TD, Sinsky CA, Awad KM, Dyrbye LN, Fiscus LC, Trockel M, Goh J. Estimating the attributable cost of physician Burnout in the United States. Ann Intern Med. 2019;170(11):784–90. https://doi.org/10.7326/M18-1422. Epub 2019 May 28
17. Wu AW. Medical error: the second victim. The doctor who makes the mistake needs help too. BMJ. 2000;320:726–7. https://doi.org/10.1136/bmj.320.7237.726.
18. World Medical Association (WMA): Declaration on the Rights of the Patient 1981.
19. American Hospital Association (AHA): Patient's Bill of Rights 1992.
20. Riskin A, Erez A, Foulk TA, Riskin-Geuz KS, Ziv A, Sela R, Pessach-Gelblum L, Bamberger PA. Rudeness and medical team performance—randomized controlled trial. Pediatrics. 2017;139(2):e20162305. https://doi.org/10.1542/peds.2016-2305. Epub 2017 Jan 10
21. Asimov I. Runaround. I, robot. New York: Bantam Dell; 1950.
22. Gupta N, Chatterjee P, Choudhury T. Smart and sustainable intelligent systems (sustainable computing and optimization). Wiley-Scrivener; 2021.
23. McLuhan M, Powers BR. The global village: transformations in world life and media in the 21st century. Oxford University Press Inc.; 1992.
24. Bashshur RL, Shannon GW. History of telemedicine: evolution, context, and transformation. New Rochelle, NY: Mary Ann Liebert, Inc.; 2009. p. 25–76.
25. Menage J. Why telemedicine diminishes the doctor-patient relationship. Comment BMJ. 2020;371:m4348. https://doi.org/10.1136/bmj.m4348.

26. Erin Shigekawa, Margaret Fix, Garen Corbett, Dylan H. Roby, Janet Coffman. The current state of telehealth evidence: a rapid review. Rev Health Aff (Millwood) 2018;37(12):1975–1982. doi: 10.1377/ hlthaff.2018.05132.
27. Chang Y-W, Hsu P-Y, Wang Y, Chang P-Y. Integration of online and offline health services: the role of doctor-patient online interaction. Patient Educ Couns. 2019;102(10):1905–10. https://doi.org/10.1016/j.pec.2019.04.018. Epub 2019 Apr 18 PMID: 31279612
28. Yan M, Tan H, Jia L, Akram U. The antecedents of poor doctor-patient relationship in mobile consultation: a perspective from computer-mediated communication. Int J Environ Res Public Health. 2020;17(7):2579. https://doi.org/10.3390/ijerph17072579.
29. Sabesan S, Allen D, Caldwell P, Loh PK, Mozer R, Komesaroff PA, Talman P, Williams M, Shaheen N, Grabinski O. Royal Australasian College of Physicians Telehealth Working Group. Practical aspects of telehealth: doctor-patient relationship and communication. Rev. Intern Med J. 2014;44(1):101–3. https://doi.org/10.1111/imj.12323.
30. Protásio Lemos da Luz. Telemedicine and the doctor/patient relationship. Editorial Arq Bras Cardiol. 2019;113(1):100–2. https://doi.org/10.5935/abc.20190117.
31. Friedemann Schulz von Thun: Miteinander reden: Störungen und Klärungen. Psychologie der zwischenmenschlichen Kommunikation. Rowohlt, Reinbek 1981. ISBN 3–499–17489-8.
32. Bai Q, Dan Q, Zhe M, Yang M. A systematic review of emoji: current research and future perspectives. Front Psychol. 2019;10:2221. doi: 10.3389/ fpsyg.2019.02221. eCollection:2019.
33. Tasneem S, Kim A, Bagheri A, Lebret J. Telemedicine video visits for patients receiving palliative care: a qualitative study. Am J Hosp Palliat Care. 2019;36(9):789–94. https://doi.org/10.1177/1049909119846843. Epub 2019 May 7
34. Onor ML, Misan S. The clinical interview and the doctor-patient relationship in telemedicine. Telemed J E Health. 2005;11(1):102–5. https://doi.org/10.1089/tmj.2005.11.102.
35. Terrasse M, Gorin M, Sisti D. Social Media, E-Health, and medical ethics. Hast Cent Rep. 2019;49(1):24–33. https://doi.org/10.1002/hast.975.
36. Zhang W, Deng Z, Hong Z, Evans R, Ma J, Zhang H. Unhappy patients are not alike: content analysis of the negative comments from China's good doctor website. J Med Internet Res. 2018;20(1):e35. https://doi.org/10.2196/jmir.8223. PMID: 29371176
37. Pearl J, Mackenzie D. The book of why: the new science of cause and effect. Basic Books; 2017.
38. Bhaskar S, Bradley S, Sakhamuri S, Moguilner S, Chattu VK, Pandya S, Schroeder S, Ray D, Banach M. Designing futuristic telemedicine using artificial intelligence and robotics in the COVID-19 Era. Front Public Health. 2020;8:556789. https://doi.org/10.3389/fpubh.2020.556789. eCollection 2020
39. Regulation (Eu) 2016/679 of The European Parliament and of the Council—On the protection of natural persons with regard to the processing of personal data and on the free movement of such data, and repealing Directive 95/46/EC (General Data Protection Regulation) 27 April 2016.
40. Náfrádi L, Nakamoto K, Schulz PJ. Is patient empowerment the key to promote adherence? A systematic review of the relationship between self-efficacy, health locus of control and medication adherence. PLoS One. 2017;12(10):e0186458. https://doi.org/10.1371/journal.pone.0186458. eCollection
41. van Riel PL, Zuidema RM, Vogel C, Rongen-van Dartel SA. Patient self-management and tracking: a European experience. Rev Rheum Dis Clin North Am. 2019;45(2):187–95. https://doi.org/10.1016/j.rdc.2019.01.008.
42. Silverman RD. Current legal and ethical concerns in telemedicine and e-medicine. J Telemed Telecare. 2003;9(Suppl. 1):S67. https://doi.org/10.1258/135763303322196402.
43. Fogel AL, Kvedar JC. Reported cases of medical malpractice in direct-to-consumer telemedicine. JAMA. 2019;321(13):1309–10.
44. Tulchinsky TH. Marc Lalonde, the health field concept and health promotion. Case Studies Public Health. 2018:523–41. https://doi.org/10.1016/B978-0-12-804571-8.00028-7.
45. Kruse CS, Krowski N, Rodriguez B, Tran L, Vela J, Brooks M. Telehealth and patient satisfaction: a systematic review and narrative analysis. BMJ Open. 2017;7(8):e016242. https://doi.org/10.1136/bmjopen-2017-016242.

46. Hyder MA, Razzak J. Telemedicine in the United States: an introduction for students and residents. J Med Internet Res. 2020;22(11):e20839. https://doi.org/10.2196/20839.
47. Randhawa RS, Chandan JS, Thomas T, Singh S. An exploration of the attitudes and views of general practitioners on the use of video consultations in a primary healthcare setting: a qualitative pilot study. Prim Health Care Res Dev. 2019;20:e5. https://doi.org/10.1017/S1463423618000361. Epub 2018 Jun 18
48. Marino MM, Rienzo M, Serra N, Nicola Marino R, Ricciotti L, Mazzariello CA, Leonetti MP, Ceraldi A, Casamassimi F, Capocelli G, Martone AL, Caracciolo. Mobile screening units for the early detection of breast cancer and cardiovascular disease: a pilot telemedicine study in Southern Italy. Telemed J E Health. 2020;26(3):286–93. https://doi.org/10.1089/tmj.2018.0328. Epub 2019 Apr 4
49. Manta C, Jain SS, Coravos A, Mendelsohn D, Izmailova ES. An evaluation of biometric monitoring technologies for vital signs in the era of COVID-19. Rev Clin Transl Sci. 2020;13(6):1034–44. https://doi.org/10.1111/cts.12874. Epub 2020 Oct 12
50. Cabrera MF, Arredondo MT, Quiroga J. Integration of telemedicine into emergency medical services. J Telemed Telecare 2002;8(Suppl. 2):12–14. doi: 10.1177/ 1357633X020080S206.
51. Martins C, Godycki-Cwirko M, Heleno B, Brodersen J. Quaternary prevention: reviewing the concept. Eur J Gen Pract. 2018;24(1):106–11. https://doi.org/10.1080/13814788.2017.1422177.
52. Tanrikulu MA, Agirbasli M, Berenson G. Primordial prevention of cardiometabolic risk in childhood. Rev Adv Exp Med Biol. 2017;956:489–96. https://doi.org/10.1007/5584_2016_172.
53. Falkner B, Lurbe E. Primordial prevention of high blood pressure in childhood: an opportunity not to be missed. Hypertension. 2020;75(5):1142–50. https://doi.org/10.1161/HYPERTENSIONAHA.119.14059. Epub 2020 Mar 30
54. Bhaskar S, Bradley S, Chattu VK, Adisesh A, Nurtazina A, Kyrykbayeva S, Sakhamuri S, Yaya S, Sunil T, Thomas P, Mucci V, Moguilner S, Israel-Korn S, Alacapa J, Mishra A, Pandya S, Schroeder S, Atreja A, Banach M, Ray D. Telemedicine across the globe-position paper From the COVID-19 Pandemic Health System Resilience PROGRAM (REPROGRAM) International Consortium (Part 1). Front Public Health. 2020;8:556720. https://doi.org/10.3389/fpubh.2020.556720. eCollection 2020
55. Bhaskar S, Bradley S, Chattu VK, Adisesh A, Nurtazina A, Kyrykbayeva S, Sakhamuri S, Moguilner S, Pandya S, Schroeder S, Banach M, Ray D. Telemedicine as the new outpatient clinic gone digital: position paper from the Pandemic Health System REsilience PROGRAM (REPROGRAM) International Consortium (Part 2). Front Public Health. 2020;8:410. https://doi.org/10.3389/fpubh.2020.00410. eCollection 2020
56. Officer A, Thiyagarajan JA, Schneiders ML, Nash P, de la Fuente-Núñez V. Ageism, healthy life expectancy and population ageing: how are they related? Int J Environ Res Public Health. 2020;17(9):3159. https://doi.org/10.3390/ijerph17093159.
57. Williams B, Warren S, McKim R, Janzen W. Caller self-care decisions following teletriage advice—comparative study. J Clin Nurs. 2012;21(7–8):1041–50. https://doi.org/10.1111/j.1365-2702.2011.03986.x. Epub 2012 Jan 27
58. Coleman K, Austin BT, Brach C, Wagner EH. Evidence on the chronic care model in the new millennium. Health Aff (Millwood). 2009;28(1):75–85. https://doi.org/10.1377/hlthaff.28.1.75.
59. Campbell H, Hotchkiss R, Bradshaw N, Porteous M. Integrated care pathways. Rev BMJ. 1998;316(7125):133–7. https://doi.org/10.1136/bmj.316.7125.133.
60. Parry W, Wolters AT, Brine RJ, Steventon A. Effect of an integrated care pathway on use of primary and secondary healthcare by patients at high risk of emergency inpatient admission: a matched control cohort study in Tower Hamlets—Observational Study. BMJ Open. 2019;119(6):e026470. https://doi.org/10.1136/bmjopen-2018-026470.
61. Shaw S, Levenson R. Towards integrated care in Trafford. Research report—UK. London: Nuffeld Trust; 2011.
62. Frid AS, Ratti MFG, Pedretti A, Valinoti M, Martínez B, Sommer J, Luna D, Plazzotta F. Teletriage Pilot Study (strategy for unscheduled teleconsultations): results, patient accep-

tance and satisfaction. Stud Health Technol Inform. 2020;270:776–80. https://doi.org/10.3233/SHTI200266.

63. Yellowlees P, Chan SR, Parish MB. The hybrid doctor-patient relationship in the age of technology—telepsychiatry consultations and the use of virtual space. Rev Int Rev Psychiatry. 2015;27(6):476–89. https://doi.org/10.3109/09540261.2015.1082987. Epub 2015 Oct 23

64. Flodgren G, Rachas A, Farmer AJ, Inzitari M, Shepperd S. Interactive telemedicine: effects on professional practice and health care outcomes. Rev Cochrane Database Syst Rev. 2015;(9):CD002098. https://doi.org/10.1002/14651858.CD002098.pub2.

65. Hara T, Nishizuka T, Yamamoto M, Iwatsuki K, Natsume T, Hirata H. Teletriage for patients with traumatic finger injury directing emergency medical transportation services to appropriate hospitals: a pilot project in Nagoya City, Japan. Injury. 2015;46(7):1349–53. https://doi.org/10.1016/j.injury.2015.02.022.

66. Odendaal WA, Watkins JA, Leon N, Goudge J, Griffiths F, Tomlinson M, Daniels K. Health workers' perceptions and experiences of using mHealth technologies to deliver primary healthcare services: a qualitative evidence synthesis. Meta-Anal Cochrane Database Syst Rev. 2020:CD011942. https://doi.org/10.1002/14651858.CD011942.pub2.

67. Tzeyu L, Michaud JZ, McCarthy MA, Siahpush M, Su D. Costs of home-based telemedicine programs: a systematic review. Int J Technol Assess Health Care. 2018;34(4):410–8. https://doi.org/10.1017/S0266462318000454. Epub 2018 Jul 30

68. Kaplan B. Revisting health information technology ethical, legal, and social issues and evaluation: telehealth/telemedicine and COVID-19. Int J Med Inform. 2020;143:104239.

69. Ohannessian R, Duong TA, Odone A. Global telemedicine implementation and integration within health systems to fight the COVID-19 pandemic: a call to action. JMIR Public Health Surveill. 2020;6(2):e18810.

70. Lukas H, Xu C, Yu Y, Gao W. Emerging telemedicine tools for remote COVID-19 diagnosis, monitoring, and management. ACS Nano. 2020;14(12):16180–93.

71. Bokolo AJ. Exploring the adoption of telemedicine and virtual software for care of outpatients during and after COVID-19 pandemic. Irish J Med Sci (1971-). 2021;190(1):1–10.

72. Garattini L, Martini MB, Zanetti M (2020) More room for telemedicine after COVID-19: lessons for primary care?

Smart Health Monitoring System

5

Fahmi Ben Rejab ⓘ and Kaouther Nouira ⓘ

5.1 Introduction

Intensive care unit denoted by ICU can be defined as a special department in hospital which gives a special treatment and monitoring for patients who suffer from severe illnesses. In ICU, most of the patients require a complete medical assistance which justifies the necessity of an important and reliable monitoring. They are supervised through an online monitoring system over time. This latter considers several medical parameters. These latter have not to exceed a threshold which was set by the medical staff; otherwise, the patient will be in critical state. In fact, an alarm is generated each time that the measured parameter exceeds its limit [1].

Monitoring system in ICU aims to make patients safe and to help doctors to take the best decision. It is based on alarms which are important and sometimes lifesaving to detect critical states. Unfortunately, in ICU there are numerous triggered alarms. In some cases, they describe real critical states of patients, and most frequently, they are considered as irrelevant or as false alarms [2]. In addition, they do not correctly describe the patient state and they have no clinical significance. Furthermore, the current system does not consider the real link between measured parameters and the evolution of patient's state [3].

Many researchers focused on the problem of excessive alarms. Tsien and Fackler [1] concluded that 86% of false-positive alarms are generated in ICU. Many other studies proved the same problem with monitoring system where the false alarms rate exceeds 90%. The constant alarming of monitors has bad effect on patients. It can also be frightening and worrying to medical staff [1]. In fact, this highly sophisticated monitoring equipment is created to guarantee the best care. Numerous clinical but also social studies contribute to demonstrate the need for efficient

F. B. Rejab (✉) · K. Nouira
BESTMOD, Institut Supérieur de Gestion de Tunis, Université de Tunis, Le Bardo, Tunisia
e-mail: fahmi.benrejab@isg.rnu.tn; kaouther.nouira@planet.tn

T. Choudhury et al. (eds.), *Telemedicine: The Computer Transformation of Healthcare*, TELe-Health, https://doi.org/10.1007/978-3-030-99457-0_5

monitoring tools in the medical field. Many works were proposed to minimize the important number of inaccurate alarms in ICU including digital signal processing [4], trend extraction methodology, and intelligent monitoring [1]. Smart health is more and more necessary as it helps to make the right decisions at real time [5].

Through this study, we present a novel Smart health Monitoring System (SMS) using machine learning techniques and the expert knowledge (i.e., medical staff). Our main purpose is to improve the patients monitoring conditions by detecting alarms and reducing the false and/or irrelevant ones. The SMS uses machine learning techniques to help the medical staff when making decisions at real time. As a result, our new system aims to build and update an intelligent model that detects normal and critical patients states over time and store data relative to monitored patients.

We propose a system using the real-time support vector machines method (RTSVM) and data stream technology. This system needs a training phase to build the classification model. But medical staff needs a system that starts the classification task immediately when we have a new patient to be monitored. To this end, we have to use an existing model generated from training data relative to a number of patients (a group of patients) with similar conditions. These groups are built using the k-prototypes method. Hence, our RTSVM acquires and stores data using the developed data stream component. Then, it makes the classification of patients' states to detect critical ones and adjust the model parameters when new annotated data are available to be more accurate for next observations.

5.2   Health Monitoring System and False Alarms

Patient monitoring is an important task insured by systems and medical staff on which the patient life depends. In fact, monitoring system in ICU is considered as one of the most important tools used to monitor patients. It continuously measures one or several parameters (such as heart rate, saturated percentage of oxygen in the blood, and respiration rate), displays, and/or records them for the medical staff to take the best decision at real time. Hence, the monitoring system presents a fundamental tool that helps medical staff to do their works in the best conditions. The multi-parameter monitoring system indicates the state of patients, i.e., stable or critical. Each medical parameter is measured and has two limits (i.e., consisting of minimum and maximum measures). These limits are set by medical staff. If there are some values that do not respect (exceed) these limits, an alarm is triggered. An alarm informs and warns medical staff that a patient has a serious problem and needs an immediate intervention. As a result, medical staff considers triggered alarms as a warning of critical states.

5.2.1   Alarms: Causes and Results

Actually, monitoring systems in ICU allow the access to monitor parameters. Alarms mean a violation of a threshold parameter. For each monitoring parameter, two thresholds are set corresponding to a minimum and a maximum value of the threshold. The values in this interval relative to measured parameters are considered as normal (patient is in a stable state). As a result, any alarm translates an unstable value of the parameter, and thus it indicates a critical state of a patient. According to the patient's condition, his treatment, and morphology, the doctor in charge chooses these thresholds. These latter are fixed but can be always changed by the doctor during the monitoring task.

However, medical staff often keeps the default values of threshold and uses the monitoring system as a measurement tool. To make the best decision and to provide the appropriate treatment and drug, medical staff needs important data.

If a certain threshold is exceeded for a measured medical parameter, an alarm is generated. However, it is not the best solution for providing and describing the patient states. In fact, medical staff generally needs precision information describing the critical changes of the patient state. Moreover, the violation of the thresholds does not reflect the real situation of a patient since the relation between different medical parameters and their simultaneous evolution are neglected. Alarms should consider the relation between the different parameters. Studies proved that most triggered alarms are not accurate meaning that they have not always clinical relevance [6]. Siebig et al. analyze monitoring data recorded in ICU and relative to 68 patients with critical states in ICU. They recorded 5934 alarms over a period of 982 hours. They observed that 15% of all detected alarms are clinically accurate (i.e., true alarms).

In addition, researchers are working to propose new monitoring systems with a better scalability considering the overall conditions of patients [1]. They also focused on the best way to consider the patients' states and to study data in ICU.

The multi-parameter monitoring system can monitor up to 20 variables per patient in the course of time. Data is characterized by uncertainty, vagueness, and ambiguity, and can have very high frequency of acquisition (streaming data).

5.2.2 Proposed Approaches for False Alarm Reduction

In order to reduce false alarm rates in ICU, many research for reducing the rate of false alarms were presented. They focused on two main possibilities. The first one is based on the creation of more efficiency and better sensors that minimize measurement noise and notice systematic faults such as disconnected wires [7]. The second one is developing intelligent algorithms for the detection of alarms relative to monitored patients [8, 9]. Several algorithms including the neural networks, the classification trees, and the fuzzy logic have proved their efficiency to reduce false alarm rates. These artificial intelligence algorithms may also be applied for improving more general criteria when monitoring patient, such as data integration and analysis, prognosis generation, and decision support.

Researchers have reported some approaches that were developed to improve medical devices and specially to minimize the rate of false alarms. In Schmid et al. [10] study, several approaches are reported including the improvement made in the monitoring system using the signal extraction for reducing false alarms caused by artifacts. In addition, research by Borowski et al. [4] presented an overview of some artificial intelligence algorithms used in ICU for monitoring patients. In this study, they tried to interpret alarms by imitating human thinking.

Generally, monitoring patients is a complex task. Data generated by the monitoring system, the high dimensionality of data (as we can monitor multiple variables for each patient), and the relation between the measured parameters make the task of monitoring patients more and more difficult. These characteristics of the monitoring system can be the causes of the important rate of false alarms. These alarms have bad effects on both medical staff and patients.

These problems pushed researchers to develop new methods and algorithms to improve monitoring quality in ICU. Fortunately, machine learning techniques can provide efficient algorithms that overcome the problem of false alarms and improve the monitoring task.

5.3   Machine Learning Techniques

In this section, we detail our theoretical proposal, i.e., the real-time support vector machines denoted by RTSVM by providing its description and algorithm.

5.3.1   Real-Time Support Vector Machines

The support vector machines denoted by SVM [11] present one of the well-known algorithms for classification. Its main drawback is working in batch mode. In other words, adding new annotated examples means retraining from the beginning.

Researchers have proposed new versions based on the standard SVM such as the incremental and decremental SVM [12] and the LASVM [13]. These latter are considered as online methods (i.e., the update of models is needed in training phase). These proposed methods deal with the problem of large datasets by introducing the incremental learning in training phase to minimize the execution time and memory requirement. Currently, the real-time learning (i.e., the update of models is needed in test phase) is needed in many fields.

In this context, we have studied and implemented our algorithm, consisting of a real-time version of support vector machines for classification denoted by RTSVM [14, 15]. In other words, it is possible to improve the classification model, when we add new records in the test phase, without restarting the training task from the beginning.

In fact, by proposing the RTSVM, we can deal with these aspects:

- The expert (which is the doctor) interaction: His decisions can change with the evolution of patient states, i.e., with the change of the meaning of data over time.
- The improvement of the classification model over time: Adjusting the model when new annotated data are available in test phase is important. The model can improve the accuracy of new observations over time.

Thus, the real-time algorithm considers of new annotated data that are added incrementally in test phase.

In fact, incremental learning corresponds to training phase. Real-time learning allows the update of the model over time in test phase.

We build the first model using a training set. Then, it classifies new observations. After that, the current model is improved by using new annotated data set by the expert in test phase.

As follows, we give a description of the input, output, and our new algorithm.

- The algorithm inputs: The input requested from the RTSVM is described by the following pseudo-code:

INPUTS
```
    1. TrainingSet (Xi,Yi): Xi: an observation, Yi: the corre-
       sponding label of Xi, i = 1..1.
    2. W and b which are respectively the weight and the bias
       that are computed in training phase.
    3. Partition of the training set into CandidateSet (S) and
       ErrorSet (E).
    4. The cost C, KernelType, and KernelParameters are used as
       parameters and they are obtained from RTSVM training
       phase using the grid search technique.
    5. S is the set of new annotated observations (i.e. candi-
       date set) Sc = (Xc, Yc).
```

- The algorithm outputs: In test phase, we obtain the TrainingSet, parameters (W, b, C, Kernel and its parameters), CandidateSet, and ErrorSet generated by the RTSVM. Please note that all these values should be stored to train new values. When training with the support vector machines, only the training set, weight, and bias are necessary. The output contains all the updated values produced from the inputs.

OUTPUTS
```
    1. A new TrainingSet: (Xi, Yi, i = 1,..,1),
    2. The weight W and the bias b with new and
       updated values.
    3. A new CandidateSet (S) and a new ErrorSet (E).
```

RTSVM Algorithm [15]
```
BEGIN
```

$$M \leftarrow RTSVM \left(\text{The initial model} \right)$$

```
For each new observation
```
X_i

$$Y_i \leftarrow M \left(X_i \right)$$

$Y_i \leftarrow M(X_i)$ ```IF``` X_i ```is not a candidate```
```
AddErrorset
```
(X_i)
```
Else
AddCandidate
```
(X_i, Y_i) ```at the candidateSet.```
```
END IF
For each time interval.
Print CandidateSet.
Update CandidateSet from Expert Decision.
PROCESS()
REPROCESS()
```

$$M \leftarrow Update \left(M, parameters \right)$$

```
End For.
End For.
END
```

Note that PROCESS procedure attempts to insert an example K that does not belong to the set of potential support vector S into the set of current support vectors.

PROCESS Procedure
```
BEGIN
```

$$\text{Exit if } k \in S.$$
$$S \leftarrow S \cup \{K\}$$
$$M \leftarrow Update \left(M, parameters \right)$$

```
END
```

However, the REPROCESS procedure removes some elements from the set of potential support vector S with a maximal gradient. Then, it eliminates blatant non-support vectors. Finally, it calculates the bias term of the decision function denoted by b.

REPROCESS Procedure
```
BEGIN
```

$$i \leftarrow search(K;S) : first\ example$$
$$j \leftarrow search(K;S) : second\ exam3.$$
$$if\ (i,j)\ is\ not\ a\ violating\ pair\ then$$
$$Exit,$$
$$else$$
$$for\ all\ s \in S\ such\ that\ \alpha_s = 0\ do$$
$$S = S - s$$
$$end\ for$$
$$M \leftarrow Update(M, parameters)$$

```
END
```

Based on this procedure, we remark that the initial (original) model of classification is the input of the RTSVM which is generated in training phase. If a new vector is available, i.e., a set of medical variables that are measured, RTSVM algorithm associates a label to this vector that is equal to (+1) when it belongs to the first class or (−1) otherwise. The vector is considered as a candidate if it could be a support vector. In this case, RTSVM algorithm assigns it to CandidateSet. When classifying new medical information, the expert has to confirm that the CandidateSet for each predetermined interval time is correct. This validation is made by expert. He proves and may modify the label assigned by RTSVM.

After setting CandidateSet by the expert, the original model parameters are updated. This update uses the two functions of LASVM which are the PROCESS and REPROCESS. This step aims to minimize the time of execution relative to the training. The reduction of the execution time is made by only using the CandidateSet (the whole dataset is not used) for retraining the initial model. Besides, it increases the accuracy of the original model over time.

5.3.2   K-Prototypes Clustering Method

The k-prototypes method presents the second machine learning technique that will be used in this paper. The aim of this method is to make groups of similar patients and to build for each group a global classification model using the RTSVM. Then, when there is a new patient to be monitored, the model of the most similar group to this patient is selected and used to classify the states.

The k-prototypes is a method for clustering mixture data. It was proposed by Huang [16]. This algorithm deals with databases with both numeric and categorical data. It consists of the improvement of k-means algorithm. The k-prototypes clustering algorithm applies two different distances between attributes. The Euclidean distance is devoted to numeric attributes (which represents the same distance used by the k-means algorithm) and the simple matching dissimilarity measure devoted to categorical attributes (as the k-modes algorithm [17] does for calculating the distance between objects). Two objects with different values will enlarge the distance between them and the objects will be considered as different.

Assume there are X and Y two objects having mixture attributes' values, i.e., categorical and numeric, and each object has the following representation:

$$X = \left\{ A_1^r, A_2^r, \ldots, A_p^r, A_{p+1}^c, A_{p+2}^c, \ldots, A_m^c \right\} \tag{5.1}$$

where m presents the attributes number, p presents a subset of numeric attributes, the $(m\text{-}p)$ attributes present categorical data.

The dissimilarity $d(X,Y)$ between the objects X and Y is computed by applying the following formula:

$$d(X,Y) = \sum_{j=1}^{p} \left(x_j + y_j \right)^2 + \gamma \sum_{j=p+1}^{m} \delta \left(x_j + y_j \right) \tag{5.2}$$

The first part presents the Euclidean distance applied to numeric values of attributes. The second part corresponds to the dissimilarity measure which is the simple matching. It is used for categorical values of attributes. It is defined by Eq. (5.3).

$$\delta \left(x_j, y_i \right) = \begin{cases} 0 \text{ if } x_j = y_j \\ 1 \text{ if } x_j = y_j \end{cases} \tag{5.3}$$

Note that p is the number of numeric attributes and m is the number of categorical attributes. γ presents a weight used to not favor any type of attributes.

In this study, we apply k-prototypes algorithm as it provides many advantages and overcomes the main limits of the k-means algorithm. In fact, it needs less iterations to converge and it can deal with numeric and categorical attributes. This clustering method will be used to create a cluster of patients having mixed values of attributes describing medical parameters. The obtained clusters consist of several groups of patients with similar description of their states (i.e., groups of patients sharing similar characteristics or diseases).

5.4   Proposed Approach: The SMS

Our main aims in this work are reducing the rate of false alarms, collecting, and storing streaming data generated from monitoring system in order to detect critical state of patients over time. Thus, we develop a new Smart health Monitoring System (SMS) for ICU.

Current monitoring system works at real time; however, it provides many false alarms. In addition, patient states and data generated by the monitoring system (MS) change over time. Thus, the model generated during the training phase is not able to handle new data. As a result, we aim to propose a new real-time or scalable MS (i.e., able to be adapted to the change of data).

First, our new SMS uses the k-prototypes algorithm to make clusters of patients sharing similar parameters and information, i.e., suffering from similar diseases. After that, the real-time support vector machines algorithm [14] is used to collect data generated from the monitoring system using our new developed data stream component and then it stores this data stream. Finally, the RTSVM makes the classification of patient states to detect critical states.

The SMS algorithm can be adapted to new information in training and test phases without retraining from the beginning. It can provide a first model for each cluster of patients by applying RTSVM. When we have a new patient to be monitored, the SMS detects in which group the patient can belong. Then, we use the model of this group to immediately start the classification task (i.e., detecting alarms) without making the training phase. Then, for each time interval, RTSVM updates its model with new arriving values relative to the states of patients based on new annotated data by the expert, i.e., the doctor. This aspect is denoted by the self-regulation or any-time learning or real-time learning. Hence, the new system provides necessary information that facilitate the decision-making by medical staff. It also generates alarms relative to patients which are monitored in ICU. Moreover, we improve our monitoring system to be able to not only synchronize the collection of physiological signals but also clinical annotations. These latter are included in our new real-time algorithm when training and evaluating alarms.

Figure 5.1 provides a description of the SMS that uses the k-prototypes and RTSVM techniques.

Based on Fig. 5.1, we remark that the SMS follows five main steps:

1. The new system should regroup patients in different clusters using the k-prototypes technique.
2. Then, the RTSVM is applied to build an initial model for each group.
3. When we have a new patient to be monitored, the information of this patient has to be available in the MS. Then, the SMS computes the distance between this new patient and all existing groups.
4. Finally, SMS uses the model of the most similar group to the new patient. Thus, the system starts the classification of data collected from MS using the data stream component without the training phase.
5. For each interval time predetermined by medical staff, the expert validates the candidateSet (that means a vector can be defined as a support vector). He approves or changes the label of the vector. After the validation of the candidateSet, RTSVM updates and generates the new models' parameters to be more accurate in the future.

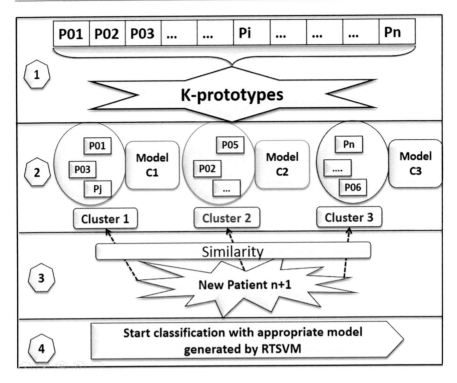

Fig. 5.1 Smart monitoring system structure

In order to get our SMS, we propose the RTSVM monitoring system (RTSVM-MS), then we make improvement to it by introducing k-prototypes.

5.4.1 Real-Time SVM for Monitoring System

In order to better interpret medical data over time, real-time systems are used. These systems are also applied to adapt the model with new information and/or new conditions. In this work, our purpose is to improve the MS in ICU by applying a new real-time monitoring system. This latter has as input a model which is produced by RTSVM method in the training phase. Finally, the current model is updated and improved by the expert opinion. In this section, we will detail our real-time monitoring system that uses the real-time SVM (RTSVM) [14].

Figure 5.2 describes the structure of our proposal using the RTSVM algorithm and the data stream component.

This system uses data describing medical parameters measured over time which dynamically change. It also uses states of patients that vary over time and are critical. It is necessary to consider new data over time in both training and test phases [18]. The proposed real-time monitoring system considers all new information

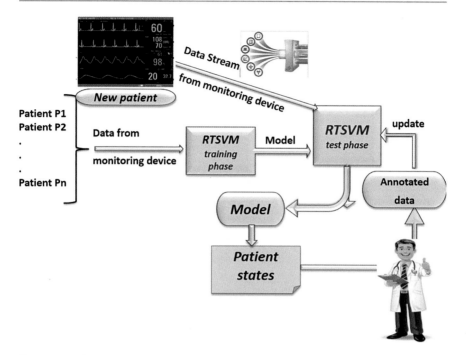

Fig. 5.2 Monitoring system using RTSVM

describing patients states over time. Besides, it updates the model generated by
RTSVM each time interval which make the model more correct and more precise.
They also overcome the problem of missing information. Hence, our proposal pro-
vides more accurate and easier monitoring.

Seven main steps are followed for reaching the results. They are illustrated as
follows:

1. Divide the dataset relative to patients into training and test sets.
2. Build the initial model using RTSVM method based on the training set.
3. In test phase, start the classification of observations using the model resulting
   from the training phase. As a result, doctors could be alerted if a patient has a
   critical state based on vectors (e.g., SPO_2, HR, RESP) generated by the monitoring system.
4. For each vector, RTSVM tests the classified vector if it is a candidate vector or
   an error vector and keeps only the candidate vectors.
5. For each interval time predetermined by medical staff, the expert validates the
   candidateSet by approving or changing the label of the vector.
6. Knowing the CandidateSet, RTSVM updates and generates the new models'
   parameters to be more accurate in the future.
7. Make the classification of the remaining observations in the test phase.

Real-time MS provides several advantages for the monitoring system through the use of the incremental learning in training phase and test phase. Besides, this new MS handles the issues detected in ICU by providing a model that considers the dynamic changing of data over time. However, the real-time MS needs the training phase before starting the classification task. Medical staff wants that the proposed SMS immediately starts the classification task when they received a new monitored patient.

5.4.2   Improvement Monitoring System Using K-Prototypes

With classical static classification techniques, a training set is needed before we start classifying the states of patient. In this study, when we have a new patient to be monitored, we should immediately start the classification task. In fact, it is not possible to wait that the model learns from the observations, then starts the classification of patients' states. To this end, we introduce the k-prototypes clustering technique that guarantees the clustering of similar patients based on their attributes (i.e., information and characteristics; see Table 5.1 [19]) in the same group. Then, we build a classification model for each cluster using RTSVM (Table 5.2).

Thus, when we have a new patient, we can compute the similarity distance between the patient and each group (see Eq. 5.2). After that, we select the most appropriate model (i.e., the model of the group for which the distance is minimized compared to the new patient) to classify the states of the new monitored patient.

5.5   Data Stream for Monitoring System

Our proposed data stream component is very important in our new SMS. The acquired signals are made available by the Data AcQuisition (DAQ) user interface in Labview for further analysis that can be designed in the block diagram panel. The interface of our proposed component of data stream is presented in Fig. 5.3. This latter describes a block diagram relative to the module of data acquisition which is generated by Labview.

After acquisition of data from the MS, we store data in a structured database designed by Oracle Stream.

Table 5.1 Example of measured parameters [19]

Medical parameters	Lower limit	Higher limit
Heart rate (HR)	50	120
Respiratory rate (RR)	5	25
Pulse rate (PR)	65	115
Saturated percentage of oxygen in the blood (SPO$_2$)	90	130

Table 5.2 Monitored patients' parameters [19]

Patient	Age	Sex	Diagnostic	Surgery	Rhythm	ART	PAPmax	PAPmin	RAP	RESP	Ventilation
P 01	80	0	Carotid	Endartarec	Unifocal	95	56	16	10	16	Spontaneous
P 02	71	1	Grafting	Graft	Graft	85	32	8	4	14	Spontaneous
P 03	47	0	Laparotomy	Obstruction	Normal	110	48	28	9	36	Spontaneous
P 04	64	0	Cholecystitis	Cholecys	Normal	90	32	16	5	18	Spontaneous
P 05	56	1	Laparotomy	Graft	Sinus	90	28	20	12	12	Controlled
P 06	72	1	Endocarditis	Sepsis	Ventricular	72	47	20	11	8	Intermittent
P 07	60	0	Trauma	Graft	Normal	92	32	18	12	16	Spontaneous
P 08	71	0	Endocarditis	Regurgitation	Ventricular	70	34	16	10	16	Spontaneous
P 09	56	1	Grafting	Graft	Sinus	26	103	26	16	20	Intermittent
P 10	56	0	Endocarditis	Regurgitation	Sinus	86	80	35	16	17	Spontaneous
P 11	70	0	Nephrectomy	Regurgitation	Unifocal	102	32	16	6	20	Spontaneous
P 12	77	0	Trauma	Regurgitation	Multifocal	95	42	20	16	11	Intermittent
P 13	73	1	Angioplasty	Graft	Ventricular	87	56	32	10	20	Spontaneous
P 14	58	1	Coronary	Graft	Unifocal	84	41	13	13	18	Spontaneous

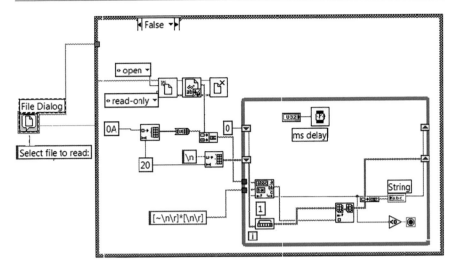

Fig. 5.3 How to synchronize and collect physiological data from monitoring system

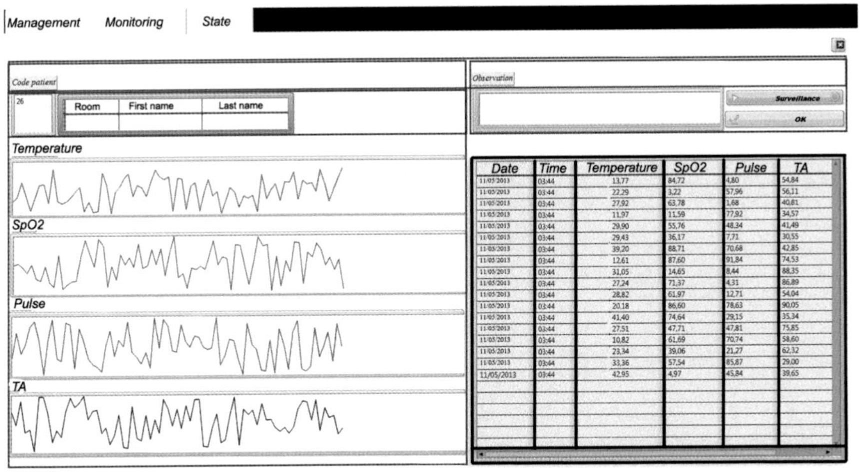

Fig. 5.4 How to present data of the new developed component for data streams

In addition, most of the devices are not using memory or relational database. We can cite the MS that is not effective for managing monitoring data. In addition, medical staff should store again data by programming another system which delays making appropriate choices. However, to make good and appropriate choices, it is necessarily to have accurate and precise data. To this end, we developed a layer presentation for medical staff to consult and monitor patient state at real time.

Figure 5.4 presents the new system output that corresponds to the report and the chart. It is possible to interpret the output from any computer and at any time.

We have used this proposed component of data stream to transfer data from data-bases to the SMS based on the RTSVM.

5.6   Experiments

This section details the experimental results of our new proposed system (SMS). For the evaluation and test of our system, we use real-world databases and different evaluation criteria.

5.6.1   The Used Databases

Table 5.3 details the real-world databases taken from Physiobank [20], which are used for the evaluation of our proposal. #Attributes defines the total number of measured parameters and #Instances presents the total number of instances for a particular database. Note that each patient presents a database with bi-classes.

The attributes used for each patient are presented in Table 5.4.

5.6.2   Evaluation Criteria

We compare our SMS to the current one and to the MS based on standard SVM. We use four evaluation criteria which are presented as follows:

1. The common performance criterion for machine learning technique is the sensitivity (S). In this work, S is the conditional probability that the monitoring system triggers relevant alarms. S informs if the system could detect true alarms (positive results) or not.

$$S = \frac{TP}{TP + FN} \tag{5.4}$$

Table 5.3 Description of the used data sets [19]

Patient	#Attributes	#Instances
P 01	6	4101
P 02	8	42,188
P 03	8	42,188
P 04	7	42,188
P 05	9	42,188
P 06	9	5350
P 07	7	11,300
P 08	7	10,600
P 09	12	5700
P 10	5	42,188
P 11	7	42,188
P 12	7	42,188
P 13	9	42,188
P 14	7	42,188

Table 5.4 The used attributes for each patient [19]

Attributes	Description
ARTmean	Arterial Revascularization Therapy
ARTsys	Systolic Arterial Revascularization Therapy
ARTdias	Diastolic Arterial Revascularization Therapy
NBPmean	Non-Invasive Blood Pressure
NBPsys	Systolic Non-Invasive Blood Pressure
NBPdias	Diastolic Non-Invasive Blood Pressure
PAPmean	Pulmonary Arterial Pressure
PAPsys	Systolic Pulmonary Arterial Pressure
PAPdias	Diastolic Pulmonary Arterial Pressure
SPO2	Oxygen Saturation
RESP	Respiratory Rate
HR	Heart Rate

2. The reduction rate of false alarm (FARR) [5]: presented the ratio of false alarms, which are removed by our proposed system, to all false alarms. More the value of the rate is high, more the results are better.

$$FARR = \frac{Suppressed\_FA}{Total\_FA} \qquad (5.5)$$

3. The error rate (ER) which corresponds to the rate of false alarms. This criterion shows the number of irrelevant alarms by a given monitoring system. More the value of the rate is low, more the results are better.

$$Error\ rate = \frac{False\ positive + False\ Negative}{Total\ Alarms} \qquad (5.6)$$

4. The true alarms rate provided by monitoring systems that proves the performance of our new system.

5.6.3 Experimental Results

Before starting the classification task, we have clustered patients in several groups using the k-prototypes.

Table 5.5 describes the resulting clusters by using the k-prototypes on datasets (detailed in Table 5.2).

We train RTSVM algorithm for all observations of cluster C_i to obtain a general model for each cluster of patients. When a new monitored patient arrives having new medical parameters (values of attributes), it is possible to categorize this patient by applying the built model of the most similar group for him. All what we need is to calculate the similarity between a new arrived patient and all available clusters (groups). We choose the most suitable model relative to the selected cluster and we classify the states of the patient using this model (without the training phase and

Table 5.5   Resulting clusters

Clusters	Patients
C01	P 01, P 03, P 07, P 12
C02	P 02, P 05, P 09, P 13, P 14
C03	P 04, P 06, P 08, P 10, P 11

Table 5.6   Sensitivity of the proposed SMS compared to different systems in percent

Databases	CS	SVM-MS	RTSVM-MS	SMS
P 01	100	86.41	97.41	99.68
P 02	100	80.76	92.28	98.14
P 03	100	68.24	95	97.70
P 04	97.77	88.63	98.66	99.20
P 05	97.34	66.32	95.73	98.09
P 06	48.36	85.87	92.88	95.56
P 07	100	94.44	94.44	96.30
P 08	23.30	81.55	93.20	94.17
P 09	4.60	67.97	91.31	96.25
P 10	87.01	87.96	96.39	99.78
P 11	36.27	85.80	95.58	96.16
P 12	95.50	77.60	93.10	96.66
P 13	100	88.12	99.50	99.69
P 14	100	63.41	98.42	98.99

building a new model of classification). This selected model will be applied to classify all observations of the new patient.

Table 5.6 illustrates a comparison between the SMS, the monitoring system using SVM, and the current system denoted by CS based on the sensitivity. Note that the sensitivity is defined as the capacity of the system to trigger only relevant alarms.

We can notice from Table 5.6 that the proposed monitoring systems have a high sensitivity compared to the current system. Although the important rate of triggered alarms, the rate of the sensitivity of the current system is low especially for patients 08 (23.3%) and 09 (4.6%). It can be explained by the bad setting of thresholds. In addition, we can remark that the SMS has an important and stable sensitivity (more than 94% for all patients' datasets).

The obtained results in Table 5.7 present the rate of suppressed alarms by monitoring systems. After the selection of the appropriate model of classification relative to the new patient, the new SMS classifies all records of this patient. Then, it computes the FARR. We have compared the obtained results of the SMS to the monitoring system using the standard SVM, MS based on RTSVM and the current system (CS), since it provided the best results.

Looking at Table 5.7, we remark that SMS has the most important rate of suppressed false alarms for different datasets. The improvement of the results can be

Table 5.7 Rate of suppressed false alarms for patients' datasets

Databases	SVM-MS	RTSVM-MS	SMS
P 01	94.54	98.84	99.325
P 02	98.80	99.75	99.918
P 03	99.23	99.95	99.96
P 04	95.87	98.96	99.25
P 05	96.51	99.55	99.69
P 06	94.62	98.83	98.92
P 07	98.84	99.64	99.79
P 08	95.72	98.68	98.94
P 09	96.22	99.59	99.79
P 10	77.49	95.35	97.65
P 11	97.59	99.31	99.68
P 12	96.703	99.00	99.99
P 13	95.314	99.60	99.74
P 14	98.20	99.89	99.95

explained by the ability of our proposal to consider the evolution of patient states over time.

Indeed, SVM-MS classifies all observations of the new patient using the same model. However, the SMS updates the initial model many times during the classification of the same patient. Thus, this latter will provide more accurate results than the SVM-MS and the RTSVM-MS. This performance is obvious for patients 1 (99,325%) and 10 (97,653%) where the SMS has successfully removed all false alarms.

Based on this first criterion, we can say that the SMS deals with the problem of health monitoring system which is the high rate of false alarms. In addition, our proposed is to decrease the error rate.

The next criterion consisting of the error rate is presented in Table 5.8.

The error rate presents the rate of irrelevant alarms triggered by the monitoring system. Thus, the aim is to minimize this rate. Through Table 5.8, we can notice the high efficiency of the SMS by providing the lowest error rate for the different patients. Besides, we can remark that the SMS has the more accurate results compared to other systems relative to all datasets. We can mention the example of patient 13 where the new SMS can reach 1%.

The false alarms reduction rate proves again the performance gain that our new SMS provides. It is obvious that there is an improvement of the current monitoring system. Besides, the SMS has 9% of error rate for all datasets compared to the error rate of the current system that corresponds to more than 83%. The proposed monitoring system based on the RTSVM and K-prototypes has the ability to decrease the number of false alarms. This is what medical staff needs in their work. We can say

Table 5.8 Error rate of the proposed SMS compared to other systems in percent

Databases	CS	RTSVM-MS	SMS
P 01	94.92	21.86	11.52
P 02	98.93	30.10	8.88
P 03	99.51	16.95	9.83
P 04	88.50	8.86	6.01
P 05	94.83	13.58	6.93
P 06	100	19.65	13.91
P 07	98.62	26.15	18.03
P 08	100	27,049	22.22
P 09	100	22.40	8.89
P 10	72.99	14.46	4.42
P 11	100	16.15	11.98
P 12	95.18	13.12	3.52
P 13	83.62	2.50	1.60
P 14	98.35	7.91	4.07

that the smart monitoring system responds to the expectations of medical staff, and it can simulate the human reasoning. Indeed, the reduction of irrelevant alarms is very important, but it is also necessary to keep a high level of sensitivity. In fact, if true alarms are missed, it can be a real threat for patients since their lives depend on detected alarms.

In addition, we verify the similarity between trigged alarms by the new proposed system and the expert opinion. As a result, a comparison is made between detected alarms (true positive alarms) by the SMS and the expert opinion (a doctor). In our work, we define true alarms as alarms generated by the monitoring system and that indicates a real critical state of the patient. Figure 5.5 presents the results relative to this last criterion.

It is obvious from Fig. 5.5 that the SMS provides very similar results to the opinion of the expert (the doctor). This latter mentions the cases where alarms should be trigged, i.e., where there are real critical states. The new SMS is close to the expert opinion by 97% as the average for all datasets. The high sensitivity is reached by training data from some patients that share similar conditions. The hypothesis is that models built by using a large number of patients are more accurate than model created from only limited amount of data and relative to a particular patient.

Besides, we can remark that the new SMS has not a trouble to detect true positive alarms such as the current system. This is obvious especially for patients number 06, 08, and 09. The new SMS is better than the other systems because it considers the evolution of data and patient states over time.

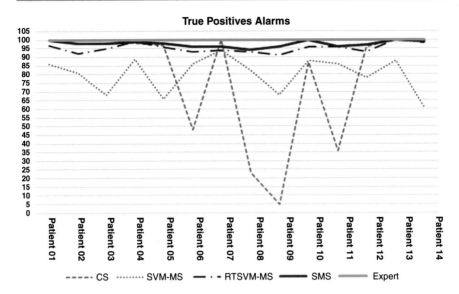

Fig. 5.5 Number of true positive alarms of the proposed SMS compared to other systems and the expert

5.7   Conclusion

In this work, we overcame the main issues of the current monitoring system in intensive care unit (ICU) by proposing a new system. This latter consists of the Smart health Monitoring System (SMS) which combines an improved version of the support vector machines and the k-prototypes clustering technique and used a new data stream component.

The SMS is able to make several updates of the initial classification model using new observations and, hence, follow patient states evolution over time (known as the self-regulation). Hence, the new system offers to the medical staff the possibility to detect true alarms and to improve the working conditions in ICU. Furthermore, it makes medical staff able to analyze the patients states and make the best decisions. The SMS has successfully proved its effectiveness compared to the SVM monitoring system, the monitoring system using only the RTSVM, and the current monitoring system.

The new system was tested at the Hospital of Children in Tunisia and it has significantly improved the working conditions in ICU through the detection of true positive alarms, the decreasing of the rate of false alarms, and increasing the sensitivity.

Acknowledgments The authors would like to thank Noomen Kadri doctor at the Hospital of Children in Tunisia for stimulating discussions on the role of monitoring and to explain us medical knowledge and practice.

References

1. Cvach M. Monitor alarm fatigue: an integrative review. Proc Biomed Instrum Technol. 2012;46:268–77.
2. Baumgartner B, Rodel K, Knoll A. A data mining approach to reduce the false alarm rate of patient monitors. In: Proc. International Conference of the IEEE Engineering in Medicine and Biology Society; 2012. p. 5935–8.
3. Liu L, Stroulia E, Nikolaidis I, Miguel-Cruz A, Rios Rincon A. Smart homes and home health monitoring technologies for older adults: a systematic review. Int J Med Inform. 2016;91:44–59.
4. M. Borowski, S. Siebig, C. Wrede, M. Imhoff, Reducing false alarms of intensive care online-monitoring systems: an evaluation of two signal extraction algorithms. Comp Math Methods Med 2011, 2011.
5. Leroy G, Chen H, Rindflesch TC. Smart and connected health. IEEE Intell Syst. 2014;29:2–5.
6. Siebig S, Kuhls S, Imhoff M, Langgartner J, Reng M, Scholmerich J, Gather U, Wrede C. Collection of annotated data in a clinical validation study for alarm algorithms in intensive care-a methodologic framework. J Crit Care. 2010;25:107–94.
7. Qiao L, Clifford G. Signal processing: false alarm reduction. Secondary analysis of electronic health records. Springer International Publishing; 2016. p. 391–403.
8. Siebig S, Kuhls S, Imhoff M, Langgartner J, Reng M, Scholmerich J, Gather U, Wrede CE. Collection of annotated data in a clinical validation study for alarm algorithms in intensive care-a methodologic framework. J Crit Care. 2010;25:128–35.
9. Nouira K, Trabelsi A. Intelligent monitoring system for intensive care units. J Med Syst. 2011;36:2309–18.
10. Schmid F, Goepfert M, Reuter D. Patient monitoring alarms in the ICU and in the operating room. Crit Care. 2003;17(2):1–7.
11. Vladimir V. Statistical learning theory. Wiley-Interscience; 1998.
12. G. Cauwenberghs, T. Poggio, Incremental and decremental support vector machine learning. In: Proc. Advances in Neural Information Processing Systems (NIPS*2000), vol. 13, 2001, pp. 409–415.
13. Bordes A, Ertekin S, Weston J, Bottou L. Fast kernel classifiers with online and active learning. J Mach Learn Res. 2005;6:1579–619.
14. Ben Rejab F, Nouira K, Trabelsi A. Real time support vector machines. In: Proc. Science and Information Conference (SAI); 2014. p. 496–501.
15. Ben Rejab F, Nouira K, Trabelsi A. Incremental support vector machines for monitoring systems in intensive care unit. In: Proceedings of the Science and Information Conference (SAI); 2013. p. 496–501.
16. Huang Z. Clustering large data sets with mixed numeric and categorical values. In: Proc. 1st Pacific-Asia Conference on Knowledge Discovery and Data Mining; 1997. p. 21–34.
17. Huang Z. Extensions to the k-means algorithm for clustering large data sets with categorical values. Data Mining Knowl Discov. 1998;2:283–304.
18. De Georgia M, Kaffashi F, Jacono F, Loparo K. Information technology in critical care: review of monitoring and data acquisition systems for patient care and research. Scientific World J. 2015;2015:1–9.
19. Ben Rejab F, Nouira K, Trabelsi A. Health monitoring systems using machine learning techniques. Intell Syst Sci Inform Stud. Comput Intell. 2014;542
20. Goldberger A, Amaral L, Glass L, Hausdorff J, Ivanov P, Mark R, Mietus J, Moody G, Peng C, Stanley H. PhysioBank, PhysioToolkit, and PhysioNet: components of a new research resource for complex physiologic signals. Circulation. 2000;101:215–20.

Machine Learning Techniques for Big Data Analytics in Healthcare: Current Scenario and Future Prospects

6

Shahid Mohammad Ganie, Majid Bashir Malik, and Tasleem Arif

6.1 Introduction

6.1.1 Big Data

Many definitions are floating around which have raised some confusion, but big data can be defined only based on characteristics, dimensions, classification along with the analytical framework for storing and processing data [1]. According to the Gartner IT Glossary [2] *"Big data is a collection of high-volume, high-velocity and high-variety information assets that require advanced tools and techniques in order to store and process the data for building superior insight and decision making."* Big data is also defined as a collection of complex and voluminous data that are being generated from different sources including the healthcare system, social networking sites, smart meters, sensors, online transactions, and administrative services [3]. Among all sectors, healthcare industry data is increasing faster due to the advancement of smart devices and well-equipped labs [4].

6.1.2 Inclination Towards the Study

The growth of the data can be understood from the fact, Internet Users produce 2.5 quintillion bytes of data each day, 90% of all data today was shaped in the last two years, in 2016 there was 7.5% of internet population in the world and now estimated to 3.7 billion people according to recent research cited by Domo [5]. 300+ hours of videos are being uploaded on YouTube every minute [6]. 40,000 search queries are being posted every second, 350,000 tweets per minute, and 171 million emails per

S. M. Ganie · M. B. Malik (✉) · T. Arif
BGSB University, Rajouri, Jammu and Kashmir, India
e-mail: majidbashirmalik@bgsbu.ac.in

© The Author(s), under exclusive license to Springer Nature
Switzerland AG 2022
T. Choudhury et al. (eds.), *Telemedicine: The Computer Transformation of Healthcare*, TELe-Health, https://doi.org/10.1007/978-3-030-99457-0_6

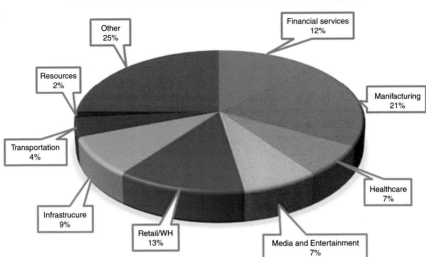

Fig. 6.1 Generation of "Global Datasphere"

minute [7]. Healthcare data is increasing at a rate of 48% annually, and by 2020, the Stanford University study projection is that 2314 Exabytes of data will be formed per year [8]. As represented in Fig. 6.1, most of the data is being generated by different organizations [9].

6.1.3 Characteristics of Big Data

According to the existing literature, characteristics of big data in healthcare give a brief description of 42 V's, 17 V's, 10 V's, 7 V's [10] so on and so forth, but it summarizes and divides the concepts into five dimensions as presented in Table 6.1 [11].

6.2 Literature Review

Different approaches have been carried out by researchers/practitioners using machine learning techniques in order to integrate, manage, analyze, interpret, etc. big data in healthcare industry. Technological advancement can be used for better healthcare outcomes, reducing the cost and complexity of hospitals, and to centralize the large volume of data to expand the superiority of the existing healthcare system [12]. If healthcare data is being created from varied sources with a heterogeneity of data formats, to analyze and drive actionable insights is very highly essential to predict future health conditions. The research work presents the state-of-the-art examination of data mining techniques using big data in healthcare informatics

Table 6.1 V's of big data in healthcare

V's of big data	Definition
• Volume	It can be defined as the parameter that describes the quantity of the data being generated and stored from different health sources.
• Velocity	The rate at which data is being generated and processed along with the speediness at which data changes especially in case of streaming.
• Variety	It is the type and nature of the data. Type refers to different data formats and generating sources, while nature defines different forms like structured, semi-structured, and unstructured data.
• Veracity	It is all about the quality of the data. The data that is submitted can either be incorrect, may have noise or even missing values. How can this data be confided for its truthfulness?
• Value	It refers to the identification and extraction of valuable information for analysis. Data incorporates information of great benefit and insight for users.

[13]. Prediction of the clinical outcomes using gene expression data and tissue-level data has been presented for smart healthcare systems. Also, ICU readmissions using patient-level data, HER's, etc. have been discussed; social media data regarding healthcare has been also presented using population-level data for better prediction of different diseases. In [14], a probabilistic data acquisition mechanism and stochastic prediction framework are designed and implemented for analyzing healthcare data using big data analytics. Intra-cluster correlation evaluation (IaCE) and inter-cluster correlation evaluation (IeCE) have been developed for healthcare big data. Besides, the future health condition prediction (FHCP) algorithm is used to predict the health conditions of a patient based on current status. MapReduce tool has been used for processing of big data on cloud architecture. The prediction model gives an accuracy rate of 98% for predicting the current health status correlated with a patient. The framework has been developed through extensive simulations in the cloud architecture and 90% of it utilizes the resources efficiently to reduce analysis time. The research work provides the detailed, complete, and organized study of recent methodology of big data healthcare applications in five sections including ML, heuristic-based, agent-based, and hybrid approaches [15]. The work surveys 205 research articles from different reputed publishing houses that have been presented and discussed for big data analytics in healthcare domain. Big data security and privacy are considered big challenges to secure the information of the patients in healthcare [16]. The security and privacy issues are discussed and addressed so that the floating information of different sources can be secured from the third parties in healthcare. Anonymization and encryption techniques have been designed and implemented in this study. Different stages of big data lifecycle in the healthcare domain like data collection, aggregation, analyze, interpretation, information gain, etc. are to be protected and encrypted from the end-users by applying different privacy preservation techniques. The paper highlights the vast impacts of big data in healthcare system [17]. The different stakeholders like medical practitioners, patients, physicians, clinicians, pharmaceuticals, and health insurers are taken into account while dealing with big data lifecycle in healthcare informatics. Big data technology like Hadoop architecture has been used for different tasks, viz. data

collection, data processing, big storage, and data analysis. Also, some of the prominent big data applications in healthcare have been discussed. Big data was categorized into four types: descriptive, prescriptive, predictive, and discovery analytics. In [4], classification of big data in healthcare along with varied sources is discussed. Big data is being generated from sources like HER's, EMR's, clinical reports, Omics, etc. and to integrate this large volume of data in healthcare analytics to promote the personalized treatment of different diseases. Various platforms for healthcare data analytics like Hadoop, spark, etc. are being used for the management of big data. To develop a sophisticated framework for a healthcare system that will integrate diverse fields like bioinformatics, chemoinformatics, etc. to provide better decision making in scientific and social science. This will facilitate healthcare by new treatments of epidemics, provide early alarming of diseases, and will help the healthcare providers in drug and medicine discoveries.

6.3   Big Data Healthcare Analytics (BDHA)

In a big data environment, data analytics is a step to perform actionable insights over data with the help of highly scalable distributed platforms and technologies that are capable of storing and processing the big data from varied sources [18]. *It is the overall organization of the whole data lifecycle from collection, integration, storing, analyzing, and leading data so that meaningful information is generated and presented in the form of reports or visualization for decision support or even decision-making* [19]. The different stages of big data for healthcare analytics include identifying the problem, data aggregation, preprocessing of data, performing analytics over data, and then visualization of the results as shown in Fig. 6.2 [20].

BDA helps to make healthier decisions, optimize business operations by analyzing customer behavior, cost reduction, and making smarter and more efficient support systems in the organizations [21]. For instance, a healthcare provider uses big data from various repositories for the better prediction of disease by making actionable insights from raw data [4]. There are four general categories of big data analytics [22]. As depicted in Fig. 6.3, as we go upwards from descriptive to prescriptive analytics, we add to the value of the results generated but at the same time complexity also increases proportionally [22].

6.4   Various Big Data Platforms for Healthcare Analytics

This fast-growing and tremendous amount of health data has far exceeded the bounds of human interpretation and analytical capabilities [23]. Powerful and versatile DM and ML techniques are the dire need of time so that they can automatically excavate and organize information from heterogeneous and complex healthcare data [24]. The goal is to link the computational power of the technology to automate the capability of ingestion, processing, and visualization of results from the huge volume of data for the betterment of public health [25]. The big data platforms for

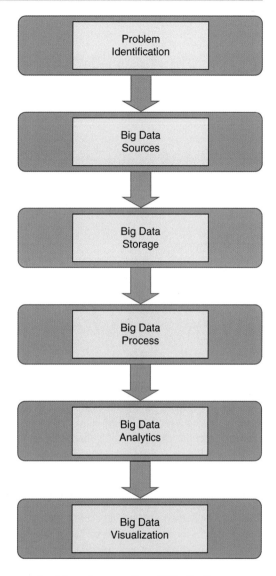

Fig. 6.2 Big data lifecycle for healthcare

healthcare analytics have been categorized based on scaling [26]. Scaling means adapting to cumulative demands of the system in terms of processing requests. Scaling can be horizontal scaling and vertical scaling.

6.4.1 Horizontal Scaling Platforms

Horizontal scaling or "scale-out" is distributed data processing that shares workload among multiple nodes. This increases the processing capability up to a great extent. The most popular horizontal scale-out platforms are as follows [26]:

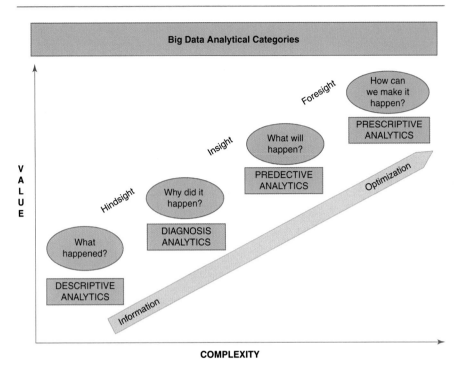

Fig. 6.3 Big data analytics at different phases

6.4.1.1 Peer-to-Peer Networks

One of the decentralized and scattered network architectures having millions of nodes interconnected with each other [27]. In this architecture, the machines (called peers) provide as well as ingest resources. Peer to peer is the oldest distributed network platform used for computing big data. Usually the Message Passing Interface (MPI) standard is the communication system deployed to communicate, transfer, and exchange the data between the machines (peers) [26]. In addition to this, it is suitable for iterative processing and capable of storing data instances over a limitless boundary (can be millions of nodes). MPI acts as a master as well as a slave to utilize the resources when deployed in the master-slave model.

6.4.1.2 Apache Hadoop

Hadoop ecosystem [28] is a batch processing open-source software framework that permits to storage and processes large and complex data sets that cannot be handled by traditional approaches. Hadoop works in a decentralized environment across a cluster of computers. It is particularly developed to scale up from single servers to hundreds and even thousands of machines [17]. Apache Hadoop framework is highly faulted tolerant with the feature of replicating data [26]. The Hadoop ecosystem comprises an array of related software, which is collectively used for collection and aggregation of big data up to analysis of required results [17].

Data Collection

- *Sqoop:* An open-source framework comprised of SQL and Hadoop systems [29]. Sqoop is designed to provide a command-line interface that is used to transfer data to-and-fro between HDFS and relational database servers.
- *Flume:* Flume is a robust tool used for data ingestion in HDFS. It is used to collect, aggregate, and transpose a large volume of real-time data such as log-based files, social media, and email [30]. It also operates by capturing the real-time/ streaming data from different web services to HDFS.
- *Kafka:* It is an open-source disseminated platform that communicates the publish-subscribe messaging system. Originally it was developed at LinkedIn and later it became part of the Apache project and is now used by many organizations because of its scalability, durability, and fault tolerance [31].
- *Chukwa:* It is distributed data collection and rapid processing system. Chukwa is a powerful and flexible platform with different core components as Agents, Collectors, MapReduce Jobs, and Hadoop Infrastructure Care Center (HICC) [17].

Data Processing

- *MapReduce:* Dean and Ghemawat proposed MapReduce at Google technology [32]. MapReduce takes care of processing and computing data present in HDFS. The working principle of MapReduce is mainly divided into two parts, called Mappers and Reducers [33]. The Map module takes input data from HDFS and translates it into some intermediate results to the reducers. The reduced task is based on map task; it takes the output of Mappers as input and then generates the final results by aggregating the intermediate sets which are again reflected in HDFS [34].
- *YARN:* Yet Another Resource Negotiator is a framework that provides job arrangement and cluster resource organization, i.e., the jobs across the cluster [35]. It is a global scheduler that handles both batch and stream processing [36]. It is also known as MapReduce version 2 and is compatible with MapReduce, having master-slave architecture with the full support of the virtual distributed system.
- *Storm:* An open-source computing system used for real-time processing of big data analytics [28]. The storm is distributed, reliable, and fault-tolerant in nature, used for extract, transform, and load (ETL) operations, online machine learning, and continuous computation [37].
- *Flink*: It is a data ingestion tool in HDFS [38], which came into the picture for gathering, combining, and transport a large amount of streaming data. The main idea behind flink is to capture a large amount of data from varied sources into HDFS [39].
- *Spark:* It is a cluster computing framework used for both batch and real-time processing [40]. Spark was developed at the University of California and is next-generation big data processing engine. It is a cluster computing framework particularly designed for the speed up (100 times more than the speed of Hadoop MapReduce for data that resides in main memory and around 10 times faster when data is in disk) in terms of processing [41].

Big Data Storage
- *HDFS:* Hadoop Distributed File System (HDFS) [7] is the main module of Hadoop ecosystem that is used to store big data files across various clusters of the cost-effective system (commodity hardware) while providing high availability and fault tolerance [42].
- *HBase:* Apache HBase is a NoSQL non-relational distributed columnar database that is being used to store unstructured and semi-structured data easily and also provides a real-time read/write access mechanism [43].
- *Hcatalog:* It is a table storage management system for Hadoop and provides a shared schema and data type mechanism to read and write data for various tools of Hadoop ecosystem [17].

Big Data Analysis
- *Pig:* Pig is a high-level data flow system developed by yahoo, used to write simple queries that are converted into the MapReduce program and then executed over Hadoop cluster [44]. It has been used to overcome the complexity of Map and Reduce Stages; Pig helps to process bulk large data sets by spending less time in writing MapReduce programs.
- *Hive:* It is a tool for big data analytics made on the top of Hadoop, used to analyze structured and semi-structured data. It runs an interface mechanism for performing many queries transcribed in HQL (Hive Query Language) that are alike to SQL declarations [45].
- *Mahout:* Apache Mahout is meant for machine learning that runs on Hadoop ecosystem, extracts insight from a large volume and complex data [46]. It is used for various machine learning tasks like clustering, classification, collaborative filtering, and text mining in a scalable and distributed fashion [46].

Hadoop ecosystem comprises a bunch of tools that are used together by various organizations to handle big data. So, it provides all the services that are required to process big data for accomplishing the different tasks. The pictorial representation of Hadoop ecosystem is shown below in Fig. 6.4 [17].

6.4.2 Vertical Scaling Platforms

Vertical scaling or "scale up" is achieved by enhancing the processing and storage capability of a single server by increasing the number of processors or cores and enhancing the memory and other required resources. The most popular vertical scale-up platforms are as follows [26]:

- *HPC clusters:* The blades of high-performance computing with a big number of processing cores have a dynamic memory organization, different levels of cache, and communication mechanisms that are optimized for diverse user requirements [47]. To achieve the scalability of such systems is much costlier than

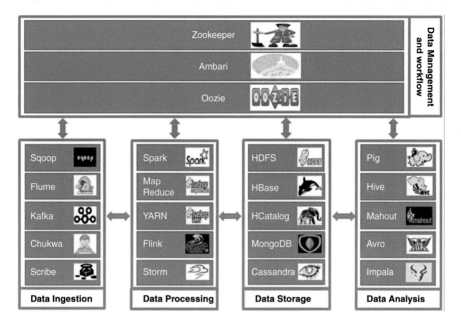

Fig. 6.4 Hadoop ecosystem for healthcare analytics

Hadoop or Spark. The Message Passing Interface (MPI) is usually used for communication and sharing information in such systems [48].

- *Graphics Processing Unit (GPUs):* They are used for accelerating the graphic operations for pictorial representation on display using frame buffer [26]. General-purpose computing on graphics processing units is the result of advanced enhancements in hardware and algorithms in GPU-like parallel architecture.
- *Field Programmable Gate Arrays (FPGA):* Field Programmable Gate Arrays are specialized and custom-built hardware units that can be optimized for high speed and throughput for a particular application [49]. The customization and development cost is typically very high, as compared to other platforms also its feature of programming using Hardware Descriptive Language (HDL) increases the overall development cost [26].

6.5   Materials and Methods

Machine learning techniques are being used broadly for the health data to provide the diagnosis and prognosis of several diseases [50]. Implementation of sophisticated computer algorithms in the area of healthcare is an old story but there are still some areas in healthcare where advanced computing, scientific methods, and perfect visualization by using machine learning and deep learning paradigms can make a difference [51]. ML techniques play a dynamic role in the early prediction of

Fig. 6.5 Machine learning techniques for healthcare analytics

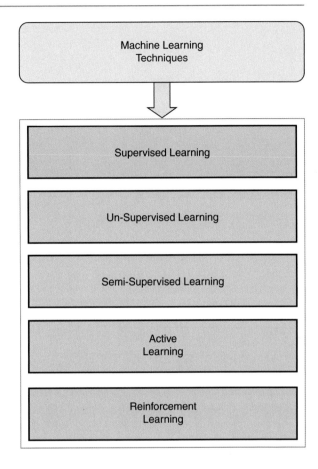

diseases and their complications to reduce costs and readmissions in hospitals. Machine learning techniques can be categorized based on learning mechanisms as shown in Fig. 6.5 [52].

6.5.1 Machine Learning Techniques

Machine learning techniques are built on the basic principles and concepts of statistics that are being used to solve data mysteries. Machine learning algorithms are used successfully for data analytics by different organizations, especially in healthcare [53]. The ML algorithms used for data analysis following are some most prominent ML classifiers that are being widely used in big data healthcare analytics to provide better solutions to health problems [54]. Machine learning techniques can be explored for various real-world problems and also these problems can be modeled to produce optimal solution [28].

- *Logistic Regression:* It is a supervised ML model for classification that produces the dichotomous output in terms of binary format which is used to probabilistically forecast the outcome of categorical variable by using a sigmoid function [55]. It forecasts the probability of the event based on the logarithmic function decided by some threshold. *"Suppose there are 'N' input independent variables with their values represented by $X_1, X_2, X_3, ...X_n$. Let us assume that Y is the probability of Yes (1) and 1 − Y is the probability of No (0). Then the final logistic regression equation is given as"* [56]:

$$\log\left[\frac{Y}{1-Y}\right] ==> Y = C + B_1X_1 + B_2X_2 + B_3X_3 + \cdots\cdots B_nX_n \quad (6.1)$$

- *Naive Bayes:* It is a ML-based classifier, mostly used for predictive analytical of different real-life problems [57]. It is classification technique which is based on Bayesian theorem with an inference among predicate and target variables used for study. Its working mechanism is simple and is highly used for large datasets. "Given a hypothesis *H* and evidence *E*, Bayes theorem states that the relationship between the probability of the hypothesis before getting the evidence *P(H)* and the probability of the hypothesis after getting the evidence *P(H|E)* is" [58]:

$$P(H|E) = \frac{P(E|H).P(H)}{P(E)} \quad (6.2)$$

In simple English, we write the equation as:
P(H|E) = Posterior likelihood
P(E|H) = Probability
P(H) = Session prior likelihood
P(E) = Forecaster prior likelihood

- *Support Vector Machine*: It is a ML classifier that is designed by a separative hyper-plane [59]. Support vector machine algorithm is being used for both classification and regression analysis for different real-world problems. The basic function of this supervised classifier is to segregate or classify the given data points in the best possible and appropriate way in a multidimensional space. To work in high and complex dimensions, the SVM classifier uses different versions of the kernels like linear, polynomial, and radial basis function kernels. The equations for various kernels are [60]:

Linear Kernel Equation

$$F(X) = B(0) + Sum(ai * (x,xi)) \quad (6.3)$$

Polynomial Kernel Equation

$$K(X_1,X_2) = \left(a + X_{1^T}X_2\right)^b \quad (6.4)$$

where b = degree of kernel and a = constant term.

Radial Basis Function Kernel Equation

$$K(X_1,X_2) = \text{exponent}\left(-\gamma \|X_{1,}X_2\|\right)^2 \quad (6.5)$$

where $\|X_1, X_2\|$ = Euclidean distance between (X_1 and X_2)

- *Decision Tree:* It is a classification technique with the graphical representation of all possible solutions to a decision based on certain conditions [55]. The working principle behind the DT algorithm is decision-making for a specific classification problem. The computation procedure of the algorithm is very expensive as far as training and testing data is being concerned. In this acyclic connected graph at each node, one feature is selected to make separating decisions that lead to the prediction. The process of splitting the nodes continues unless and until the leaf node has optimally fewer data points. The decision tree classifier is shown in Fig. 6.6 [61].
- *Random Forest:* It is a well-known supervised ML classifier that is used for regression and classification problems [62]. RF algorithm is made by using many DT models where it compiles all the results of the decision trees that lead to the final outcome. The RF classifier handles the problem of overfitting that may make the results worse by creating the n number of decision trees depending upon the size and complexity of the dataset. The decision tree classifier is shown in Fig. 6.7 [63].

Fig. 6.6 The decision tree

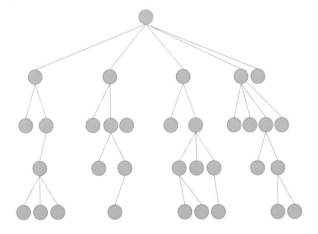

Fig. 6.7 The random forest

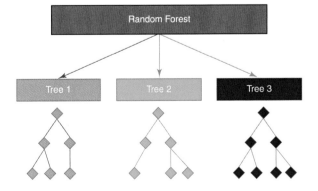

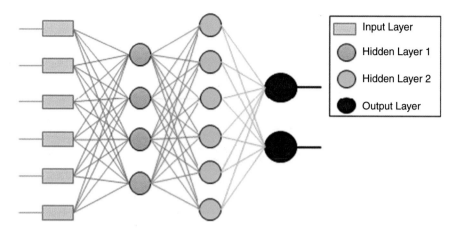

Fig. 6.8 The neural network

- *Artificial Neural Networks:* Artificial Neural Networks are algorithms inspired by human nervous system that have self-capability to produce better results on voluminous data [64]. The structure of the neural network can be divided into three layers: input (disparate sources), hidden (accountable for internal processing), and output (desired results). ANN is currently being used in healthcare analytics for better diagnosis and prognosis of various diseases because of the diversity of data sources in healthcare like EHR, clinical data, omics data, CT scans, ultrasound images, MRI images, etc. The graphical representation of the ANN is shown in Fig. 6.8 [65]:

6.5.2 Description of Dataset

The publicly available PIMA diabetes dataset has been used for the experimental study. The dataset is sourced from UC Irvine Machine Learning Repository [66]. It comprised of 768 instances and 9 attributes, 8 predicted variables and 1 target variable in order to classify whether a patient is diabetic or not. The dataset contains the rich amount of contributing parameters that can be explored to identify the severity of the diabetic disease. Different ML classifiers have developed realistic health management system for diabetes. Table 6.2 demonstrates the attribute name, description, range, and their data type used in the PIMA dataset.

6.5.3 Proposed Framework

The proposed framework shown in Fig. 6.9 presents the working principle of developing ML techniques for forecast of various chronic diseases showcasing diabetes. In this framework, ML models have been developed using the PIMA dataset for forecast of diabetes. The preprocessing techniques have been used to perform various

Table 6.2 Parameter description used for the analysis

S. No	Attribute name	Description	Range	Data Type
1	Pregnancies	Number of times an individual is pregnant	[0–17]	int64
2	Glucose	Plasma glucose concentration	[0–199]	int64
3	BloodPressure	Diastolic blood pressure of an individual	[0–122]	int64
4	SkinThickness	Triceps skin fold thickness (mm)	[0–99]	int64
5	Insulin	2-hour serum insulin (mu U/ml)	[0–846]	int64
6	BMI	Body Mass Index of individual (kg/m2)	[0–67.10]	float64
7	DiabetesPedigreeFunction	Diabetes Pedigree Function	[0–2.42]	float64
8	Age	Age of the individual	[21–28]	int64
9	Class	Diabetic or Non-diabetic	[0/1]	int64

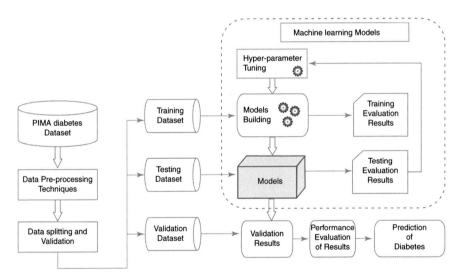

Fig. 6.9 The proposed framework for prediction of diabetes

statistical measurements over the dataset to improve the quality assessment of the data. Feature engineering has been done to identify the contribution of the parameters towards the prediction of disease. Data transformation was performed before building the various ML models. K-fold cross-validation, where K = 10, has been incorporated to validate the performance evaluation of various statistical measures of ML models.

6.6   Case Study and Application

The machine learning paradigm is a highly sophisticated technological application that is being applied almost in every sphere of engineering and science domains, especially in healthcare [67]. In healthcare domain, the analysis of healthcare parameters and based on these parameters predicting the future health conditions of different chronic diseases are still in the informative stage [14, 68]. Machine learning libraries help in implementing the whole end-to-end ML process, which includes building a statistical model that predicts a precise outcome. Different supervised machine learning algorithms, viz. *logistic regression (LR), Naive Bayes (NB), support vector machine (SVM), decision tree (DT), random forest (RF), and artificial neural network (ANN)*, have been developed by using the PIMA diabetes dataset. These classifiers were executed using Jupyter and Spyder (Integrated Development Environment) along with python 3.8 in windows operating system [69].

Exploratory data analysis (EDA) is used to describe the dataset for different tasks based on inferential statistics that need to be executed before building the ML models. The report of attributes used in the dataset is depicted in Fig. 6.10. The statistical measurements of parameters in dataset like count, mean, std., min, max, etc. have been calculated. The describe() function on pandas DataFrame has been used to list the statistical measures of each parameter in the dataset.

The data exploratory analysis has been performed to identify the relationship among the attributes used in the dataset as shown in Fig. 6.11. Different packages for data visualization like Matplot, Seaborn, etc. have been used to draw the correlation matrix plot between the set of attributes. The association between the reliant on and autonomous variables lies in between −1 and +1.

The predictive machine learning models, viz. *LR, NB, SVM, DT, RF, and ANN*, were employed. The algorithms were developed by splitting the PIMA diabetes dataset into an 80:20 ratio, i.e., 80% of data has been used for training the classifiers and 20% of data for testing the developed models. Also, ten-fold cross-validation has been applied to validate the building models for better prediction of diabetes

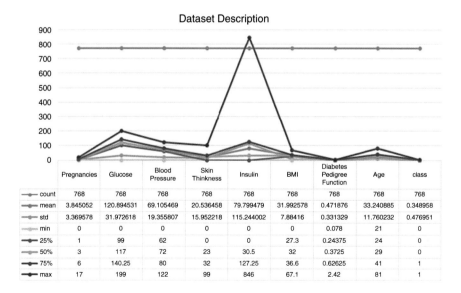

Dataset Description

	Pregnancies	Glucose	Blood Pressure	Skin Thinkness	Insulin	BMI	Diabetes Pedigree Function	Age	class
count	768	768	768	768	768	768	768	768	768
mean	3.845052	120.894531	69.105469	20.536458	79.799479	31.992578	0.471876	33.240885	0.348958
std	3.369578	31.972618	19.355807	15.952218	115.244002	7.88416	0.331329	11.760232	0.476951
min	0	0	0	0	0	0	0.078	21	0
25%	1	99	62	0	0	27.3	0.24375	24	0
50%	3	117	72	23	30.5	32	0.3725	29	0
75%	6	140.25	80	32	127.25	36.6	0.62625	41	1
max	17	199	122	99	846	67.1	2.42	81	1

Fig. 6.10 Dataset description used in the experimental study

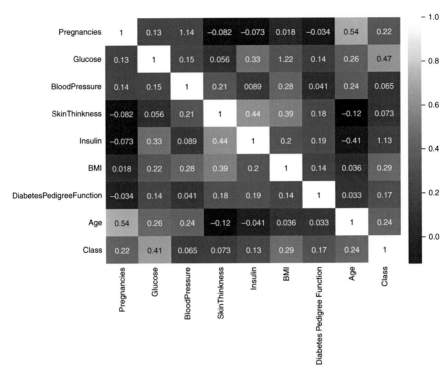

Fig. 6.11 Correlation matrix plot of attributes

Table 6.3 Accuracy of machine learning classifiers

Model	Training accuracy	Testing accuracy
Logistic regression	**76.50%**	**80.51%**
Naïve Bayes	76.01%	74.67%
Support vector machine	76.34%	79.87%
Decision tree	83.36%	75.32%
Random forest	84.99%	79.22%
Artificial neural network	71.94%	70.77%

diseases. The aggregation accuracy results using ten-fold cross-validation of different algorithms are shown in Table 6.3.

Figure 6.12 shows the accuracy results achieved by various classifiers used for prediction of diabetes. Among all the classifiers, Logistic Regression happened to be the best model with a testing accuracy rate of 80.51%, followed by support vector machine model with an accuracy rate of 79.87%, random forest with an accuracy rate of 79.22%, decision tree with an accuracy rate of 75.32%, Naive Bayes with an accuracy rate of 74.67%, and lastly artificial neural network with an accuracy rate of 70.77%.

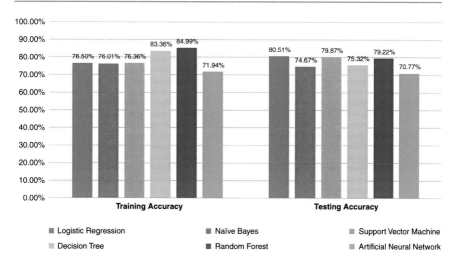

Fig. 6.12 Accuracy of various algorithms

Table 6.4 Various statistical measures of algorithms

Algorithm	Precision (%)	Recall (%)	Specificity (%)	FPR (%)	FNR (%)	F1-score (%)
LR	0.880	0.819	0.755	0.224	0.180	0.851
NB	0.845	0.773	0.687	0.312	0.226	0.807
SVM	0.876	0.817	0.760	0.240	0.182	0.845
DT	0.855	0.775	0.702	0.297	0.224	0.813
RF	0.876	0.801	0.750	0.250	0.198	0.837
ANN	0.835	0.736	0.636	0.363	0.236	0.782

The other statistical measures are shown in Table 6.4. The various measurements have been used to evaluate the performance evaluation of different classifiers towards the prediction of diabetic disease. However, in terms of precision, LR model predicts best with the highest precision rate of 0.88%, whereas in terms of false positive rate and false negative rate, LR predicts with the lowest rate of 0.224% and 0.180%, respectively.

6.7   Conclusion and Future Scope

This chapter began with a brief outline of big data, its classification, and its characteristics. The procedure of BDA in healthcare from data acquisition up to the generation of required results is presented in this study. Then various platforms for big data and BDA in healthcare have been discussed, through which we can store, manage, analyze, filter, and distribute healthcare data for further analytical procedures to provide better solutions to real-world healthcare problems. Different challenges regarding BDA in healthcare have been also discussed. These challenges must be taken into account while dealing with big data analytics life cycle. In this chapter, various ML classifiers have been discussed that play a significant role in healthcare industry. The study has presented and implemented the framework by using the PIMA diabetes dataset to forecast whether a patient is diabetic or not. The results achieved by the framework are accuracy, recall, precision, f1-score, false positive rate, false negative rate, etc. The classifiers used in this model have been validated by using k-fold cross-validation technique. To extend the current study, these ML models shall be used for other related diseases which share communality of data with diabetes. Also, for efficiency and reliability of the framework used in this study ensemble and hybridization ML techniques shall be used for the forecast of various diseases in early stages to save human lives. Similarly, new mining techniques should be developed so that sensitive information can be extracted from the huge volume of health data.

References

1. Wasson M, Buck A, Robe J., Wilson M. Big data architecture style. Azur. Appl. Archit. Guid. | Microsoft Docs, 2018, pp. 1–7.
2. Gandomi A, Haider M. Beyond the hype: Big data concepts, methods, and analytics. Int J Inf Manag. 2015;35(2):137–44. https://doi.org/10.1016/j.ijinfomgt.2014.10.007.
3. Oracle. Oracle: Big Data for the enterprise Oracle White Paper—Big Data for the enterprise, An Oracle White Pap., no. June, 2013.
4. Dash S, Shakyawar SK, Sharma M, Kaushik S. Big data in healthcare: management, analysis and future prospects. J Big Data. 2019;6(1) https://doi.org/10.1186/s40537-019-0217-0.
5. How much data do we create every day? The mind-blowing stats everyone should read.
6. 300 Hours of video are uploaded to Youtube every minute..
7. Google Search Statistics—Internet live stats.
8. Infographic: How Big Data will unlock the potential of healthcare.
9. Saracco R. Another shift in content production, 2020. pp. 2019–2020
10. Shafer T. The 42 V's of Big Data and Data Science, kdnuggets.com Elder Res., pp. 1–3, 2017, [Online]. Available: https://www.kdnuggets.com/2017/04/42-vs-big-data-data-science.html.
11. Hameed Shnain A, Jasim Hadi H, Hadishaheed S, Haji Ahmad A. Big data and five V'S characteristics. Int J Adv Electron Comput Sci. 2015;2:393–2835. Available: https://www.researchgate.net/publication/332230305
12. Ganie SM, Malik MB. Comparative analysis of various supervised machine learning algorithms for the early prediction of type-II diabetes mellitus. Int J Med Eng Inform. 2021;1(1):1. https://doi.org/10.1504/ijmei.2021.10036078.
13. Herland M, Khoshgoftaar TM, Wald R. A review of data mining using big data in health informatics. J Big Data. 2014;1(1) https://doi.org/10.1186/2196-1115-1-2.
14. Sahoo PK, Mohapatra SK, Wu SL. Analyzing Healthcare Big data with prediction for future health condition. IEEE Access. 2016;4:9786–99. https://doi.org/10.1109/ACCESS.2016.2647619.
15. Pashazadeh A, Navimipour NJ. Big data handling mechanisms in the healthcare applications: a comprehensive and systematic literature review. J Biomed Inform. 2018;2017(82):47–62. https://doi.org/10.1016/j.jbi.2018.03.014.
16. Abouelmehdi K, Beni-Hessane A, Khaloufi H. Big healthcare data: preserving security and privacy. J. Big Data. 2018;5(1):1–18. https://doi.org/10.1186/s40537-017-0110-7.
17. Bahri S, Zoghlami N, Abed M, Tavares JMRS. BIG DATA for Healthcare: a survey. IEEE Access. 2019;7:7397–408. https://doi.org/10.1109/ACCESS.2018.2889180.

18. Chong D, Shi H. Big data analytics: a literature review. J Manag Anal. 2015;2(3):175–201. https://doi.org/10.1080/23270012.2015.1082449.
19. Tsai CW, Lai CF, Chao HC, Vasilakos AV. Big data analytics: a survey. J Big Data. 2015;2(1):1–32. https://doi.org/10.1186/s40537-015-0030-3.
20. B. T. Erl, P. Buhler, and W. Kha, Big Data adoption on and planning considerations LiveLessons (Video Training) Big Data analytics lifecycle. This chapter is from the book Business Case Evaluation This chapter is from the book, 2019, pp. 1–19.
21. Yaqoob I, et al. Big data: From beginning to future. Int J Inf Manag. 2016;36(6):1231–47. https://doi.org/10.1016/j.ijinfomgt.2016.07.009.
22. Delen D, Ram S. Research challenges and opportunities in business analytics. J Bus Anal. 2018;1(1):2–12. https://doi.org/10.1080/2573234x.2018.1507324.
23. Mazumdar S, Seybold D, Kritikos K, Verginadis Y. A survey on data storage and placement methodologies for cloud-big data ecosystem. J Big Data. 2019;6(1):1–37. Springer International Publishing
24. Winter G. Machine learning in healthcare. Br J Heal Care Manag. 2019;25(2):100–1. https://doi.org/10.12968/bjhc.2019.25.2.100.
25. Ganie SM, Malik MB, Arif T. Various platforms and machine learning techniques for Big Data analytics: a technological survey. Int J Scientific Res Comput Sci Eng Inform Technol. 2018;3(6):679–87.
26. Singh D, Reddy CK. A survey on platforms for big data analytics. J. Big Data. 2015;2(1):1–20. https://doi.org/10.1186/s40537-014-0008-6.
27. Irestig M, Hallberg N, Eriksson H, Timpka T. Peer-to-peer computing in health-promoting voluntary organizations: system design analysis. J Med Syst. 2005;29(5):425–40. https://doi.org/10.1007/s10916-005-6100-x.
28. Landset S, Khoshgoftaar TM, Richter AN, Hasanin T. A survey of open source tools for machine learning with big data in the Hadoop ecosystem. J Big Data. 2015;2(1):1–36. https://doi.org/10.1186/s40537-015-0032-1.
29. Mehta S, Mehta V. Hadoop ecosystem: an introduction. Int J Sci Res. 2016;5(6):557–62. https://doi.org/10.21275/v5i6.nov164121.
30. Bhagavatula VSN, Raju SS. A survey of hadoop ecosystem as a handler of bigdata, no. August 2016, 2017.
31. Leang B, Ean S, Ryu GA, Yoo KH. Improvement of kafka streaming using partition and multi-threading in big data environment. Sensors (Switzerland). 2019;19(1) https://doi.org/10.3390/s19010134.
32. Dean J, Ghemawat S. MapReduce: simplified data processing on large clusters. In: OSDI 2004—6th Symp. Oper. Syst. Des. Implement.; 2004. p. 137–49. https://doi.org/10.21276/ijre.2018.5.5.4.
33. Sun P, Wen Y. Scalable architectures for Big Data analysis. Encycl Big Data Technol. 2019:1446–54. https://doi.org/10.1007/978-3-319-77525-8_281.
34. Kaur I, Kaur N, Ummat A, Kaur J, Kaur N. Research paper on big data and Hadoop. Int J Comput Sci Technol. 2016;8491(1):50–3.
35. Mathiya BJ, Desai VL. Apache Hadoop Yarn Parameter configuration challenges and optimization. In: Proceedigs of the IEEE International Conference on Soft-Computing and Networks Security (ICSNS). IEEE; 2015. https://doi.org/10.1109/ICSNS.2015.7292373.
36. Perwej Y, Kerim B, Adrees MS, Sheta OE. An empirical exploration of the Yarn in Big Data. Int J Appl Inf Syst. 2017;12(9):19–29. https://doi.org/10.5120/ijais2017451730.
37. Alkatheri S, Abbas SA, Siddiqui MA. Big Data frameworks: a comparative study. Int J Comput Sci Inf Secur. 2019;17(1)
38. Perwej DY, Omer M, Kerim B. A comprehend the Apache Flink in big data environments. IOSR J Comput Eng (IOSR-JCE). 2018;20(1):48–58. https://doi.org/10.9790/0661-2001044858.
39. Rabl T, Traub J, Katsifodimos A, Markl V. Apache Flink in current research. IT Inf Technol. 2016;58(4):2–9. https://doi.org/10.1515/itit-2016-0005.

40. Benbrahim H, Hachimi H, Amine A. Comparison between Hadoop and Spark. In: Proceedings of the International Conference on Industrial Engineering and Operations Management, vol. 2019; 2019. p. 690–701.
41. Qureshi NM, et al. Dynamic container-based resource management framework of spark ecosystem. In: 2019 21st International Conference on Advanced Communication Technology (ICACT). IEEE; 2019. p. 522–6. https://doi.org/10.23919/ICACT.2019.8701970.
42. Basu P. HDFS for big data. J Chem Inf Model. 2013;53(9):1689–99. https://doi.org/10.1017/CBO9781107415324.004.
43. Jin C, Ran S. The research for storage scheme based on Hadoop. In: Proceedings of the 2015 IEEE International Conference Computer and Communications (ICCC) 2015. IEEE; 2015. p. 62–6. https://doi.org/10.1109/CompComm.2015.7387541.
44. Swarna C, Ansari Z. Apache Pig—a data flow framework based on Hadoop map reduce. Int J Eng Trends Technol. 2017;50(5):271–5. https://doi.org/10.14445/22315381/ijett-v50p244.
45. Fuad A, Erwin A, Ipung HP. Processing performance on Apache Pig, Apache Hive and MySQL cluster. In: Proceedings of the 2014 International Conference on Information, Communication Technology and System (ICTS), 2014. IEEE; 2014. p. 297–301. https://doi.org/10.1109/ICTS.2014.7010600.
46. Eluri VR, Ramesh M, Al-Jabri ASM, Jane M. A comparative study of various clustering techniques on big data sets using Apache Mahout. In: 2016 3rd MEC Int. Conf. Big Data Smart City, ICBDSC 2016. IEEE; 2016. p. 374–7. https://doi.org/10.1109/ICBDSC.2016.7460397.
47. Kumar D, Ali L, Memon S. Design and implementation of high performance computing (HPC) cluster design and implementation of high performance computing (HPC) Cluster, no. January, 2018.
48. Yeo CS, Buyya R, Eskicioglu R, Graham P. Handbook of nature-inspired and innovative computing. In: Handbook nature inspired innovative computing, June 2014; 2006. p. 0–24. https://doi.org/10.1007/0-387-27705-6.
49. Ruiz-Rosero J, Ramirez-Gonzalez G, Khanna R. Field programmable gate array applications—a scientometric review. Computation. 2019;7(4):63. https://doi.org/10.3390/computation7040063.
50. Lai H, Huang H, Keshavjee K, Guergachi A, Gao X. Predictive models for diabetes mellitus using machine learning techniques. BMC Endocr Disord. 2019;19(1):1–9. https://doi.org/10.1186/s12902-019-0436-6.
51. Guleria P, Sood M. Intelligent Learning analytics in healthcare sector using machine learning. 2020.
52. Sarwar MA, Kamal N, Hamid W, Shah MA. Prediction of diabetes using machine learning algorithms in healthcare. In: ICAC 2018–2018 24th IEEE Int. Conf. Autom. Comput. Improv. Product. through Autom. Comput., September; 2018. p. 1–6. https://doi.org/10.23919/IConAC.2018.8748992.
53. Doupe P, Faghmous J, Basu S. Machine learning for health services researchers. Value Heal. 2019;22(7):808–15. https://doi.org/10.1016/j.jval.2019.02.012.
54. Ferdous M, Debnath J, Chakraborty NR. Machine learning algorithms in healthcare: a literature survey. In: 2020 11th International Conference on Computing, Communication and Networking Technologies (ICCCNT). IEEE; 2020. https://doi.org/10.1109/ICCCNT49239.2020.9225642.
55. Patil R, Tamane S. A comparative analysis on the evaluation of classification algorithms in the prediction of diabetes. Int J Electr Comput Eng. 2018;8(5):3966–75. https://doi.org/10.11591/ijece.v8i5.pp3966-3975.
56. Celine S, Dominic MM, Devi MS. Logistic regression for employability prediction. Int J Innov Technol Explor Eng. 2020;9(3):2471–8. https://doi.org/10.35940/ijitee.c8170.019320.
57. Kaviani P, Dhotre S. International journal of advance engineering and research short survey on Naive Bayes algorithm. Int J Adv Eng Res Dev. 2017;4(11):607–11.
58. Elkan C. Naive Bayesian learning. 2007, pp. 1–4.
59. Jegan C, Kumari VA, Chitra R. Classification of diabetes disease using support vector machine. Int J Eng Res Appl. 2018;3(2):1797–801. Available: https://www.researchgate.net/publication/320395340

60. Abdillah AA, Suwarno S. Diagnosis of diabetes using support vector machines with radial basis function kernels. Int J Technol. 2016;7(5):849–58. https://doi.org/10.14716/ijtech.v7i5.1370.
61. Tree D. Decision trees tutorial (https://opendatascience.com/decision-trees-tutorial/), 2020, pp. 1–11.
62. Chari KK, Chinna Babu M, Kodati S. Classification of diabetes using random forest with feature selection algorithm. Int J Innov Technol Explor Eng. 2019;9(1):1295–300. https://doi.org/10.35940/ijitee.L3595.119119.
63. Lateef Z. A comprehensive guide to Random Forest in R, pp. 1–14, 2019 [Online]. Available: https://www.edureka.co/blog/naive-bayes-in-r/.
64. Santhosh KV, Nayak S. Engineering vibration communication and information processing, vol. 478. Springer; 2019. p. 523–35. https://doi.org/10.1007/978-981-13-1642-5.
65. Is W, Learning D. what is a neural network? Introduction to artificial neural networks. 2020, pp. 1–7.
66. View ALL Data Sets Citation Policy. 2021, p. 2021.
67. Malik MM, Abdallah S, Ala'raj M. Data mining and predictive analytics applications for the delivery of healthcare services: a systematic literature review. Ann Oper Res. 2018;270(1–2):287–312. https://doi.org/10.1007/s10479-016-2393-z.
68. Nissa N, Jamwal S, Mohammad S. Early detection of cardiovascular disease using machine learning techniques an experimental study. Int J Recent Technol Eng. 2020;9(3):635–41. https://doi.org/10.35940/ijrte.c46570.99320.
69. Anaconda Inc., Anaconda Distribution, Anaconda, 2019, [Online]. Available: https://www.anaconda.com/distribution/.

Efficient Analysis in Healthcare Domain using Machine Learning

7

Ashish Joshi ⓘ, Isha Pant ⓘ, and Yashikha Dhiman ⓘ

7.1   Background and Driving Forces

The increasing rate of newly emerging diseases and ailments has brought the need of new developments in healthcare and medical sciences. Machine learning is creating its way into every domain. It has many strong applications in medical sector. Machine learning algorithms may learn from the data we supply. As fresh data is added, the model's accuracy and efficiency in making judgments improves with consecutive training. Machine learning's capacity to automate numerous decision-making activities is a highly valuable utility. This clears up a lot of time for engineers to put to better use. Machine learning is altering the world by automating practically everything we can think of. This benefit is self-evident [1].

Using this technique, we uncover distinct trends and patterns in massive amounts of data. Machine learning is now employed in every area, from defense to education. Companies make profits, lower expenses, automate, forecast the future, evaluate trends and patterns in historical data, and many other things. Machine learning provides several algorithms that help in analyzing the medical conditions of different patients [1]. Moreover, it provides a predictive approach to keep an eye on the medical conditions of patients that may occur in future. This predictive approach can save a number of patients from severe health conditions. The numbers of efficient algorithms available in machine learning are proved to be very helpful in the healthcare domain. What is the way in which machine learning works? In this

A. Joshi (✉)
BOSCH, Bangalore, Karnataka, India

I. Pant
Department of Computer Science, THDC Institute of Hydropower Engineering & Technology, Tehri, Uttarakhand, India

Y. Dhiman
TCS, Noida, Uttar Pradesh, India

© The Author(s), under exclusive license to Springer Nature
Switzerland AG 2022
T. Choudhury et al. (eds.), *Telemedicine: The Computer Transformation of Healthcare*, TELe-Health, https://doi.org/10.1007/978-3-030-99457-0_7

approach a dataset is chosen, this data set is provided to the machine, the machine applies a particular algorithm on the data, a model is created. This model is further used to classify similar data and to make future predictions. What is this dataset? The dataset is a collection of similar type of relevant information that can be used to learn about a particular scenario.

7.1.1 The Machine Learning Realm

A division of artificial intelligence is machine learning. The goal of artificial intelligence is to build machines that can learn and think like human brains. The phrase can also point to a machine that demonstrates criteria associated with the human mind, such as learning and problem-solving [2]. For this to happen efficiently, machines need to analyze data, learn from it, and apply it in the future scenarios. This process of making machines intelligent is like the way a human brain analyzes from its surroundings, makes meaningful learning from there, and uses that learning in solving future scenarios. In data science, an algorithm is a series of statistical processing processes. Machine learning algorithms are qualified to detect patterns and characteristics in huge volumes of data to make judgments and predictions based on fresh data. The stronger the algorithm, the more accurate the judgments and forecasts will become as it processes more data. There are number of algorithms used in machine learning. The machine learning algorithms can further be alienated into three categories. These are supervised form, unsupervised learning and reinforcement learning. In the Supervised learning approach, labeled datasets are used. In this approach, the input and output are known to the machine; it only must define the rules and relations between both input and output.

Supervised learning form takes fewer training datasets than other machine learning approaches and simplifies training by allowing the model's findings to be compared to actual labeled outcomes. However, properly labeled data is expensive to produce, and there is a risk of overfitting [3] or developing a form that is so strongly attached and biased to the training data that it does not handle variances in new data effectively. The unsupervised learning approach uses unlabeled datasets; it has the input and the rules known to it and needs to generate the relevant output classes. Unsupervised machine learning consumes large amounts of unlabeled data and uses algorithms to extract significant characteristics required to label, sort, and classify the data in real time, without human interaction. Unsupervised learning is less concerned with automating judgments and predictions and more concerned with detecting patterns and correlations in data that people might overlook. In the reinforcement learning [4] the algorithms ought to choose the outcome which increases the number of rewards. The training data must be properly prepared, including being randomized, de-duped, and examined for imbalances or biases that may affect the training. Reinforcement machine learning is a behavioral machine learning approach that is like supervised learning, except the algorithm is not taught using sample data. This model learns through trial and error. A series of good results will be reinforced to generate the optimal suggestion or policy for a specific situation.

7.1.2   Inception of ML for m-Health Domain

From the very beginning machine learning has been a part of medical diagnoses. Since the 1950s, when the computer emerged into general use, they have been used to implement such algorithms that worked on large datasets. Those algorithms were sufficient to analyze and train on large datasets. The classical symbolic method, the neural networks and the statistical method were the most popular machine learning techniques that were in trend in those early times. Since then, machine learning has provided several tools, techniques, and methods that can be used to enhance the medical diagnosis in healthcare sector. The collection of prospective data is planned to be done along with the same. The morbidity can be mitigated through the integration of this model into the rapid response workflow. The child mortality rate can also be improved with the same process. Another application of machine learning in the field of medical sector can be seen in the predicting if a patient will buy the medicine in the future or not. On the pattern of medicines bought by a patient can reveal the future trends of health conditions of that patient [5]. Machine learning in medical imaging is commonly used to diagnose cardiovascular irregularities, diagnose musculoskeletal problems, and screen for malignancies. Machine learning can increase the precision of surgical robotic equipment by using real-time data, knowledge from prior successful surgeries, and historic medical records. Reduced human mistake, assistance during more difficult treatments, and less invasive operations are among the advantages. Surgical robots can also provide more than just automated aid to surgeons by helping them design workflows and execute procedures. Robots can directly aid boost patient capacities. Examples include assisting paraplegic people with regaining walking capacity and doing activities such as monitoring blood pressure and reminding patients of medication. Robots can also be used to give companionship to sick or elderly folks.

A health practitioner does not have enough time in a day to evaluate all of the data required to treat patients with precision medicine. However, machine learning's capacity to harness large data and predictive analytics opens prospects for researchers to develop individualized therapies for ailments such as cancer and depression. So, what about the security and integrity of patient's data? Machine learning's advancements in healthcare efficiency and patient care delivery raise ethical problems. Health informatics specialists may play a critical role in solving AI issues as well as the ethics of AI in healthcare, such as those discussed in the following sections. Data is the foundation of good machine learning. Nonetheless, privacy and confidentiality rules are intended to safeguard patient information from threats such as a data breach. Clinical information cannot be shared between clinicians unless it is for medical reasons, such as when a doctor discusses medical information on a patient with an oncologist or a cancer expert to enhance health outcomes. There are also difficulties with patient autonomy. Many elderly and mental patients are unable to make their own healthcare decisions. On the other hand, an automated method should not completely replace patient autonomy. Machine learning, on the other hand, has the potential to be a helpful tool in medical decision-making. Erroneous or faulty data might jeopardize system dependability, calling into question whether data-driven judgments are correct or incorrect. Another issue with faulty data is that it might result in a lack of cultural competency. For example, because data often underrepresents minority communities, persons may be overdiagnosed or underdiagnosed. The bottom line is that worries about system dependability and a lack of cultural competency caused by incorrect data that machine learning algorithms may employ might yield erroneous outputs, lead to misguided medical decision-making, and ultimately harm patient safety and results.

7.1.3 Python's Role in mHealth

Python is high-level programming language that can be used for anything, for instance, web development, data science, mobile apps, machine learning, etc. For the implementation of telemedicine, python is chosen because it efficiently handles large amount of data. Telemedicine involves data visualization and analysis, which can be effortlessly performed using the inbuilt libraries available in python.

Python is not only useful for tailoring mobile apps, but it is moreover invaluable in building new healthcare platforms that are foundation to reshape healthcare narratives. Python programming can be used in healthcare by institutions and doctors to create dynamic and scalable solutions that improve patient outcomes. In the healthcare industry, patients and facilities are now generating massive amounts of data. By making the best use of this data, doctors can predict better treatment options and improve the entire healthcare delivery system. One of the most significant advantages of Python in healthcare is that it may assist in the interpretation of data by collaborating with artificial intelligence and machine learning. Python development services are the finest choice for a powerful language that offers computing capabilities to generate significant insights from data for healthcare applications. Artificial intelligence will undoubtedly be one of the most transformational technologies and enablers for human society in the twenty-first century, which is only two decades old (AI). The assumption that AI and related services and platforms would revolutionize global productivity [3], working patterns, and lifestyles, as well as create massive wealth, is well established.

The reasons for using Python in the healthcare sector accumulate many factors. For instance, Python and its frameworks are based on principles that are equally grounded in the HIPAA checklist. A comprehensive examination of big data healthcare enables organizations to exchange information in the pursuit of better patient outcomes. The most significant advantage of Python programming in healthcare is disease prediction. Python can be used effectively by developers to create machine learning models that can predict diseases before they become severe. Predicting the outcome of any disease is also difficult. Most systems today are inefficient at predicting what will happen next. Google's deep learning and machine learning algorithms, for example, can detect cancer in patients based on their medical data and history.

Machine learning models can quickly scan MRIs, ECGs, DTIS, and other images to identify any pattern of disease that may be developing in the body. Data analysis in healthcare Python depicts the inner workings of the human body perfectly. Python programming in healthcare has a number of advantages that healthcare facilities cannot afford to overlook in today's world. It, along with its frameworks such as Django and Flask, provides numerous benefits that can lead to improved healthcare outcomes. It is a dynamic programming language that allows for the creation of feature-rich web apps and mobile applications. Aside from that, wearable devices enable users to update their health data online, allowing healthcare facilities to easily access it. Python is the way to go. AI initiatives are not the same as regular software initiatives. The distinctions are found in the technological stack, the talents necessary for an AI-based project, and the requirement for extensive research. To realize your AI ambitions, you need to select a programming language that is robust, adaptable, and comes with tools. Python generates code that is both succinct and understandable. While machine learning and AI rely on complicated algorithms and varied workflows, Python's simplicity allows developers to create dependable systems.

Python's strong technological stack includes many libraries for artificial intelligence and machine learning. Python's appeal stems in part from the fact that it is a platform-independent language. It is a well-known fact that the Python AI community has expanded all around the world.

Predictive analytics for illnesses are the most major advantage of Python programming in healthcare. Python may be used effectively by developers to construct machine learning models that can predict illnesses before they become serious. Predicting how any illness may develop is similarly difficult. Today, most systems are ineffective in predicting what will happen next. Doctors may use healthcare data analytics using Python to forecast the best treatment plan or mortality based on EHR data. Google's deep learning and machine learning algorithms, for example, may identify cancer in individuals based on their medical data and history. It expedites the therapy procedure, allowing professionals to prevent any major issues that may arise in the future. Python healthcare projects including data science applications can aid in making an accurate diagnosis through picture analysis. While conventional picture-based diagnostics provided several pictures that might be difficult to read, Python code for healthcare assisted in the development of algorithms that provide a single picture for delivering the diagnosis.

7.2   The Rise of Telemedicine: Machine Learning Methodology to the Rescue

7.2.1   Integrating Machine Learning Aid to Telemedicine Trends

Any point in time you've ever communicated with your doctor for any medical reasons via email or had any medical piece of information shared with you or your other care provider online, you were actually taking part in *telemedicine.* Speaking of telemedicine at the present time, we are often referring to *m-health,* the Observance of medicine using the wireless and mobile technologies. There are a noteworthy number of mobile applications that offers a diversity of services, including the aspects of mental healthcare and medical healthcare to the community, reminders notification well-timed and healthiness tips, and also tracking of vital signs remotely by making use of personal gadgets. Unsurprisingly, countless of these services are looking to machine learning (ML) to endow with solutions to issues that have plagued the healthcare ever since its inception. At the moment we did stumble upon varied sectors in medical sciences in which the healthcare system unit has historically struggled to afford the utmost quality of care, and how the booming ML methodologies can be taken into account to promote the conducts in which healthcare is delivered at desirable times. To lay it succinctly, the professionals in medicine nowadays are long-drawn-out thin. Foremost of all, there are widespread shortages of both the concerned doctors and the other staff. On top of that, the doctors simply do not have an adequate amount of time to spend with the patients. They are not able to amass ample patient medical histories, which in turn can be critical for appropriate diagnostics and treatment of the clause. Furthermore, doctors are unable to commit the necessary amount of their spare time to keep up with the latest events, discoveries, and research in medicine.

As a matter of fact, some studies showed that it would adequately take a primary care physician working extensively for 29 hours straight per weekday to assess all significant and up-to-date literature work [1]. The healthcare firm has been one of the last foremost industries to take up machine learning. Data has been valued and utilized for long by the healthcare providers to enlarge their facts beyond their own experiences in clinical research. The rule-based course of action for the care units have been a common place for over a decade. Presently, the industry of health comprises chiefly of communication tools that helps the patients to tie with the concerned doctors. However, as the sector develops, AI and machine learning are becoming more widely used. Chatbots, diagnosis, and therapy recommendations are the most common use cases. Machine learning algorithms are also being used by certain companies to decide virtual appointment scheduling and even to connect patients with doctors who have had the best results for other patients with comparable symptoms.

They are well suited to replace or supplement people in collecting data, sending reminders, and encouraging messages, and providing a sense of security when a doctor cannot be reached right away. The most basic and widely used chatbots are rule-based, which means that the responses that a user can provide are limited. These chatbots can be strong if they are programmed with properly set principles, but they lack the natural sense of a discourse.Telehealth has traditionally been classed as either synchronous or asynchronous, depending on whether it uses real-time electronic communication or store-and-forward transmission. Remote (tele) monitoring, which incorporates information collecting through dispersed devices such as the Internet of Things, has recently been recognized as a third form (IOT). The Fundamentals of Telemedicine and Telehealth endorse four methods for providing telemedicine. To contact the patient, real-time communication employs any communication technology. This practice is known as asynchronous communication because it assists doctors in later data analysis. Natural language processing (NLP) is used by the most capable chatbots to both interpret and respond to input. The bot must determine the human's intent and the entity to which they are referring for each message sent [5]. The usage of telemedicine trends in medical research and academic trainings or consultations is magnificent and is called to be as information analysis and collaboration. Using the technology to connect medical individuals from different nations will foster collaboration on medical data as well as insights and information for diagnosis.

7.2.2   ML: The Care Model for m-Health Intelligence

Telemedicine is a dynamic process with limitless development opportunities. An application could imply accommodating more patients or discovering the finest technique for a medical procedure, both of which will have a significant impact on many people's lives. It may be said that telemedicine has caught up to the latest artificial intelligence trends, although there are still certain obstacles to overcome. Even though it's uncertain how each diagnostic software employs machine learning techniques, a simple app will almost likely include the specific procedure:

1. Make use of a massive dataset of patients' symptoms as well as doctor-informed or doctor-verified diagnosis.
2. Develop a model that can anticipate diagnosis.
3. Use the model to come up with possible diagnoses for the patient you're concerned in.

While artificial intelligence (AI) in telemedicine is still in its beginning stages, its applications are already prevalent. This wouldn't be strange to see it used in every facet of both traditional and contemporary life. In the not-too-distant future, it's not surprising to see this again in all domains of traditional and digital medicine. AI in the telemedicine realm is actively supporting breakthroughs in numerous places; according to the WHO's eHealth observatory survey, the cost of telemedicine programmers and devices is one of the most significant roadblocks to their introduction. Despite the development of cost-effective models, hospitals and facilities will need to invest time and money in installation and training in order to fully implement. There is also a dilemma with connection status or bandwidth to generate a rapid and consistent transmission of superior telemedicine information since improvements in infrastructure may be required [6], which is difficult to do, especially in rural and remote or underdeveloped facilities. Because of the current challenges with confidentiality and security in performing telemedicine consultations and operations, there has been a huge area of outlook artificial intelligence directions in the domain of healthcare information. There is still a danger of security and confidentiality while employing satellite connections in the domain of healthcare information technology. Another difficulty, analogous to other therapeutic relationships and gear, is malpractice, which has led to the requirement of training and licenses to operate telemedicine devices properly. This may hamper facility implementation by increasing the cost and project duration of the project. Patients' consistency and preferences might be influenced by malpractice and a lack of education, which can lead to dissatisfaction.

7.2.3 Adopting ML for Telemedicine

The synergies between AI and telehealth are exciting healthcare organizations. The global burden of chronic diseases has increased significantly. This, combined with an aging population with multiple morbidities, means that existing healthcare delivery models are overstressed and unsustainable. Telehealth provides promising alternatives for maximizing the use of ICT for remote healthcare diagnosis, monitoring, and delivery of care.

The advent of computer-based creation and understanding of dialogue to enable computer-to-human connection is a natural evolution from human-to-human engagement in telehealth. The development of computer-based creation and understanding of discourse to enable computer-to-human connection is a natural evolution from human-to-human engagement in telehealth. We are in the early stages of computer intelligence development, a technology that can far exceed the capabilities of manual methods and even existing technology. An AI system has been around for decades and has been involved in a variety of fields. The technology can be used in a variety of ways in healthcare, including delivering a system to evaluate medical data to identify sources of problems and generate solutions based on the existing procedure results, as well as improving processes by using computers intelligence. Finding the proper protocol and decisions for medical operations is greatly aided by the ability to detect patterns quickly and with calculated precision. Patterns discovered in the outputs of medical operations can lead to optimization and early detection of potential problems. Hospitals are now incorporating this technology to better and more effeciently harness Medial Specialists and staff. The adoption of varied machine-based learning will change the way pharmaceutical research is done. A Predictive Model for Assistive Technology Adoption for People with Dementia, for example, employs neural networks to predict the patient's ability to accept assistive technology [5]. Telepresence robots in recent designs have been built to be able to just walk through halls and rooms autonomously utilizing a software interface that connects the user to the robot over a Wi-Fi connection. This concept has recently been refined by including the use of artificial intelligence and vision technologies to aid navigation and obstacle detection. The ease with which machine learning technology may be applied has allowed it to be of considerable service in a variety of sectors, and these findings from the literature demonstrate the importance of its application in the field of medicine.

The table (Table 7.1) below lists the current research being done in the machine learning for telemedicine trends.

Table 7.1 Recent adoption of ML for telemedical trends

Journal article	Year	Trends/ technology used	Findings/summary
Disease Detection Using ML in Vital SignData Tele monitoring [2]	2020	Patient Monitoring	These findings suggest that using machine learning (ML)-based methods, it is possible to detect acute chronic disease-related symptoms more precisely
A Data Enhancement Approaches to Improve Machine Learning Performance for Predicting Health Status Using Remote-Healthcare Data [7]	2020	Healthcare Information Technology	With 95.33% accuracy, the Random Forest Classifier emerges as the winner. The results of eight alternative supervised learning algorithms in terms of existing encoding mechanism are presented in a comparison chart
Adaptive Treatment Assisting System for Patients Using Machine Learning [8]	2019	Patient Monitoring	This study recommends using a monitoring system incorporated in wearable gadgets to provide updates on the patient's condition to the doctor or family members. Fuzzy systems were used to calculate the best course of action in a particular circumstance
Wireless Continuous Patient Monitoring System for Dengue [4]	2017	Patient Monitoring	The results reveal that the suggested system is capable of picking the optimal mode of message that will direct the patient to the correct medicine box through interactions with the patient of simulated physical and mental skills
Mobile Cyber Physical Sys. for Health Care: Functions, Ambient Ontology and e-Diagnostics [9]	2016	Patient Monitoring	This study incorporated a wireless monitoring system for patients who require continuous monitoring, based on the Wireless Body Area Network (WBAN) concept, according to the research conducted
Effective Telemed. Security Using Wavelet Based Watermarking [10]	2016	Healthcare Information Technology	To ensure anonymity, this work presents a technique for embedding and reading digital wavelet watermarks on medical photographs.

7.3 Summary

The "last-mile" difficulty is always implementation, so our focus should be on building methodologies for integrating AI into society rather than building new AI tools or algorithms. The chapter is focused on the measures of performance by machine learning for the healthcare domain, as well as providing accurate results for the prediction of the patient's condition using the healthcare dataset in Python. Predictive modeling makes use of premise or off premise data to forecast an output variable. Machine learning applications have foreseen a patient's disease with a positive response. The healthcare domain has evolved with machine learning features that aid in data analysis and prediction. Machine learning achieves intelligence analytics by breaking down data and using it for prediction.

References

1. How much effort is needed to keep up with the literature relevant for primary care? https://www.ncbi.nlm.nih.gov/pmc/articles/PMC521514/
2. Kobayashi N, Ishikawa M, Hinako O, Homma S. Disease detection using machine learning in vital sign data telemonitoring. IEEE. 2020;
3. https://healthinformatics.uic.edu/blog/machine-learning-in-healthcare/
4. Hastie T, Ibshirani T, Friedman J. Elements of statistical learning: Springer Series. Statistics. 2001;
5. Morguet A, Kühnelt P, Kallel A, Jaster M, Schultheiss HP. Impact of tele-medical care monitoring on morbidity in mild to moderate chronic-heart-failure. Telemedicine and e-Health. 2021;111:134–9.
6. Huai Zhang S, Cleland I, McClean I, Nugent C, Donnelly M, Galway L, Scotney BW. IEEE J Biom Informatics. 2014;18(1):375.
7. Tabassum S, Sampa M, Islam R, Fumihiko Y, Nakashima N, Ahmed A. Data enhancement approach to improve machine -learning performance for predicting health status using remote healthcare data. IEEE. 2020;
8. Naeem C. Paragliola. IEEE: An adaptive treatment assisting sys. for patients using machine learning; 2019.
9. Costanzo A, Faro A, Giordano D, Pino C. Mobile cyber physical systems for health care: functions, ambient ontology and e-diagnostics. In: 2016 13th IEEE Annual Consumer Communications & Networking Conference (CCNC), (Las Vegas, NV, 2016), pp. 972–975.
10. Singh J, Patel A. An effective telemedicine security using wavelet based watermarking. In: IEEE International Conference on Computational Intelligence Computing Research, 2016.

Choice of Embedded Processor for IoT-Based Teleradiology Applications and a Pilot Study on Need for Portable Teleradiology System in Rural Areas

8

S. N. Kumar ⓘ, A. Lenin Fred ⓘ, H. Ajay Kumar ⓘ,
R. Melba Kani ⓘ, Parasuraman Padmanabhan ⓘ,
and Balázs Gulyás ⓘ

8.1 Introduction

Teleradiology improves the accessibility of medical services and medicines in remote areas [1]. The transmission of medical images from an isolated location to a radiologist in a super-speciality hospital is carried out for better diagnosis. The mobile technology advancement enables the volume rendering of large data sets [2]. The multimedia-based systems were found to be efficient in medical education [3]. Advances in technology and the availability of higher bandwidth connections have amplified the use of multimedia in healthcare for clinical diagnosis [4]. The advanced teleradiology system supports user interaction [5], collaboration [6] and advanced visualization [7]. The IoT-based system is found to be proficient in the data exchange between physicians and radiologists [8]. The field-programmable

S. N. Kumar (✉)
Department of EEE, Amal Jyothi College of Engineering, Kanjirapally, Kerala, India

A. Lenin Fred
Department of CSE, Mar Ephraem College of Engineering and Technology,
Marthandam, Tamil Nadu, India

H. Ajay Kumar
Department of ECE, Mar Ephraem College of Engineering and Technology,
Marthandam, Tamil Nadu, India

R. M. Kani
Department of Mechanical Engineering, Mar Ephraem College of Engineering and
Technology, Marthandam, Tamil Nadu, India

P. Padmanabhan · B. Gulyás
Lee Kong Chian School of Medicine, Nanyang Technological University,
Singapore, Singapore
e-mail: ppadmanabhan@ntu.edu.sg; balazs.gulyas@ntu.edu.sg

T. Choudhury et al. (eds.), *Telemedicine: The Computer Transformation of
Healthcare*, TELe-Health, https://doi.org/10.1007/978-3-030-99457-0_8

gate arrays (FPGAs) are cost-effective and can perform parallel computing with low power [9, 10]. The FPGA processor offers high data rates compared with the digital signal processor (DSP) and it is better for image and video processing, FPGAs outperform over DSPs [11].

The performance of GPU was found to be superior for image and video processing applications [12]. Ultrasound (US) image enhancement algorithms were implemented in the Kintex-7 FPGAs platform and MATLAB Simulink [13]. The reversible medical image watermarking technique based on discrete wavelet transform was implemented in FPGA [14]. The hardware implementation of 3D medical image compression was done in NVIDIA GPU, the context-based adaptive binary arithmetic coder generates proficient results when compared with the H.264/AVC technique [15]. The hardware implementation of filtering of 3D medical images using discrete wavelet transform on an FPGA processor generates satisfactory results [16]. The FPGA implementation of medical image reconstruction based on a probabilistic model was found to generate successful results [17].

Section 8.2 discusses the need for telemedicine in India, choice of an embedded processor for telemedicine application and pilot study undergone for the choice of IoT-based system for teleradiology application. The conclusion is justified in Sect. 8.3.

8.2   Materials and Methods

8.2.1   Need for Telemedicine in India

India is a country with 65.53% rural area. Telemedicine refers to the technology of transferring medical data and consultation by physicians for disease diagnosis through a cloud network. The features of telemedicine are summarized as follows:

- Transfer of medical data in the secured path by obeying the medical ethics; the rural area doctors will send the medical data to the expert physicians in super-speciality hospitals for expert opinion and treatment planning.
- Improving the living standards of people by imparting a healthy environment through technology.

The top telemedicine benefits are depicted in Fig. 8.1. In the current COVID 19 scenario, taking into a concern of social distance and avoidance of unnecessary travel, teleconsultation for preliminary treatment gains importance.

The different modes of teleconsultation are depicted in Fig. 8.2. The videoconferencing allows the patients to interact with the physicians and they can express their health problems. The physicians from different hospitals can also interact with each other through videoconferencing. A scan centre in a rural area can transmit images to super-speciality hospitals through teleradiology applications. The patient's reports are transferred to their mobile phones or emails from super-speciality hospitals for future reference. The nursing call centre aids the

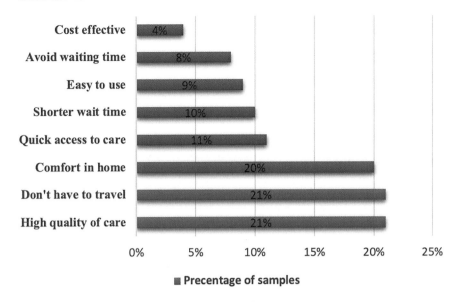

Fig. 8.1 Top telemedicine benefits

Fig. 8.2 Different modes
of telemedicine
consultation

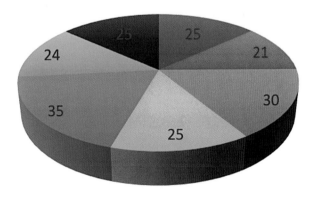

public health enquiry; e-Health portals and continuing education are also other merits of telemedicine. Figure 8.3 depicts the global telemedicine market revenue. Telemedicine is gaining much prominence in foreign countries owing to its merits. The patients don't want to go to a hospital for minor health problems, because through teleconsultation, physicians will provide guidance. The medical data will be transferred to an expert physician for obtaining a better diagnosis or a second expert opinion. Figure 8.4 depicts the global IoT healthcare market size and forecast.

There are two modes of telemedicine: synchronous and asynchronous. The synchronous model involves both the patient and the physician at the same time and a real-time interaction takes place. The asynchronous mode does not involve the simultaneous interaction of patient and physician; the data are acquired and transmitted to the receiver, and the data can be accessed at a convenient time. The survey results of Mckinsey indicate that there is a dramatic shift in usage of telehealth from 11% to 76% as a result of the outbreak of COVID 19. India being a country with many villages in rural areas, there is an urge to set up telemedicine facilities for improving healthcare.

Fig. 8.3 Global telemedicine market revenue (2016–2022)

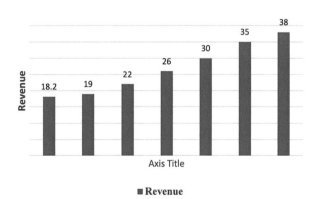

Fig. 8.4 Global IoT healthcare market size and forecast (2015–2024)

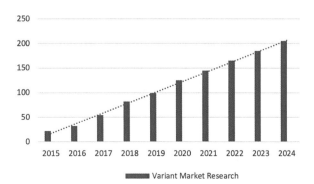

8.2.2   Choice of an Embedded Processor for Telemedicine Application

The role of medical image processing is vital in telemedicine for the transfer of medical data. Image preprocessing, segmentation, compression and classification are the main process used for the analysis of medical images. In most cases, the algorithms are implemented in MATLAB software and simulated on a PC. However, a dedicated portable embedded system is needed for the analysis and transfer of medical data through a secured cloud network. Some of the related works in the hardware implementation of image processing algorithms are also described in this section.

Embedded system-based products had revolutionized modern technology. An embedded system is a PC-based system dedicated to a specific purpose. The heart of the embedded system is the microprocessor/microcontroller. The merits of an embedded system are low cost, portable and speed in operation. The classical model of data transmission and communication using Email, and USB portable drives is not applicable as per medical ethics. The transfer of information in CD/DVD through a registered postal service will consume time. Teleradiology provides a solution for the transfer and analysis of medical data.

The wavelet transform plays a vital role in image preprocessing, segmentation and compression, and in [18], TMS320C50 DSP processor was deployed for the implementation of wavelet transform for image processing application. The FPGA architecture-based board was utilized for the image compression in [19], and the less computational complexity algorithm LOCO-I was also implemented in FPGA-based system [20]. The authors of [21] suggest the implementation of image compression techniques (wavelet-based image compression algorithms) in iPaq devices with the Linux operating system. The SPIHT image compression algorithm is an improved version of the EZW algorithm, the algorithm was implemented in FPGA [22]. The work [23] also put forward the efficient implementation of the SPIHT algorithm in FPGA. The article [24] reports the proficient implementation of JPEG 2000 in FPGA and the article [25] reports the JPEG implementation in Xilinx XSA 100 board. The Nios II processor was utilized in [26] for the implementation of the JPEG 2000 algorithm. The NVIDIA graphics processor was deployed for MR image processing and a system called PUMA was put forward in [27].

A real-time study was done before the selection of a processor for telemedicine application based on the discussion with the industrial experts. Table 8.1 below represents the response from the industry indicating the choice of processor for telemedicine application.

The analysis of choice for an embedded processor for telemedicine application reveals the following: expert's opinion E2 and E4 focus on the DSP processors; however the programming is complex and the standard size of LCD interface is small. The expert opinion E5 focus on the FPGA architecture, the VHDL or Verilog programming for medical image processing is crucial and representation of output as the image requires additional software, expert opinion E3 favours the usage of MATLAB Simulink integrated with Raspberry Pi processor. The expert opinion E1

Table 8.1 Choice of embedded processor based on the real-time discussion with the experts

SI No	Experts	Opinion from industry	Cost per board
1	Expert 1	Beagle Bone Black - AM335x 1GHz ARM Cortex-A 8 (Processor), 512 MB memory, Ethernet and HDMI ports, programming can be done in C++, Java or Python.	3367 Rs
2	Expert 2	Panda Board 4500- SoC-based board with programmable DSP processor, integrated graphics processor, 1GB of memory.	15,714 Rs
3	Expert 3	Raspberry Pi B + − 64-bit quad-core processor. The Raspbian operating system is compatible with Python, Java, Matlab Simulink, and C++ language.	2899 Rs
4	Expert 4	TMS 320C6416- Multilevel cache memory, 6 ALU, 2 multipliers, 5760 MIPS, 1.39 ns instruction cycle, with programming by Code Composer Studio.	43,783 Rs
5	Expert 5	Zynq-7000 ARM/FPGA SoC- ARM Cortex A9 Dual-core processor 1GHz, ARTIX- 7 FPGA.	14,877 Rs

favours the usage of Beagle Bone Black embedded board. The MATLAB Simulink on Raspberry Pi processor is proficient for simple image processing applications, and complex applications like ROI extraction and compression on DICOM images are not advisable. Based on the physician requirement and application, specific hardware configuration and software can be used for the telemedicine application.

The key objective of the proposed project sanctioned by the Department of Science and Technology (DST) was to develop a portable embedded system for teleradiology applications. The objectives of the project are as follows:

1. A computer-aided filtering algorithm for the minimization of noise in CT/ MR images.
2. Computer-aided segmentation algorithm for the extraction of the region of interest.
3. Computer-aided algorithm for the classification of anomalies.

The pilot study was prepared based on the above-mentioned objectives; the objectives of the pilot study are as follows:

1. To investigate the need for a portable embedded system for teleradiology application in rural areas.
2. To fetch the requirements from users for the product development.
3. To promote the role of telemedicine and its need in rural areas.

8.2.2.1 Hypothesis of Study

H0: There is no need for a portable embedded system for authenticating data transfer in rural areas for teleradiology applications.

H1: There is a need for a portable embedded system for authenticating data transfer in rural areas for teleradiology applications.

A questionnaire was prepared, the response was collected and the summary of the response is as follows:

Q1. Whether the telemedicine or PACS facility will be available in a rural area hospital or scan centres?

(a) It is highly available in all rural areas ().
(b) It is available in all rural areas ().
(c) Available, but not in all rural areas ().
(d) Availability is very rare in rural areas ().

Q2. When a system is developed primarily for medical image transfer, whether it will be helpful for rural area hospitals and scan centres?

(a) The system will be highly beneficial ().
(b) The system will be beneficial ().
(c) The system may be beneficial ().
(d) Not beneficial ().

Q3. Whether dedicated equipment or a PC-based system is needed for transferring medical images?

(a) Dedicated equipment is needed ().
(b) Can be a dedicated equipment or PC-based system ().
(c) A PC-based system is highly needed ().
(d) Dedicated equipment is highly needed ().

Q4. What is the opinion in sending the medical images by CD/DVD/Pen drive through courier or in person, Is it favourable or not

(a) Highly favourable and I recommend ().
(b) It's favourable but I don't recommend ().
(c) It's favourable but only at some instances ().
(d) It's not favourable ().

Q5. Whether the system needs a facility for the transfer of the medical diagnostic report of a patient?

(a) Yes it needs a dedicated system ().
(b) It needs a system but not necessarily be a dedicated one ().
(c) Any channel transmission is acceptable ().
(d) Not necessary ().

Q6. What type of display the user will prefer

(a) Dedicated LCD Display ()
(b) Any display but necessarily not needed to be a dedicated one ()
(c) HDMI/VGA display ()
(d) Television display ()

Q7. What size of display do you prefer when a dedicated LCD is used?

(a) 15 inch and above ()
(b) 10 inch ()
(c) 5 inch ()
(d) Any dimension ().

Q8. Whether USB port facility is required in the system?

(a) Mandatory ()
(b) Needed but not necessarily be a compulsion ()
(c) Not to be considered ()
(d) Not needed ()

Q9. Whether the system should be integrated with Hospital Information System (HIS)?

(a) Definitely it should be integrated with HIS ()
(b) May or may not be ()
(c) Not necessary ()
(d) No comments ()

Q10. Whether the system needs the transmission of medical video data?

(a) Yes ()
(b) Probably ()
(c) Optional ()
(d) No ()

Q11. Whether the system needs to transmit the patient information to the consultant doctor mobile phone?

(a) Yes, it's highly recommended ()
(b) May be recommended ()
(c) It's not recommended ()
(d) Wish of the concerned doctor ()

Q12. Whether video chat is required in the system for the communication of rural area hospitals and super-speciality hospitals?

(a) It's highly necessary ()
(b) Necessary but not concerned ()
(c) Optional ()
(d) Not necessary ()

The response was collected from 120 respondents comprising 70 respondents from urban and 50 from rural areas. The response from the respondents is listed in Tables 8.2 and 8.3. Questions Q1, Q2 and Q4 are grouped in Table 8.2; the response represents the need for telemedicine in rural areas. Questions Q3, Q5, Q6, Q7, Q8, Q9, Q10, Q11 and Q12 are grouped in Table 8.3; the response represents the features required in the design and development of a portable embedded system for data transfer in teleradiology.

A detailed survey has been conducted with physicians and radiologists based on the following criteria:

- Awareness level of teleradiology in rural area hospitals and scan centres.
- The intention of rural area hospitals and scan centres in using teleradiology services.
- Reasons for not adopting the teleradiology services.

Based on the maximum voting strategy, the response is analysed. The following inferences are made: Q1—Availability is very rare in rural areas, Q2—The system will be highly beneficial, Q4—It is not favourable (sending medical data by CD/DVD/Pen drive).

The following inferences are made: Q3—A dedicated equipment is highly needed, Q5—It needs a system but not necessarily be a dedicated one, Q6—Dedicated LCD Display, Q7—10 inch, Q8—Mandatory, Q9—It should be integrated with HIS, Q10—Yes (video transmission is needed), Q11—Yes, it is highly recommended, Q12—optional (video chats and videoconferencing). After the analysis of response, a portable embedded system was developed for the transmission of medical images in DICOM format and is highlighted in Sect. 8.3. The survey results

Table 8.2 Response analysis of Q1, Q2 and Q4

Questions/responses	a	b	c	d
Q1	5	10	35	70
Q2	70	20	30	0
Q4	0	10	20	90

Table 8.3 Response analysis of Q3, Q5, Q6, Q7, Q8, Q9, Q10, Q11 and Q12

Questions/responses	a	b	c	d
Q3	30	30	20	40
Q5	30	50	30	10
Q6	50	20	20	30
Q7	15	70	15	20
Q8	80	20	10	10
Q9	70	30	15	5
Q10	60	30	30	0
Q11	80	20	5	15
Q12	30	20	60	10

show that telemedicine facility is rare in rural areas. The intention level to use tele-medicine facilities is depicted in Fig. 8.5.

Though telemedicine is much beneficial for rural area hospitals and scan centres, Fig. 8.6 depicts the reasons for not adopting teleradiology services. The cost is a vital factor that many hospitals and scan centres in rural areas are not affordable, efficiency in the data transfer and analysis is also a factor considered by 15% of physicians and internet connectivity issues accounts for one of the reasons for not adopting teleradiology services.

Fig. 8.5 Pie chart representing rural area hospitals and scan centres in using teleradiology services

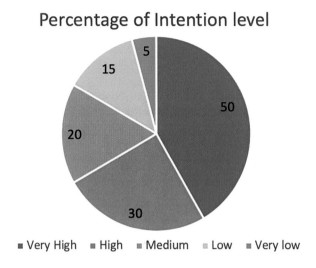

Fig. 8.6 Reasons for not adopting the teleradiology services

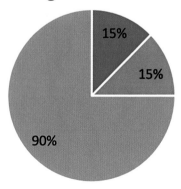

8.3   Hardware Implementation of Medical Image Processing Algorithms for Telemedicine Applications

The role of preprocessing, segmentation and compression is vital in medical data transfer. Preprocessing refers to the technique of filtering noise in images. Segmentation is the process of extraction of the desired ROI (region of interest) and compression is the technique of reducing the cost of storage or transmission. Figure 8.7 below depicts the flow diagram of the embedded system for the telemedicine application.

The proposed developed system for teleradiology is depicted in Fig. 8.8. The system comprises the following modules: preprocessing, segmentation, compression and classification.

Figure 8.9 depicts the preprocessing and segmentation output and Fig. 8.10 represents the final prototype for teleradiology application.

For preprocessing, a nonlinear tensor diffusion filter was employed and for segmentation, improved fuzzy c-means clustering based on crow search optimization was employed [28]. The compression of DICOM medical images was done by the least square algorithm based on an improved prediction Scheme [29]. The IoT

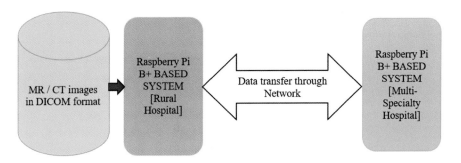

Fig. 8.7   Flow diagram of the embedded system for teleradiology application

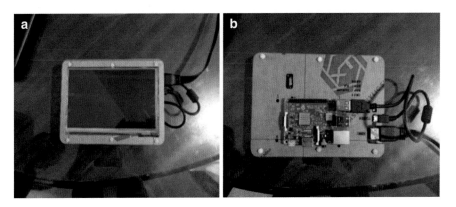

Fig. 8.8   (**a**) Front view of the portable system, (**b**) rear view of the portable system

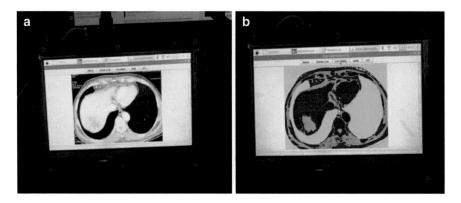

Fig. 8.9 (a) Preprocessing output, (b) segmentation output

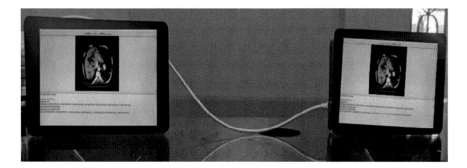

Fig. 8.10 Embedded device for telemedicine application

device is capable of accessing and recovering the DICOM images from cloud databases. The future work will be focusing on the parallel processing of algorithms that will minimize the computational complexity and hence can accommodate more DICOM images for analysis.

8.4 Conclusion

This chapter focuses on the benefits of telemedicine and highlights the urge for telemedicine service in India for healthcare. The selection of embedded processors is a crucial task in the design of IoT-based systems for teleradiology applications and this work discusses the various types of processors that can be employed for teleradiology applications. The ARM processor-based IoT system implementation for teleradiology application is also discussed in this chapter. The outcome of this research work paves the way for the researchers working on the hardware implementation of medical image processing algorithms for telemedicine applications.

Acknowledgements The authors would like to acknowledge the support provided by DST under the IDP scheme (No. IDP/MED/03/2015). Parasuraman Padmanabhan and Balázs Gulyásalso acknowledge the support from Lee Kong Chian School of Medicine and Data Science and AI Research (DSAIR) centre of NTU (Project Number ADH-11/2017-DSAIR and the support from the Cognitive NeuroImaging Centre (CONIC) at NTU. The author S.N Kumar would also like to acknowledge the support provided by the Schmitt Centre for Biomedical Instrumentation (SCBMI) of Amal Jyothi College of Engineering.

References

1. Hosteler S. PACS and teleradiology, analysis of market status and industry trends. San Francisco, CA: Miller Freeman; 1994.
2. Hachaj T. Real time exploration and management of large medical volumetric datasets on small mobile devices—evaluation of remote volume rendering approach. Int J Inform Manage. 2014;34(3):336–43.
3. Mayer RE. Applying the science of learning to medical education. Med Educ. 2010;44(6):543–9.
4. Barratt J. A focus group study of the use of video-recorded simulated objective structured clinical examinations in nurse practitioner education. Nurse Educ Pract. 2010;10(3):170–5.
5. Kinosada Y, Takada A, Hosoba M. Real-time radiology—new concepts for teleradiology. Comput Methods Prog Biomed. 2001;66(1):47–54.
6. Lee J-S, Tsai C-T, Pen C-H, Lu H-C. A real time collaboration system for teleradiology consultation. Int J Med Inform. 2003;72(1–3):73–9.
7. Evers H, Mayer A, Engelmann U, et al. Extending a teleradiology system by tools for visualization and volumetric analysis through a plug-in mechanism. Int J Med Inform. 1999;53(2–3):265–75.
8. Yoo SK, Kim KM, Jung SM, Lee KJ, Kim NH. Design of multimedia telemedicine system for inter-hospital consultation. In: Proceedings of the 26th Annual International Conference of the IEEE Engineering in Medicine and Biology Society (EMBS & 39;04), vol. 2, pp. 3109–3111, San Francisco, CA, USA, September 2004.
9. Kim S, Sohn H, Chang JH, Song T, Yoo Y. A PC-based fully-programmable medical ultrasound imaging system using a graphics processing unit. IEEE Int Ultrason Symp. 2010:314–7.
10. Ahmad A, Krill B, Amira A, Rabah H. 3D Haar wavelet transform with dynamic partial reconfiguration for 3D medical image compression. In: 2009 IEEE Biomedical circuits and systems conference, vol. 1, IEEE, 2009, pp. 137–140.
11. Kehtarnavaz N, Mahotra S. FPGA Implementation made easy for applied digital signal processing courses. In: 2011 IEEE International Conference on Acoustics, Speech and Signal Processing (ICASSP); 2011. p. 2892–5.
12. Zhang N, Wang J, Chen Y. Image parallel processing based on GPU. In: 2nd International conference on advanced computer control; 2010. p. 367–70.
13. Akkala V, Rajalakshmi P, Kumar P, Desai UB. FPGA based ultrasound backend system with image enhancement technique. ISSNIP Biosignals Biorobotics Conf. 2014;
14. Jana P, Phadikar A. Low-power FPGA-based hardware implementation of reversible watermarking scheme for medical image. In: Computational advancement in communication circuits and systems. Singapore: Springer; 2020. p. 287–96.
15. Ahmad A, Muharam A, Amira A. GPU-based implementation of CABAC for 3-dimensional medical image compression. J Telecommun Electron Comput Eng (JTEC). 2017;9(3–8):45–50.
16. Lyakhov PA, Valueva MV, Nagornov NN, Chervyakov NI, Kaplun DI. Low-bit hardware implementation of DWT for 3D medical images processing. In: 2020 IEEE Conference of Russian Young Researchers in Electrical and Electronic Engineering (EIConRus) 2020 Jan 27. IEEE; 2020. p. 1396–9.

17. Ravi M, Sewa A, Shashidhar TG, Sanagapati SS. FPGA as a hardware accelerator for computation intensive maximum likelihood expectation maximization medical image reconstruction algorithm. IEEE Access. 2019;7:111727–35.
18. Vlcek K, Vlcek J, Kucera R. DSP implementation of image compression by multiresolutional analysis. Radio Eng. 1998;7(1):7–9.
19. Mosqueron R, Dubois J, Paindavoine M. Embedded image processing/compression for high-speed CMOS sensor. In: 14th IEEE European signal processing conference, Italy, Sep 4, 2006, pp. 1-5.
20. Klimesh M, Stanton V, Watola D. Hardware implementation of a lossless image compression algorithm using a field programmable gate array. TMO Prog Rep. 2001:42–144.
21. Image Compression Application on Battery-aware Embedded Systems. http://mesl.ucsd.edu/gupta/cse237b/PastProjects/Compression.pdf.
22. Fry TW, Hauck SA. SPIHT image compression on FPGAs. IEEE Trans Circ Syst Video Technol. 2005;15(9):1138–47.
23. Corsonello P, Perri S, Zicari P, Cocorullo G. Microprocessor-based FPGA implementation of SPIHT image compression subsystems. Microprocess Microsyst. 2005;29(6):299–305.
24. Al Muhit A, Islam MS, Othman M. VLSI Implementation of Discrete Wavelet Transform (Dwt) for image compression. In: International Conference on Autonomous Robots and Agents, New Zealand, Dec 13, 2004, pp. 391–395.
25. Mike Dyer, Amit Kumar Gupta, and Natalie Galin Nios II processor-based hardware/software co-design of the JPEG2000 Standard. Nios II Embedded processor design contest—outstanding designs, 2005, pp. 24–36.
26. Singh SN, Kumar J, Ranjan R, Panigrahi S. Hardware image compression with FPGA. Int J Recent Trends Eng. 2009;2(8):33–5.
27. Dasika G, Fan K, Mahlke S. Power-efficient medical image processing using Puma. In: IEEE 7th Symposium on Application Specific Processors, USA, Jul 27, 2009, pp. 29–34.
28. Fred AL, Kumar SN, Padmanaban P, Gulyas B, Kumar HA. Fuzzy-crow search optimization for medical image segmentation. In: Applications of hybrid metaheuristic algorithms for image processing. Cham: Springer; 2020. p. 413–39.
29. Kumar SN, Fred AL, Kumar HA, Varghese PS. Lossless compression of CT images by an improved prediction scheme using least square algorithm. Circ Syst Signal Process. 2020;39(2):522–42.

Providing Efficient Healthcare System: Web-Based Telemedicine System

9

D. Mahima

9.1 Introduction

To give proficient healthcare services to the underprivileged in the underdeveloped and developing countries in the world, the main aim is to develop an efficient e-Healthcare system with the help of utilizing telemedicine for the needy in the society [1]. Telemedicine has clear benefits in rural or remote areas where it deters the requirement for travel for healthcare workers and patients and improves access to medical care services.

While in urban areas, telemedicine usage can lead to improvement in access to information and healthcare services. It has appeared to make improvisation in the quality and consistency of medical care. This is less expensive as compared to conventional practice despite the fact of just discovering telemedicine applications [2].

Ubiquitous health systems which are web based and can give healthcare to citizen anyplace/whenever using internet technologies is becoming increasingly significant. Since they are web based, they can also be opened on PDAs and smartphones, thus making it more convenient for healthcare delivery.

9.2 Background and Problem Definition

World Health Organization (WHO) has expressed confronting humanity in this twenty-first century so as to provide them with great well-being as one of the greatest difficulties. The main reasons for facing this challenge are socioeconomic conditions, increase in expectations for health, and burdens imposed by old as well as new diseases on the growing world population [3]. The progressing propels in

D. Mahima (✉)
College of Engineering & Applied Science, University of Cincinnati, Cincinnati, OH, USA
e-mail: dahiyama@mail.uc.edu

© The Author(s), under exclusive license to Springer Nature
Switzerland AG 2022
T. Choudhury et al. (eds.), *Telemedicine: The Computer Transformation of Healthcare*, TELe-Health, https://doi.org/10.1007/978-3-030-99457-0_9

information and communication technologies have given the possibility to improve healthcare facilities in both developed nations and developing nations.

But this commitment is only considered by those who have the financial means to do so. For instance, the government of the UK aiming to improve and modernize the NHS (National Health Stack) by utilizing information technology which also includes telemedicine [4].

From an economical perspective, it is imperative to highlight the fact that the private clinics arrange all the equipment by overcharging the necessary things by the doctor for the surgery. In a government hospital, all the medications and drugs are to be organized by the patient's family members. In the event of a crisis, it turns into mayhem as one doesn't have the foggiest idea where in the city so much stuff will be accessible [5, 6].

It has interdisciplinary pertinence in the setting that it is an e-Health initiative to improve healthcare service for all sections of society in developing and developed countries in the world. It has great importance in the government health sector as it allows the layout of medical facilities for the patient.

Further, the chapter is organized as follows: Section 9.3 imparts a brief summary of what is telemedicine and traces its history and evolution; Section 9.4 discusses the part of e-Health and telemedicine in the development of healthcare while Sect. 9.5 briefly spells the advantages of telemedicine. Further, Sect. 9.6 highlights how in this interconnected world coordination and networking play an important role in telemedicine. An in-depth review of literature, its significance, aim and objectives of this study is carried out in Sect. 9.7. Finally, the chapter discusses on different e-Health/telemedicine frameworks, example case studies, and other current initiatives undertaken amidst the corona pandemic. At the end, Sect. 9.9 summarizes all the above and lists the advantages of the e-Health / telemedicine system.

9.3   What Is Telemedicine

One of the principal issues that are overlooked by humanity in this twenty-first century is access to top-caliber healthcare facilities. This problem can be solved with the help of telemedicine as it helps the patients connect with healthcare specialists and experts over a distance. This is also made possible with the advancements in technologies. With more inventions taking place, more features can be provided to the patients and healthcare experts. Telemedicine is basically characterized as delivering health services and remote medical expertise with the help of data advancements and telecommunications technologies over a distance, regardless of what the location of information and patient is. Due to this, telemedicine is also considered an important part of health telematics [7].

Usage of telemedicine will allow suburbanization and the effort recently could be seen in the secondary and primary care sector, respectively (Fig. 9.1). These changes would allow providing access to better therapeutic and diagnostic services, better analytic, improved correspondence between medical care laborers, and quicker access to medical information in the rural or remote areas [7].

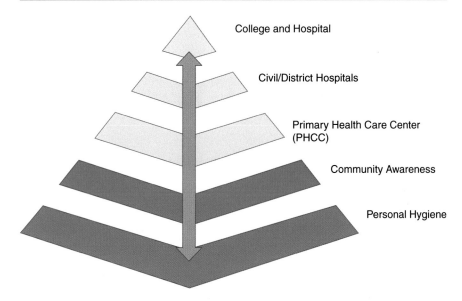

Fig. 9.1 Enhance transmission up and down theihealthcare pyramid via usage of telemedicine

Telemedicine also serves an important role in remote or rural areas for the cases of emergencies where there is a probability that the patient won't be able to get medical care on time. With the help of telemedicine, countries having weak economies can also gain access to healthcare services that are otherwise not accessible to them.

An instance of this is the arrangement of medical services to the different parts of the district out of the town of Arkhangelsk present in the northwest Russia and the trading of experience or information between northwest Russia and the University Hospital of Tromsø [7, 8].

Although there's always a scope of improvement in terms of solving barriers like social, language, culture, etc., it also needs to be seen that the underdeveloped countries should have access to telemedicine by improving infrastructure, technical factors, etc.

9.3.1   History of Telemedicine

One early instance for the usage of medicine over a distance was in Middle Ages where communication across Europe took place by using bonfire for the information about bubonic plague.

Then in the mid-nineteenth century, with the establishment of postal services the physicians could provide instructions for cure and diagnosis over a distance. Here telegraphy also began with which planning for medical care could quickly be delivered. It was majorly used in the USA and Europe for communication, for instance, in the American Civil War for communicating casualty, requesting medical supplies, etc.

In the late nineteenth century came the telephone which could be used to deliver health services and amplified voice from a stethoscope. The next important development was the radio which took place towards the end of the nineteenth century. Institute of Seaman's Church situated in New York was among the earliest associations for using the radio to deliver medical care in 1920. In 1935, CIRM (Centre for International Radio Medical) situated in Rome, Italy, became the biggest organization globally to deliver seafarers access to healthcare by using telemedicine [7].

9.3.2   The Birth of Present-Day Telemedicine

The latest evolution for telemedicine was made in two ways:

1. Advancement in electronic strategies of transmission.
2. Spearheading endeavors of a few individuals and organizations.

A significant impact on the improvement of telemedicine occurred with the presentation of television in the United States. A two-way circuit that was closed was set up between the state mental hospital present in Norfolk and Nebraska Mental Institute situated in Omaha for television. This system allowed communications between general practitioners and experts and also encouraged schooling and training at distance [9].

This was made possible with the help of enhancements in computerized interchanges and low-priced computing; a large number of video conferencing systems are presently being founded on personal computers.

Advancements in satellite communications and mobile phones have provided mobile telemedicine. For instance, in Canada, the Memorial University situated in Newfoundland program was set up in the year 1977 to give long-distance schooling and medical care to Canadians [10].

9.4   e-Health/Telemedicine for Development of Healthcare

Since the mid-1990s, programs for telemedicine/e-Health have gotten common all through the world in almost every zone of medical services.

With the help of telemedicine, many problems can be solved, such as:

1. In contrast with the economic growth, healthcare expenditures are increasing rapidly.
2. With the development of new technologies and a growing population, healthcare expenses are increasing.
3. Ensuring that the medical services are available to all people.
4. Progression of medical care [11].

In 2006, International Business Machines Corporation (IBM) conducted a survey asking 150,000 people from 104 countries to tell which all technologies will be popular in the future. According to the results, there were 5 significant innovations. One amid them was e-Health. Many scientific studies prove that various fields of healthcare have gradually started accepting applications of e-Health [12].

One more advantage of using telemedicine/e-Health is cost-effectiveness. One such example which showcases cost-effectiveness is the studies conducted in countries like Russia and Brazil which have large territories. As per the assessments done by the physicians in West Siberian, the patients financed around forty times less via online consultation as compared to visiting the same doctor in Moscow. Tele-cardiology service operating since June 2006 at the State of Minas Gerais in Brazil is another example that depicts cost-effectiveness. According to the results, there has been an increase in savings to 1.5%. This can then be utilized to manage the operational cost of the system [11, 13].

e-Health applications can be used at any place. A study was conducted in Parma, a small region in Italy, from first January 2001 to 31 December 2006. In this, all youngsters and youths with type 1 diabetes were provided with a 24/7 toll-free telephone service. The total number of participants was 421. With the help of this, the number of patients admitted to the hospital was reduced from a normal of 10 cases for every 100 kids in a year to 3 cases for every 100 youngsters yearly. Hence, reducing the expenses for confirmation diminished by 60% [14].

9.5   Advantages of e-Health/Telemedicine

The main advantages of telemedicine/e-Health that also prove what it is capable of are:

1. Improving healthcare delivery and making it speedier, ideal, high quality, and budget friendly for all at any place and anytime.
2. Diminishing the difference in healthcare services between the economically developed and growing countries.
3. Enhancing the work of staff in the field of healthcare.
4. Reducing the gaps between the demands in the healthcare and existing services.
5. Reduction in the budget of healthcare.

In spite of undoubted e-Health/telemedicine benefits, humankind is still distant from the world of digital healthcare and from broad utilization of e-Health/telemedicine to help all. Specialists admit that e-Health/telemedicine has immense and still undiscovered potential.

9.6   Coordination and Networking

In the world of telemedicine/e-Health, it's important for everyone to know more about what is happening globally. Thus, cooperation and networking are the two major factors that are going hand in hand.

Initiatives taken to enable networking:

1. The International Society for Telemedicine and e-Health (ISfTeH).
2. Med-e-Tel (Annual Event conducted for International Society for Telemedicine and e-Health).

ISfTeH is a non-profit community corporation and also a global assignee committee of public and worldwide telemedicine and e-Health associations and advances telemedicine/e-Health globally. Its main point is to spread information, data, and encounter and to give entry to perceived specialists in the e-Health domain around the world.

Med-e-Tel is a top-notch specialized occasion that brings together the purchasers, medical service experts, and decision and policymakers from various nations with the providers of specific equipment and service providers. This gives them an idea and hands-on experience with the present-day accessible products, technologies, and applications. It is a gathering which takes place for presenting and discussing the thoughts, projects, etc.

The two of them are cooperating for what is happening worldwide along with the recent trends in the area of e-Health. The two of them lead the path in practical applications, education for work, science, practitioners, and the general public talking about genuine issues, real accomplishments, and products.

9.7   Literature Review

Many countries such as the USA, Norway, and Finland have produced the largest number of publications in comparison to the population in the domain of e-Health/telemedicine. The main aim for doing such rigorous analyses for telemedicine was to improve the health of people in certain well-defined scenarios and provide access to healthcare facilities to all sections of society in the world.

During the study of e-Health/telemedicine, they have looked up various separate attributes such as sustainability, feasibility, safety, acceptability, cost, and viability while developing an efficient system using telemedicine, and the significance of studying every one of these factors will systematically change from one application to another depending on the functionalities required.

At the international gathering, with a populace of more than 1.3 billion India not just requires a viable and effectively available healthcare system yet in addition also requires one which can provide access to healthcare services to the majority. It is a test for both developing countries and developed countries who are as yet attempting to plan a viable healthcare prototype that will fulfill the necessities of different groups inside their population [15].

Research studies related to the utilization of wireless communications technologies to expand the mobility of medical facilities applications, reach, and range have been reported. Some other research works that focus on demonstrating the efficiency, achievability, and comfort of utilizing handheld gadgets in upgrading medical care delivery in zones, for example, electronic messaging systems [16], moving clinical information have likewise been broadly revealed.

Technology integration inside the health sector can possibly advance to promote healthy ways of life, improve choices by healthcare experts and also patients, and upgrade medical care quality by refining admittance to health and medical data [17]. In July 2018, NITI Aayog, GoI, suggested the making of NHS which would coordinate all the health areas at state and national levels and also plans to make computerized records related to health for Indian residents before the year 2022. The Union spending plan in India for the year 2020–2021 suggested the utilization of machine learning and artificial intelligence in the Ayushman Bharat scheme for focusing on infection by planning a suitable preventive regime [18].

The utilization of different groundbreaking e-Health developments is advancing completely, however at an exceptionally decent steady and furthermore at various speed in various countries [19]. With the expanded utilization of innovation in medical care, there has been an incredible accentuation on tele-Health in light of the fact that it can stretch out the services of suppliers to distant areas and exploit the accessibility of medical experts and conquer the hindrance of proximity. Advancing development in tele-Health systems would help extend access and making medical care benefits more helpful for patients, particularly those in remote or rural areas having small kids or mobility limitations [20].

e-Health systems are arising as a promising tool for utilizing developing technologies like the internet, PDAs, interactive televisions, CD-ROMs, etc., to empower medical care facilities and improvement. Despite the fact that it is still in the beginning phase of development, these systems provide the possible reach like the underserved populations at moderate ease, time efficiency, versatility; and the ability to offer customization to consumers and patients on the basis of their necessities. Regardless of these expected advantages, there are hurdles like quality measures, health, restrictions of access, and technology literacy that still need to be addressed [21].

In the year 2002, a foundation known as Robert Wood Johnson developed the drive for Health e-Technologies, a public program office zeroed in on increasing the collection of data regarding the adequacy, effective price, and applications quality in the domain of e-Health for chronic infection management and change in health behavior. To build up a firm arrangement of financing needs, it was fundamental for plan to think from various points of view from a wide scope of areas while tending to disputes and comparing spaces of intersection [21].

After the initiation of ICT (Information and Communication Technologies) in e-Health, a big impact has taken place in all aspects of medical care, going from giving the data, the people need to know so as to live a healthy lifestyle and giving new apparatuses so as to make it accessible in the future of medication. Along these lines, ICTs ensure more effective and responsive medical care systems provided to the patients by giving at home and mobile technologies. It isn't just that electronic cards were used instead of e-Health Systems, yet ICTs likewise empower better-customized care. This is done to make medicines more powerful and allow specialists to analyze issues quicker, and even to predict issues before they show up, thus proving that ICTs can refine medical care by permitting the examination of the patients in real time, i.e., during transportation or from home, and hence playing a vital part in various processes [22].

The ongoing surge of Covid-19 has given rise to a national calamity and there is growing proof that if appropriate steps were taken to limit its dangerous effect in the early phase by the government and the people, it could have not drastically raised. Apart from this, the lack of preparation in case of the next covid wave hits has caused utter chaos with the shortages of beds, oxygen cylinders, medicines, etc. in hospitals. With India now accounting for more than half of new cases in the world every day, the state and national government have taken initiatives so as to diminish the present threat and overcome the barriers of shortages of healthcare equipment and medicines. For example, e-education and e-Health by utilizing digital platforms, digitalization of public services in districts, urban, and rural communities and policy implementation, developing new applications that diminish the spread of COVID-19, and upheld the slow lifting of confinement measures by educating residents if by chance they were close to individuals contaminated by the infection and assuming this is the case, urging them to inform health authorities, isolate themselves and request support from the medical staff and tracking apps so as to bring timely and correct reporting.

Various steps have been contemplated by numerous nations to inspect and supervise the COVID-19 pandemic. One of them being virtual software and telemedicine system platforms. Given the high risk of communication of the disease via contact from one individual to another individual, telemedicine can be productive in diminishing uninterrupted exposure and aids for patient follow-up. This platform would help access medical care and doctor consultation, connect with family and friends in the middle of isolation, maintaining social distancing and stay-at-home requests. Likewise, a few hospitals have turned to virtual software like Skype, Apple Facetime, zoom, etc. to work with telemedicine care during the pandemic. Apart from these, voice-interface systems like Apple Siri, Google Voice, etc. or mobile sensors like smartwatches, oxygen monitors, etc. are also on the rise [23].

In the midst of covid, telemedicine facilities have extended from giving medical care facilities at hospitals to delivering care at patients' homes, for instance, usage of a telemonitoring system for people with congestive cardiovascular breakdown at home to ameliorate their general ailment, which would lessen their danger of getting admitted in the hospital because of its capacity to engage a self-care for a patient, inspiration, self-administration, and education [24].

9.7.1 Significance of the Study

It has been observed from the study that the government of India is working hard not only to provide a successful and effectively available medical care system yet additionally one which can convey medical care facilities to the majority. Registries are relied upon to be the critical innovation for beating obstructions to deliver healthcare facilities to the masses and also will interest service providers (like pharmacists and pharmaceutical companies) as it promotes global online business.

Its prosperity is intently attached to an expected return from putting resources into innovation for Internet online business and the expected worldwide electronic market [25].

9.7.2   e-Healthcare System: Aim and Objectives

The aim and objectives of the e-Healthcare system is to provide:

1. A platform where all the service providers, i.e., chemists and pharmaceutical company, can register themselves and provide the list of all the facilities they provide.
2. Service providers who can maintain a list of precious lifesaving drugs and equipment they provide.
3. Facility to the end-user who will be the patient's family members can use the web service to locate the service providers who supply the equipment he is looking for.
4. Comparison feature to the end-user who can make a comparative search among all the service providers and choose the best according to his requirements and locate his address and thereby able to contact him for the service.
5. Raising a drug not available request so that the end-user can directly communicate to the Pharmaceutical Company through the hub to deliver the medicine or medical equipment's direct to the hospital by charging the amount by credit card/cash on delivery / Demand Draft and issuing an invoice in the name of the patient admitted to the hospital.
6. It will also reduce the chaos among the patient's family and also free the doctors from the patient requesting/pleading for medicine trauma that they often have to face and thereby being now more focused on the main task of saving the life of the patients.
7. Probable stakeholders include patient's family, chemists/ service providers in the city, pharmaceutical companies, NGOs, and others.

9.8   Various Telemedicine System Frameworks

Due to the increase in demand for e-Health facilities, many telemedicine systems have been designed, developed, and also prompted for research efforts. Many of them are utilized in special zones, for example, injuries, neurosurgery, cardiology, and many more. While some of the e-Health systems are utilized for specific purposes like checking patients, marine purposes, crises, and so on. With the benefits of wireless technologies, there are likewise numerous web-based and mobile-based e-Health systems emerging [26].

The utilization of wireless technology for medical services delivery is incredibly affecting the medical services area all around the world. Due to the portability and flexibility provided by the technical devices like laptops, smartphones, and PDAs for healthcare to the doctors as compared to the computational PCs, there has been a significant increase in the adoption of wireless technology.

This technology also remains a top choice for providing a budget-friendly high-quality healthcare facility. With the development taking place in this technology, it can contribute widely in the field of healthcare in not so developed countries where there is a consistent scarcity of healthcare staff. The WHO organization is motivating the countries to work on producing methods for appropriate plan and execution of telemedicine system. With the help of this, the governments would have the option to profit from health surveillance, information sharing, research, and education on medical among others.

In light of the discussion in Sect. 7 and employing the tools and technologies of service-oriented architecture (SOA) like XML, SOAP, WSDL, WS-REST, and UDDI [27, 28], the authors propose a general architecture of a telemedicine system as depicted in Fig. 9.2.

Any discussion of these technologies is outside the scope of this chapter, but interested readers may like to refer [27, 28]. In the sub-sections below, we briefly discuss web-based and mobile-based telemedicine systems.

9.8.1 Web-Based Telemedicine System

e-Health is an upcoming field for addressing the issues of patients, healthcare experts, and medical care providers by utilizing the available data and communication technologies. The medical care industry is going through essential changes, for instance, shift to the ambulatory system from hospital services [26]. With the

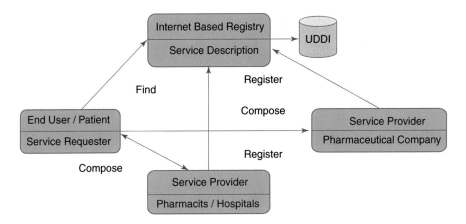

Fig. 9.2 General architecture for a telemedicine system

advancements in technology, web-based telemedicine systems can give the general public easier access to their medical data and facilities.

9.8.1.1 Web-Based Telemedicine System Based on Languages

The first step while designing and developing a telemedicine system is to know what are the important necessities required by the healthcare experts, nurses, and patients so as to provide them with those. For this, studies and surveys can be conducted for different staff members at different locations. For instance, a research study was conducted where data from two hospitals—Mulago and Nsambya hospitals situated in Kampala, Uganda, was collected. Here they made two questionnaires separate for IT staff and non-IT, staff. There was a total of 200 participants, i.e., 100 from each hospital. The group from each hospital comprised 20 doctors, 20 patients, 20 nurses, and 20 ICT staff belonging to both senior and junior staff category [29].

The quantitative data received was then analyzed using SPSS's descriptive statistics and content analysis method to give out the factors which were then used as design requirements [29].

There are no specific guidelines and standards while developing a telemedicine system. With the help of research, three guidelines came to be known: operational, clinical, and technical as stated by Loane and Wooten [30].

e-Health services support healthcare significantly, anyway from the viewpoint of interaction between healthcare experts and patient, they are advantageous but, in many cases, communication tools provided by the system are more beneficial. Understanding medical terms are one difficulty that is often faced by multinational patients in terms of intonation, clarity, pronunciation in speech, technical words, and pitch. In such cases, patients with not that good communication skills in the foreign language would find it better to understand the instructions in written form by the medical staff better than speech [31].

Some EU projects like Khresmoi and UniversalNurseSpeaker aim to improvise the prospects of medical care given by the governments of the countries around the world which tend to be the most well-known destination for travel [31].

9.8.1.2 Case Study: Khresmoi: A Web-Based Telemedicine System

Khresmoi is a multilingual search engine system created under the EU FP7 project which aims at facilitating medical information search. This system mainly addresses two end user-end clients: medical experts such as nurses, medical staff and students, experts and biomedical researchers, and the general public most importantly multinational users (as shown below in Fig. 9.3). This system is used for medical image analysis, machine translation, and more intricate interaction between the patients and radiologist. The best part is that the users can use this system as a mobile application or web interface [32].

This search engine system permits an approach to biomedical information by analyzing and ordering the 2D and 3 D medical pictures from various sources with the help of improved search capabilities because of the incorporation of

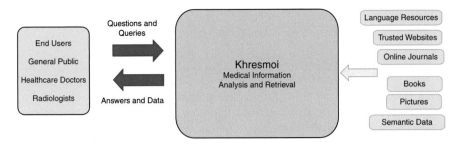

Fig. 9.3 Khresmoi search engine system

technologies for linking pictures and texts to facts in a multilingual climate, thus developing trustable outcomes for the clients to understand.

This web-based system consolidated different information sources and knowledge got from different information sources which also includes books, image sources from radiology departments, i.e., PACS (Picture Archiving and Communication Systems), online journals, and trusted websites.

Advantages of using this system are:

1. Provides doctors with correct answers rapidly.
2. Providing the patients with understandable and trustable information related to medicines and drugs.
3. Manages the images so as to prevent the radiologist from drowning in images as multiple images as created every day.

As seen in Fig. 9.4, the architecture uses an IDL interface as the frontend and RESTful web services for permitting simple connections and distributing the services on a basic level. The content search depends on Lucene while the image search utilizes ParaDISE (Parallel Distributed Image Search Engine). This search engine utilizes Hadoop implementation for parallelizing the ordering of the visual highlights. The plug-in-like blueprint permits indexing strategies and simple expansion of features [33].

The 3D picture search aims at supporting clinical radiologists during the evaluation of radiology information. Here the radiologist marks a district of interest in the data given for imaging after which the system searches for a related image content in the enormous database. The search list made comprises ranked cases for regions having an alike appearance as a query. A radiology report is shown for each case with the pathological observations highlighted in the image. A fragment registration-based localization engine is used by the model for indexing.

After indexing, feature vocabularies and indices are made for every anatomical structure. While entering a query, the anatomy structure for the query region is recognized, then the nearest neighbors. The main motive is to radiologists with efficient data in the image storage of the hospital along with the reports even before they determine an observation or make a diagnosis [33].

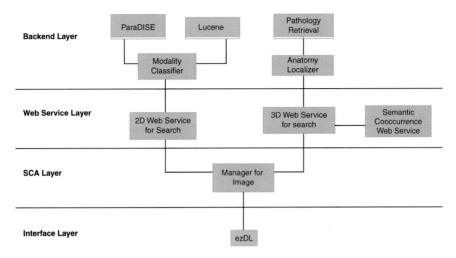

Fig. 9.4 Architecture of Khresmoi search system [33]

9.8.2   Mobile-Based Telemedicine System

Pervasive health systems which center around mechanized applications that can give Healthcare to a resident at any place and whenever with the help of utilizing wired and remote mobile technologies are getting progressively significant.

Thus, handheld gadgets particularly cell phones and PDAs have been accounted for to turn out to be progressively prevalent for medical facilities delivery [34]. Apart from this, smartphones also support users from far off or remote areas to synchronize their personal information and give access to organize services provided by mobile devices, for instance, email using wireless technology, internet access, and web browsing subsequently meeting the portability needs of clinical experts or patients who are consistently moving. The development and explosive growth of mobile technology, no doubt, have a significant impact on the manner in which we get things done. Furthermore, handheld gadgets and the applications packaged inside them are essentially less expensive and require almost no preparation, not at all like most PC-based options.

But despite the development in portable healthcare services, there have often been circumstances where patients with certain ailments are reluctant or unfit to dependably go to a doctor. Taking a common medical issue for instance AIDS is an illness achieved by an infection called HIV (human immunodeficiency infection). HIV can infect anybody irrespective of their age, sex, race, or sexual orientation. In such scenarios, humankind is normally encouraged to occasionally visit their physicians for scheduled clinical inspection and lay hold of the advised medication consistently [35].

One significant reason for death every year in the world is due to the wrong prescription or wrong dosage or drug is given by caregivers to the clients due to befuddling drug names, messy handwriting, and measurement mistakes. By using cell phones like smartphones and personal digital assistants, these blunders can be eliminated to the extent of the fact that they permit information related to prescription to be viewed in SMS. For example, basic medications like Zidovine, Abacavir, and Lamivudine for HIV/AIDS should be consumed as per the doctor's prescriptions [35].

9.8.2.1 Case Study: Mobile-Based Alert System for Healthcare

The mobile-based medical alert system is a system made for alerting the patients and healthcare workers via text messages about crisis and information on handheld gadgets like PDAs and cell phones. It is also utilized for managing diseases by updating the patients regarding the medications and the scheduled appointment to follow up that will work with their treatment processes.

The plan and organization of a medical system used for alerting are such that they would refine the facilities of healthcare facilities on a worldwide scale. It supports real-time transfer through SMS for the information regarding the prescription of the patients. This system incorporates the working of the Ozeki SMS server with an e-Health-based system. For the production of the system, an incremental way to deal with software development is used. Thus, allowing the system to deteriorate into various parts, where each part is planned and constructed independently which permits every part to be conveyed to the customer when it is finished. This is done to permit fractional usage of products and at the same time dodges a long time for the development of the system.

Using the Ozeki SMS server, the mobile alert system can forward alert message which includes the time to take medications for a disease to the patient's phone. As seen in Fig. 9.5, the system is divided into three parts:

1. Database (MySQL).
2. Device used by the client such as mobile phone, PDA, etc.
3. Three Servers: Application, Web, and Ozeki SMS Server.

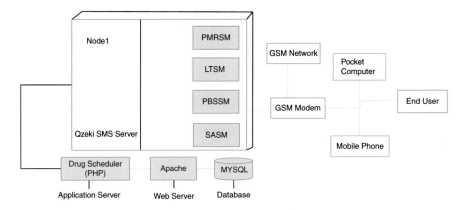

Fig. 9.5 Architecture for mobile-based alert system [35]

The system contains a module known as security and authentication which is used in a hospital setting where multiple users like specialists, pharmacists, doctors, laboratory personnel, etc. can view the patient's details at the same time to make positive changes in the medical facilities provided to the patients. The permit is given to the hospital staff on the basis of their roles in terms of specialty and profession.

A research was conducted to evaluate the MAS by using a cognitive walk-through strategy where the evaluators have to assess the system by undergoing various assessments. In this study, they tried to cover numerous types of end-users including age and gender. A series of tasks were provided to the evaluators so as to ensure no major assessment was ignored and they were asked to evaluate the performance of the system on the basis of this. The result achieved on evaluating all the questionnaires was that the model MAS introduced has a decent convenience. This investigation makes a commitment in the field of medical care services using mobile [35].

The advantages of Mobile Alert System are:

1. The design of the system is simple with no communication architecture or perplexing framework.
2. It is budget friendly as the arrangement comprises some low-price parts.

9.8.3   Other Initiatives

UniversalNurse Speaker is a joint venture to allow healthcare specialists, medical staff, and nurses to interact with patients who speak different languages. It is a translation tool where the phrases are verified by the healthcare specialist after being translated by the native speakers. The patients can then try to understand the phrase said by the doctor by listening or reading them from the system screen at the same time. This also encourages the nurses and medical staff to master the language barriers while taking care of the patient when hospitalized [36].

HealthVault is a web-based e-Health system designed to support elderly people by remotely screening the elderly people's movements and well-being. This system permits the utilization of other observing equipment. It permits overseeing difficult health signals, storing information, and effectively sharing information with healthcare experts. Nonetheless, it has a major disadvantage, that is, the system is not adaptable and versatile as they cannot be utilized in outdoor conditions and also cannot be set up to get new sensorial gadgets [37].

One more initiative which has been taken is Short Message Services (SMS) which has numerous advantages in the terms of its wide reach, adaptability, widespread popularity, and expense viability in the developing world. On an overall note, mHealth activities guarantee to minimize the information gap that presently persists for information of the patient. Thus, enabling healthcare workers to change strategies and projects, distribute resources all the more proficiently, and also gauge the efficiency of healthcare programs.

9.9 Conclusions

An efficient web-based telemedicine system can be utilized to refine the nature of the e-Healthcare system and also expand the range of innovation for communication technologies among the patients and healthcare experts by giving them clinical information on the past diseases, treatment, the medications or drugs utilized by the patient, the impacts of the treatment the patients have gone through and also overcome the languages barrier.

Building an e-Health-based telemedicine system would help:

1. It will assist the clients to contact pharmacists regarding the medication/drug required as prescribed by the doctor.
2. Pharmaceutical organizations to comprehend the market interest furthermore to connect the end-user directly with on-time delivery facility and just in time inventory diminishing logistics and storage expenses essentially.
3. It will especially help the rural and semi-urban population who have to come to the city to benefit from the medical services and having no colleagues or knowledge about the city.
4. Web-based telemedicine systems are proving to be helpful in COVID-19 by strengthening the patient-focused health-related consultations in the homes and expanding their access to healthcare guidance.

References

1. Davis N, Lacour M. Saunders Foundations of Health Information Management. 4th ed. Elsevier; 2018.
2. Darkins A, Rocke LG, Dearden CH, Martin JB, Wootton R, Sibson L, et al. An evaluation of telemedical support for a minor treatment centre. J Telemed Telecare. 1996;2(2):93–9. https://doi.org/10.1177/1357633X9600200205.
3. World Health Organization. Health-for-all Policy for the 21st Century, HQ (document EB101/8). Geneva: WHO; 1997.
4. NHS Executive. Information for health: an information strategy for the modern NHS. London: The Stationery Office; 1998.
5. Averill RF, Grant TM, Steinbeck BA. Preparing for theoutpatient prospective payment system. J AHIMA. 2000;71:35–43.
6. Schraffenberger LA, Keuhn L. Effective management of codingservices. 3rd ed. Chicago: American Health Information Management Association; 2007.
7. Craig J, Patterson V, et al. Introduction to the practice of telemedicine. J Telemed Telecare. 2005;11(1):3–9. https://doi.org/10.1177/1357633X0501100102.
8. Sørensen T, Rundhovde A, Kozlov VD. Telemedicine in north-west Russia. J Telemed Telecare. 1999;5:153–6.
9. Benschoter RA, Wittson CL, Ingham CG. Teaching and consultation by television: I. Closed-circuit collaboration. J Hosp Commun Psychiatry. 1965;16:99–100.
10. Elford R. Telemedicine activities at Memorial University of Newfoundland: a historical review, 1975–1997. Telemed J. 1998;6:207–24.
11. Jordanova M, Lievens F. Lievens global telemedicine and e-Health. In: Proceedings of the 3rd International Conference on E-Health and Bioengineering—EHB; 2011.
12. Boyle A. Five-Tech forecast. Retrieved September 18, 2009 from http://cosmiclog.msnbc.msn.com/archive/2006/12/28/23418.aspx

13. Selkov AI, Stolyar VL, Atkov OU, Selkova EA, Chueva NV. Development conception of E-diagnosis departments of small towns and villages clinics for developing regions and countries. In: Jordanova M, Lievens F, editors. Med-e-Tel: The International Educational and Networking Forum for eHealth, Telemedicine and Health ICT, Electronic Proceedings. Luxembourg: Publ. Luxexpo; 2008. p. 395–414.
14. Bernardini AL, Chiari G, Vanelli M. Telephone hotline service (THS) for children and adolescents with type 1 diabetes as a strategy to reduce diabetes-related emergencies and costs for admittance. In: Jordanova M, Lievens F, editors. Global telemedicine/eHealth updates: knowledge resources, vol. 1. Luxembourg: Publ. Luxexpo; 2008. p. 26–9.
15. Mansi Shah (2008) Waiting for health care: a survey of a public hospital in Kolkata. https://ccs.in/internship_papers/2008/Waiting-for-Healthcare-A-survey-of-a-public-hospital-in-Kolkata-Mansi.pdf. Accessed on April 26, 2021.
16. Wojceichowski A, Glinkowski M, Gołębiowski M, Górecki A. The use of multi-media messaging as supplement information of musculoskeletal injury cases. In: Paper presented at the XI International Conference on Medical Informatics & Technologies. MIT; 2006. p. 246–53.
17. Mohana R, et al. Optimized service discovery using QoS based ranking: a fuzzy clustering and particle swarm optimization approach. In: Paper published in the IEEE Proceedings of the 35th IEEE Computer software and applications conference, Munich, Germany (IEEE COMPSAC 2011); 2011. p. 452–7.
18. Wadhwa M. e-Governance in healthcare sector in India. Center for Sustainable Development, Columbia University; 2020. https://csd.columbia.edu/sites/default/files/content/docs/ICT%20India/Papers/ICT_India_Working_Paper_28.pdf. Accessed on 09 May 2021
19. ItohanOkunhon. A literature review on the impact of eHealth policies on the quality health care. Laurea University of Applied Science; 2016. https://www.theseus.fi/bitstream/handle/10024/120962/Thesis-%20Impact%20Of%20Ehealth%20Policy.pdf?sequence=1. Accessed on 08 May 2021
20. Kruse CS, Krowski N, Rodriguez B. Telehealth and patient satisfaction: a systematic review and narrative analysis. BMJ Open. 2017;7:e016242. https://doi.org/10.1136/bmjopen-2017-016242.
21. Ahern D, Kreslake J, Phalen J. What is eHealth: perspectives on the evolution of eHealth research. J Med Internet Res. 2006;8(1):e4. https://doi.org/10.2196/jmir.8.1.e4.
22. Domínguez-Mayo FJ, Escalona MJ, Mejías M, Aragón G, García-García JA, Torres J, Enríquez JG. A strategic study about quality characteristics in e-Health systems based on a systematic literature review. Scientific World J. 2015:1–11. https://doi.org/10.1155/2015/863591.
23. Bokolo AJ. Exploring the adoption of telemedicine and virtual software for care of outpatients during and after COVID-19 pandemic. Ir J Med Sci. 2021;190(1):1–10. https://doi.org/10.1007/s11845-020-02299-z.
24. Almathami HKY, Win KT, Vlahu-Gjorgievska E. Barriers and facilitators that influence telemedicine-based, real-time, online consultation at patients' homes: systematic literature review. J Med Internet Res. 2020;22(2):e16407. https://doi.org/10.2196/16407.
25. Cruess SR, Cruess RL, Johnston S, et al. Profession: a working definition for medical educators. Teach Learn Med. 2004;16(1):74–6. https://doi.org/10.1207/s15328015tlm1601_15.
26. Lu S, Hong Y, Liu Q, Wang L, Dssouli R. Implementing web-based e-Health portal systems. Department of Computer Science and CIISE, Concordia University; 2007.
27. Oracle. https://www.oracle.com/technical-resources/articles/javase/soa.html. Accessed on 11 May 2021.
28. Weerawarana S, Curbera F, Leymann F, Storey T, Ferguson DF, et al. Web services platform architecture: SOAP, WSDL, WS-policy, WS-addressing, WS-BPEL, WS-reliable messaging and more. Prentice Hall; 2005.
29. Mayoka KG, Rwashana AS, Mbarika VW, Isabalija SA. A framework for designing sustainable telemedicine information systems in developing countries. J Syst Inform Technol. 2012;14:200–19. https://doi.org/10.1108/13287261211255329.
30. Bhagwan V, Grobbelaar SS. Development of a telemedicine system for monitoring intensive care patients. In: Proceedings of the 2017 International conference on information system and data mining; 2017. p. 139–44. https://doi.org/10.1145/3077584.3077600.

31. Mizera-Pietraszko J, Świątek P. Access to eHealth language-based services for multi-national patients. In: In 2015 17th International Conference on E-health Networking, Application & Services (HealthCom). IEEE; 2015. p. 232–7. https://doi.org/10.1109/HealthCom.2015.7454504.
32. 7th Framework Programme (2010) Khresmoi. http://khresmoi.eu/. Accessed 05 May 2021.
33. Kelly L, Dungs S, Kriewel S, Hanbury A, Goeuriot L, Jones GJ, Langs G, Müller H. Khresmoi professional: multilingual, multimodal professional medical search. In: European Conference on Information. Cham: Springer; 2014. p. 754–8. https://doi.org/10.1007/978-3-319-06028-6_89.
34. Wickramasinghe N, Misra SK, et al. A wireless trust model for healthcare. Int J Electron Healthc. 2004;1(1):60–77. https://doi.org/10.1504/IJEH.2004.004658.
35. Ikhu-Omoregbe NA, Azeta AA. Design and deployment of a mobile-based medical alert system. In: Watfa MK, editor. E-Healthcare systems and wireless communications: current and future challenges. 1st ed. United States of America: IGI Global; 2012. p. 210–9.
36. UniversalNurses (2014) UniversalNurse Speaker. http://www.u-nurses.com/. Accessed on 23 April 2021.
37. Pires P, Mendes L, Mendes J, Rodrigues R, Pereira A. Integrated e-Healthcare system for elderly support. Cogn Comput. 2016;8(2):368–84. https://doi.org/10.1007/s12559-015-9367-3.

Potential of Blockchain in Telemedicine 10

Avita Katal, Vitesh Sethi, and Tanupriya Choudhury

10.1 Introduction to Telemedicine

The World Health Organization defined telemedicine as providing the services related to healthcare at a distance by utilizing the electronic means for "prevention of injuries and disease, diagnosis of treatment, evaluation and research, medical care professional education [1]" to enhance health. While there are several classifications of telehealth, telehealth is commonly used as an umbrella word to include telemedicine (healthcare delivery) as well as other operations such as study, training, public healthcare awareness, and care planning.

Telemedicine by the use of video technology and the telephone has been utilized from the 1960s in the areas of space and military [2]. The utilization of broadband access technologies has advanced significantly during the last several decades and internet and cell phone users have become nearly ubiquitous. There has been a steady rise in the use of technical modalities to promote remote healthcare delivery.

Telemedicine is the combination of cordless and connected medical data delivery in which medical pictures, impulses, and films are sent to remote places for diagnosis. This minimizes the doctor's workload and the distance between caregivers and consumers. It provides the modern healthcare facilities through the use of electronic communication that enhances the patient's healthcare. This mechanism minimizes the expense related to the infrastructure and provides services related to healthcare in understaffed areas like ships, rural health centres, airplanes, and trains. This m-health is based on 4 A's that is "Anywhere, anytime Access with the best characteristics of connection Always" that leads to the rise in network technologies and

---

Avita Katal, Vitesh Sethi and Tanupriya Choudhury contributed equally to this work.

A. Katal (✉) · V. Sethi · T. Choudhury (✉)
School of Computer Science, University of Petroleum and Energy Studies (UPES),
Dehradun, Uttarakhand, India

© The Author(s), under exclusive license to Springer Nature
Switzerland AG 2022
T. Choudhury et al. (eds.), *Telemedicine: The Computer Transformation of Healthcare*, TELe-Health, https://doi.org/10.1007/978-3-030-99457-0_10

wireless communication, facilitating the delivery of healthcare through the heterogeneous infrastructure. It optimizes the monitoring of health and gives an alternative and assistance to the existing means of delivery of healthcare which is followed by some countries [3].

The characteristics of the telemedicine network are security, fault tolerance, transparency, etc. These properties allow the patient and doctor that are thousands of kilometres away to see and talk to each other. The doctor is able to identify the mental and physical state of the patient and do the required treatment. A modern technique of hospital digital networking technology emerges as a result of the systemic use of different techniques to practise healthcare quickly and expand the reach of the healthcare system. Through this technique, telephone, internet, and satellite communication networks may link primitive healthcare centres in rural areas to well advanced modern healthcare centres in urban areas in order to provide the good consultancy and better diagnosis to the needy people. This device has two modes of operation: basic and advanced. The basic mode does have a reduced broadcast bandwidth and data transfer frequency, so it can be used to transfer health records, while the sophisticated mode has an elevated stream broadband and transmitting frequency. The system's usefulness is determined on the basis of various medical equipment that can be used to capture the information of the patient and the infrastructure of the telecommunications with the desired Quality of Service (QoS). The data of the patient can be collected either in store-and-forward mode or in real-time mode where it can be transferred by utilizing the mobile communication technologies like fourth generation(4G), etc.

10.2 Integration of Blockchain with Telemedicine

Blockchain is the fastest growing technology for securing the various applications. Blockchain technology can be used for various implementations among the stakeholders. The system of bitcoin was presented by Satoshi Nakamoto on the basis of the cryptology proofing rather than trust, which enables two or more parties to do the transactions without a mediator. These parties are called "trusted third party" (TTP).

The blockchain technology is a secure, transparent, and trustworthy system for the exchange of information in a decentralized manner, so the validation and coordination efforts for the decentralized database become easy [4]. The records are designed in such a way that they can be updated regularly.

Blockchain technology has a significant impact in the domain of telemedicine. Due to its distributed system and decentralized nature, the blockchain technology provides various services in the telemedicine sector. It gives better replacement for widespread digital transformation with the technology that will grow rapidly in the future. There is markable commitment with 5G, 6G and IoT. Among various medical services, it is not secure with the ongoing telemedicine services with the centralized design which has many problems including delay in accessing and leakage of information. There is a chance that medical information of the patient can be easily accessed without the knowledge of the patient. The ongoing system of telemedicine for distance medical opinions leads to various issues related to securely accessing data within a network. The Electronic Health Record (EHR) system has a significant impact in storing and maintaining the data. The information of the patient is stored as a ledger in blockchain technology which accesses and monitors the patients and their details. The above-mentioned reasons lead to the development in blockchain technology in the telemedicine field. Figure 10.1 shows the flow of the transaction in the blockchain network. Blockchain has multiple applications in financial services, management of data, IOT, cybersecurity and healthcare. It has gained the attention of researchers to work in aforementioned fields. For the secure and safe delivery of data in telemedicine, data transmission applications of blockchain have become a remarkable interest area. The main features of blockchain technology for telemedicine are:

- Immutability: The personal health records and the EHRs cannot be changed. The consensus protocols and the asymmetric key cryptography make sure the immutability of the medical records.
- Anonymity: The identities of participants in the telemedicine network are not disclosed. They remain anonymous.

Fig. 10.1 Transaction flow in blockchain

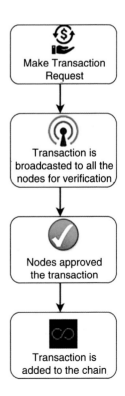

- Open-Source Access: The patients are able to check the profile of the physician before scheduling an appointment for the remote consultancy.
- Decentralization: The electronic health records of the patient are accessed, stored, and managed at the multiple locations. The consensus protocols are responsible to govern the network.
- Auditability: The drug administrative authorities can trace the provenance of a drug. The medical records are protected in order to assure the regulatory compliance operations.
- Transparency: The transparency facilitates the remote patient-centred data control to share and enquire about the suspicious activities by the users. Figure 10.2 shows the features of integration of telemedicine with the blockchain. Traditional methods in medical applications have been reformed by blockchain for safe data transmission and for effective diagnosis and treatment. The blockchain is the future technology that supports the secure, authentic, and personalized healthcare application that contains the merged database of up-to-date data of a patient in a secured manner.

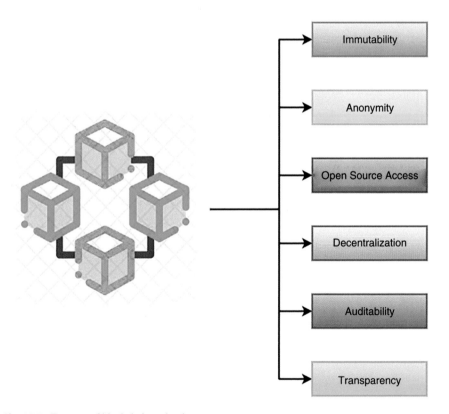

Fig. 10.2 Features of blockchain technology

10.3   Dependencies of Blockchain Technology

10.3.1 Smart Contract

It is a self-executing, self-checking, and tamper-proof type of code and remains on the blockchain, with configurable application logic. It creates the relationships and rules that govern the entities and resources in the blockchain, as well as the ability to build bespoke programme logic that is performed directly on the blockchain rather than through intermediaries.

Ethereum [5] is a pioneer blockchain that is expressly intended to provide a framework for smart contracts. With the help of smart contracts, laws and real-world rules can be enforced and embedded into the blockchain which helps in the easy development of decentralized applications. Besides the Ethereum, there are various other platforms for blockchain that support smart contracts: NEM [6], Hyperledger Fabric [7], Stellar [8], NEO [9], etc.

10.3.2 Consensus

The blockchain consensus process may be described as the method for agreeing on a consistent status or edition of the chain that can be regarded the blockchain's trustworthy truth. This avoids double spending. The attempt to spend a previously spent transaction causes a collision with the existing state, leading in the event being rejected and not being joined to the chain. Consensus protocols also hold the rules of the validation of the transaction, accepting the block that is created newly inside the chain and the selection of the fork/partition where there are partitions in the network.

10.3.3 InterPlanetary File System (IPFS)

The InterPlanetary File System (IPFS) [10] is a decentralized platform for the sharing of files that is capable of identifying the files through their content. The IPFS system is based on a distributed hash table that can extract file locations as well as information about node connectivity. Whenever a file is uploaded to the IPFS system, it is divided into the chunks which contain the maximum of 256 kilobytes of data and/or links to other chunks. A cryptographic hash, also known as a content signature, is computed from the content of each chunk to identify it. The Merkle directed acyclic graph (Merkle DAG) explains the file as a whole and can be used to rebuild any file from its chunks since the listed links often have content identifiers. An entire file can be found using the Merkle DAG by only using the root hash. Once a node has split the file into chunks and created the Merkle DAG, the node uses the Distributed Hash Table (DHT) to register as a provider.

10.4   Application of Blockchain in Healthcare

The application of blockchain in the medical field for transformation and wide-ranging exchange of medical data has been lauded owing to its open, irrevocable, decentralized, and secure operations. Through merging already dysfunctional processes to deliver holistic perspectives and improved treatment, the blockchain is responsible for reducing institutional conflict. Figure 10.3 shows the blockchain use cases in the healthcare sector.

10.4.1 Sharing of Data in Traditional Care and Telemedicine

Traditionally, telemedicine has provided services to users who live far from nearby health centres or in areas where emergency personnel are in short supply. Telemedicine is becoming more common with patients who want to receive medical treatment at their convenience. Patients that are connected save time in the doctor's office and get prompt care for mild but critical symptoms. Due to the growing accessibility of telemedicine devices and smart mobiles, companies are able to provide access to medical care entire day. In addition several user-friendly programmes are developed to administer patients, analyse, and evaluate their health reports [11]. In comparison to conventional physical health systems, telemedicine is normally fitted with more modern technology and is much more effective. As a result of these on-demand systems, it is normal for clinicians from various areas or networks to serve patients, resulting in a loss of treatment consistency. Patients and primary care providers do not have access to healthcare data gathered during telemedicine care incidents, resulting in an inaccurate medical history and putting the general level of care at risk. Blockchain technology is able to fill the communication gap between these services by eliminating the need for a third-party regulator and empowering direct

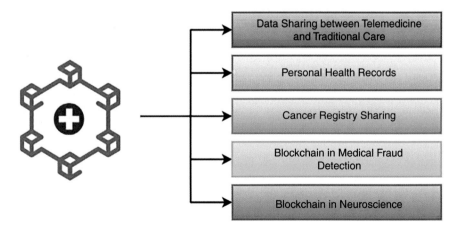

Fig. 10.3 Blockchain use cases in the domain of healthcare

communications between the participants involved. The dynamic data sharing problem cannot be solved by blockchain technology alone; it should be included into the present patchwork of medical facilities and clinical research requirements.

10.4.2 Personalized Medical Documents for Comprehensive Medical Information Ownership and Manage

Personal Health Records (PHRs) are software used by individuals, the real data proprietors, to maintain and retrieve medical records, as opposed to the existing normal practice of utilizing supplier Electronic Health Records (EHR) for the preservation and administration of patient data. PHRs are designed to assist patients in tracking, collecting, and controlling their full health information compiled from a variety of sources, such as provider visit reports, immunization history, drug records, physical activity data gathered from sensors, and more. PHRs provide people discretion in how their health history is used and communicated, as well as the accuracy of their medical reports and the ability to correct data errors [12]. Since centralized techniques do not address the root of the data exchange issue, they pose the same challenges as current disparate EHR structures. Decentralization facilitated by consensus algorithms allows blockchain to distribute power to individuals. It helps people to compile their medical records without having to obtain a copy from each physician. They have achieved success by developing a publicly accessible and dependable data delivery platform that connects to current health systems. Links with connected phones are also possible since blockchain removes distrust among health workers and third-party patient monitoring applications and sites.

10.4.3 Cancer Registry Sharing

Data interchange is critical in cancer therapy, since situations are diverse and treatments are always one-size-fits-all [13]. Sharing cancer data not only preserves the integrity of clinical trial results by allowing participant confirmation and explanation, but it also has the ability to compile information gathered to minimize unwarranted clinical trial duplication. It allows scattered drug studies to have a large batch size, which accelerates the identification of even more efficient cancer treatments. PBCRs (Population-Based Cancer Registries) provide for the collection of very basic data on cancer incidences across regional areas and the coordination of population-wide cancer prevention [14]. Cancer registries, like EHRs, are frequently walled and isolated, but Blockchain technology may help them as well for quicker data exchange. Because of the increased availability of better data gathered from numerous patients, artificial intelligence may now be utilized to construct prospective and predicting models to aid medical physicians with choice assistance. A learning network may be built using blockchain technology to trade prediction models and collectively improve the quality of acquired health findings.

10.4.4 Blockchain in Medical Fraud Detection

The medical sector, which encompasses medical drug supply chain monitoring, is increasingly adopting blockchain technology. Supply chain management is critical in all industries, but it is particularly critical in the healthcare industry due to its growing sophistication. This is due to the fact that every fault in the medical supply chain has an impact on a physician's well-being. Since supply chains contain a large number of individuals and pieces, they are vulnerable to malicious attacks. By adding higher data integrity and improved product traceability, blockchains are responsible for offering a stable and safe network to eradicate the above issue and deter fraud from occurring.

10.4.5 Blockchains in Neuroscience

The quantity of study and news dedicated to blockchain uses is increasing, and neuroscience is undoubtedly involved [15]. Current brain developments aim to build new paradigms that eliminate technology contact with the surroundings and allow humans to operate equipment and information via brain commands. This type of neural implantation can also scan trends of brain action and convert them into orders for controlling external equipment, as well as use data from brain function to analyse a person's current mental state. The blockchain idea is used by big data and powerful algorithms to record brain signals on the neural connection. The issue of confidentiality and protection is addressed by blockchain technology. By storing the user's data on a blockchain network, it becomes less vulnerable to hacker attacks and hence more valuable. According to the above use case, blockchain may be classified as a type of information technology with a variety of potential implementations capable of promoting brain augmentation, brain modelling, and brain thought. A whole human brain must be digitized, which necessitates the use of a medium to archive it, and this is where blockchain technology comes into play once more.

10.5   Blockchain Opportunities in Telemedicine and Telehealth

This section will go through the main advantages of block chain for telehealth that establish confidence among medical providers. Figure 10.4 shows the potential opportunities of blockchain in the telemedicine sector.

10.5.1 Management of Patient Consent

The effectiveness of the virtual health monitoring and virtual care is based on the integrity of the electronic health record which consists of the medical history of the patient, medication, diagnosis, and the treatment plans. The electronic health

Fig. 10.4 Potential opportunities of blockchain in telemedicine

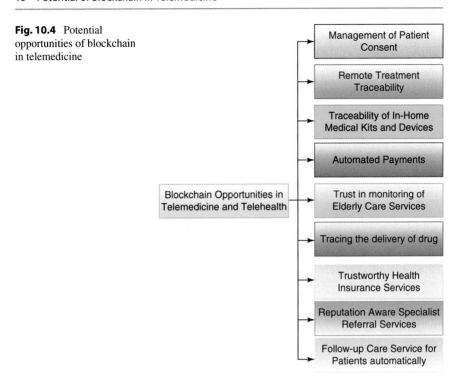

Blockchain Opportunities in Telemedicine and Telehealth

- Management of Patient Consent
- Remote Treatment Traceability
- Traceability of In-Home Medical Kits and Devices
- Automated Payments
- Trust in monitoring of Elderly Care Services
- Tracing the delivery of drug
- Trustworthy Health Insurance Services
- Reputation Aware Specialist Referral Services
- Follow-up Care Service for Patients automatically

records are highly private and sensitive information should be shared in a secured manner between the peers such as hospitals, health authorities and pharmacies to maintain the data of the patient up to date. By the use of blockchain, the management of consent is protected and assured by several peers that belong to the various organizations that take part [16].

10.5.2 Remote Treatment Traceability

Patients meet online physicians to address their health issues in the conventional model, but, in the new model, caregivers will engage directly in consultations and programmes related to medical education using resources that facilitate video and audio conferencing. Because of the insufficient data access between health providers in the current telemedicine environment, they are not able to handle the silos of patient health information. To solve this problem, blockchain technology delivers a clear and uniform picture of client electronic medical records to all relevant parties. As medical data are accurate and visible, institutions can follow a patient's medical history and provide necessary treatment. Audits are carried out using blockchain technologies to determine who accessed electronic documents and what transactions are made.

10.5.3 Timestamping of Healthcare Supplies and Equipment at Homes

Patients can do self-diagnosis in a non-clinical setting with the help of in-home equipment and diagnostic kits. The lack of clarity and data provenance of medical kits in conventional organized telehealth systems makes it difficult for patients and doctors to obtain reliable medical kits from reputable suppliers. The blockchain platform can be used to monitor transactions relating to the possession and results of research kits in a secure and immutable manner.

10.5.4 Automated Payments

The current healthcare system uses centralized services that rely on third parties for the payments among insurance companies, caregiver, and patients. The centralized methodologies for the settlement of the payment are slow, non-transparent and vulnerable to hacking. Apart from this, the centralized payment settlement system either does not accept micropayments or makes micropayments highly costly. The blockchain network supports micropayments in the telehealth domain by allowing users to pay using cryptocurrency tokens. As a result, the direct transfer of cryptocurrency tokens to the account of the person providing service presents a safe, quick, auditable, and open method that does not require a centralized payment processing infrastructure [17]. Furthermore, the digitally signed payment settlement transactions guarantee that healthcare providers and patients will not be able to back out of transactions in the future. To reduce the chances of theft, blockchain technologies will help introduce a cash-on-delivery programme. Smart contracts may be designed to pass and retain cryptocurrency tokens in the wallets of pharmacists only while the remote patient gets the medications while applying the service related to remote distribution of drugs for telepharmacy.

10.5.5 Faith in the Supervision of Aged Care Facilities

Recent advances in the Internet of Things domain aid the field of telemedicine in remotely monitoring the health of the client through the use of medical devices [18]. The health information can be linked to vital signs like body temperature and blood pressure. Therefore, the error in the data captured results in the medical errors. To overcome this issue, blockchain technology employs smart contracts to verify and record the access permissions of biosensors in order to keep the electronic health record on the network. Smart contracts can alert the doctors and health centres when there is an unforeseen emergency. In the case of home treatment, IoT-enabled blockchain systems will send a prescription refill reminder to the user.

10.5.6 Tracing the Delivery of Drug

The system of healthcare that is based on the virtual online consultancy requires the physicians to make a blockchain transaction to exchange a drug order with a nearby pharmacy. Blockchain technology can remove errors related to drugs and record changes by using the hash function [19]. Registered pharmacists have access to prescriptions held on the blockchain, which they will use to schedule, validate, and submit medications to patients. In exchange, the transporter can publish its present position on the blockchain to let doctors and pharmacies identify and monitor clients. Apart from this, the traceability and the transparency of the blockchain allows the doctors and patients to authenticate the medicine's validity via data integrity. By the use of smart contracts, prescription refill orders can be placed to the pharmacists only when the already defined criteria is met. The prescription will then be validated and refilled at the pharmacy. When a medicine refill is approved, it is shipped to the patient, and the patient's data are changed.

10.5.7 Reliable Medical Insurance Solutions

Due to the restricted benefits and stringent privacy-protection rules, a substantial percentage of people are no longer involved in disclosing their medical information. The simulated health-based law safeguards the patient's entitlement to reimbursement at the same cost as physical healthcare programmes. It takes several days to determine the facts from the provided evidence in the case of insurance fraud. Through allowing insurance insurers access to a patient's records, blockchain technologies will help them minimize insurance fraud. The patients are provided with the incentives for sharing the medical data with the insurance providers. Moreover, healthcare companies provide premiums purchasers incentives in the form of cryptocurrency tokens in exchange for leading a good life, such as tracking gym attendance.

10.5.8 Professional Recommendation Solutions with a Good Experience

The blockchain-based approach enables prescribing healthcare professionals to store the referral record on an IPFS server, which returns the IPFS hash of the document, which can then be stored on the blockchain and accessed through visiting healthcare specialists. By the IPFS hash, one can verify if the stored document is altered or not. The healthcare specialists will review the patient's well-being record before doing the assessment, and then they can archive the diagnosis report on the blockchain ledger. The referring healthcare provider will change the trust ranking on the blockchain based on the satisfaction score and overall service time of the consulting health specialists.

10.5.9 Follow-Up Care Service for Patients Automatically

This programme allows medical practitioners to keep a close eye on a patient's condition until they've completed treatment. Before registering for a virtual appointment, the follow-up programme can require patients to exchange their blood and urine test results with the practitioners. The smart contracts utilization in blockchain technologies aids in the automation of patient follow-up services. The smart contracts will send a message to the patient, nursing staff, and physician, reminding them of the forthcoming follow-up appointment. The practitioner has access to the patient's immutable and open EHR to check the patient's health status that was saved at the last follow-up conference (virtual).

10.6   Comparison Between the Centralized Telemedicine System and the Blockchain-Based Telemedicine System

Table 10.1 shows the comparison between the centralized telemedicine system and the blockchain-based telemedicine system.

10.7   Proposed Framework for the Integration of Blockchain with Telemedicine

10.7.1 Background or Literature View

The authors in [18] have crafted a healthcare infrastructure that uses the blockchain and smart contracts to enable doctor and patient enrolments in a health facility, thus increasing remote patient tracking involvement. Their suggested system keeps track of patients in remote locations and sends out warnings in the event of an emergency.

Table 10.1 Comparison between the centralized telemedicine system and blockchain-based telemedicine system

Parameter	Centralized telemedicine system	Blockchain-based telemedicine system
Cost	Low	Low
Integrity and reliability	Low	High
Audit trials	No	Yes
System administration	Centralized	Decentralized
Security and privacy	Hard	Easy
Manipulation of health record	Yes	No
Transparency	No	Yes
Data provenance	No	Yes
Fault tolerance	No	Yes

The authors in [20] have used a private blockchain built on the Ethereum Protocol to develop a framework in which sensors communicate with a mobile computer that executes smart contracts and logs all activities on the blockchain. Their suggested system allows for real-time patient tracking and emergency procedures by providing alerts to patients and medical providers, as well as keeping a safe record of who has initiated these activities.

The authors in [21] have protected the personal and device-generated information by the utilization of the blockchain-based smart contracts for the management of the patients' information and medical devices. They have created a remote healthcare system that consists of various entities. Apart from this, they have designed a system for the storage of information of the medical device along with the health situation of a patient.

10.7.2 Proposed Framework

Section 10.7.1 discusses frameworks that are either insufficient or have shortcomings. The authors have not introduced the role of insurance companies and pharmacists which can hold the claim process and deliver the medicines to the patient address on time, respectively. In this section, we have proposed a model that overcomes the limitations of the previous work. Figure 10.5 shows the proposed framework of the telemedicine with the blockchain technology. In this scenario, the medical sensors are attached to the body of the patient and the medical

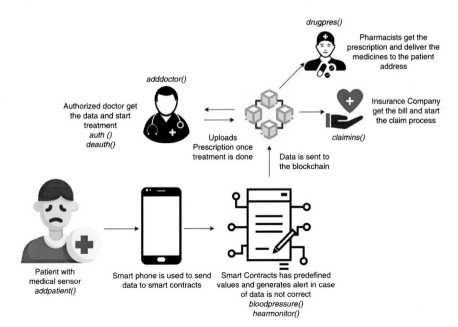

Fig. 10.5 Proposed framework

measurements are transmitted to the appropriate smart contract via a central controller, which is a phone. The healthcare centres are responsible for the registration of patients and a doctor on the system. They initialize the registration smart contract in order to initiate the registration of doctor and patient. The doctors and patients in the healthcare centre register with the help of their externally owned accounts. The registration smart contract is responsible for the registration of the doctor and the patient. The adddoctor() function registers the doctor and the addpatient() function registers the patient in the system. For the registration process, id, name and age are collected from doctors and name, age, gender, and address are collected from the patient. As a result, physicians and patients will be less hesitant to participate due to concerns over data breaches, and their enrolment in the health system will improve. Patients' and physicians' records will also be changed under the terms of the enrolment contract. A patient's health status can also be checked only by a particular doctor. Patients may also view their personal records as well as the details of their registered doctor. The health centre has the authority to approve or disallow a doctor from treating a specific patient. The functions that are used for the authorization and deauthorization are auth() and deauth(), respectively.

After the registration process, the monitoring smart contracts invokes. The data collected from the sensors is sent to the blockchain by the smart contracts. The contracts have the predefined thresholds that can be used to generate alert to the doctor and the hospital. For instance, if the SpO_2 sensor shows the oxygen level below 90, then the alert will be generated and the message will be transferred to the concerned doctor along with the location of the patient with the help of a GPS module. Each IOT device should be registered and each device will have its own smart contract for generating the alerts. For instance, the blood pressure monitor has the function bloodpressure() and the heart rate monitor has the function heartmonitor().

Once the authorized doctor gets the data values, he or she prescribes the medicines and uploads the prescription on the blockchain. The pharmacists that are registered by the patient will get the prescription and will be responsible for delivering the medicines to the patient home as soon as possible. The drug prescription has a different smart contract and the function drugpres() is responsible for the transfer of prescription to the pharmacists.

After the successful treatment, the hospital uploads the bills to the blockchain system. The insurance company gets the bill and the patient asks for the claim. The insurance starts processing the claim and pays the entire expenses to the hospital as per the norms. The claim process has a different smart contract and the function named claimins() is used for the claim process.

10.8 Case Studies

10.8.1 Medicalchain [22]

It leverages the hyperledger fabric and ethereum platforms for the implementation of remote patient-to-doctor consultation and clinical data marketplace apps are among the programmes offered. It enables patients to communicate health information with healthcare professionals in a secure manner. The EHR commerce component of the Medicalchain system enables authorized clients to confidentially accept terms of service for third-party use of personal EHR data. Medicalchain uses the permissioned Hyperledger Fabric functionality to enforce access management policies that enable access control at various levels. The Ethereum blockchain makes use of the ERC20 token to let participants use the platform resources in a straightforward manner to detect insurance fraud and resolve payments.

10.8.2 HealPoint [23]

The on-demand telemedicine programmes are implemented using the Ethereum blockchain. It allows patients to speak with clinicians about their illnesses, medical data, and vital signs through virtual medical consulting platforms. Apart from of the ethereum-based smart contracts launched by HealPoint, patients will offer a similar view from a variety of medical professionals. HealPoint is integrated into an AI-driven platform that connects and suggests appropriate doctors depending on the data of the patient. Before providing healthcare, networking experts check the physician's identification and licensing, granting or refusing the request to use the system. Finally, before even being entered on the register for auditing reasons, all client interactions are authenticated.

10.9   Research Challenges in Integration of Blockchain with Telemedicine

10.9.1 Adoption of Blockchain by Various Organizations

The old system of the telemedicine depends on outdated techniques to maintain, store, and protect the data of the patient that limits the collaboration opportunities between the healthcare providers and participants. This results in a rise of the cost of the system. Blockchain technology assures the storage of medical information of the patient in a trustworthy manner by immutable medical and transaction records. However, telemedicine patients are unable to realize the full value of blockchain technologies due to a lack of understanding, immaturity of the technology, and lack of requirements. As a result, further research is needed to establish guidelines and regulations for blockchain's widespread use in telemedicine. Furthermore, the financial benefits for participating companies to switch to blockchain technologies should be investigated.

10.9.2 Security Vulnerabilities of Smart Contracts

The smart contract's glitches and flaws have a significant effect on their daily behaviour, resulting in tampering and disruption of medical records. For example, a smart contract with exclusive rights to connect with another contract may either change a patient's EHR or obtain funds from a legal user's wallet using a re-entrancy vulnerability attack. ZeppelinOS, SolCover, and Oyente are some of the diagnostic instruments suggested by the researchers. Such tools support users in identifying vulnerable aspects in smart contracts and proposing countermeasures against external risks. However, the suggested methods are insufficient for detecting all forms of smart contract flaws and bugs. As a result, precautions need to be taken thoroughly to test smart contracts for possible bugs using a variety of test cases and techniques before deploying them.

10.9.3 Large Medical Information and Rising Transaction Rates

To minimize treatment errors, blockchain-enabled telemedicine systems need close tie-up between healthcare users and patient record to ensure a clear medical history. As a result, telemedicine systems can produce a large volume of data that requires quick analysis in order to extract insights from the medical data. The vast volume of healthcare info, on the other hand, has an effect on transaction fees and on the overall time it takes for a transaction to be validated on current blockchain networks.

10.9.4 Support for Cross-Platform Transaction Interoperability

Hospital access referral systems require that health users such as patients and doctors safely transact through blockchain networks. Interoperability functionality on blockchain systems allows users to connect with one another without the need for intermediaries to translate and forward transactions. For example, a framework that supports interoperability might help a health professional to make use of the tokens of the bitcoin to do the transactions related to business on the network of blockchain provided by Ethereum. However, owing to numerous concerns such as differences in language support and blockchain network consensus protocols, creating interoperable blockchain platforms is difficult.

10.10 Conclusion

Blockchain technology has the ability to address a number of issues that currently plague the healthcare sector. As a trust mediation, it enables creative healthcare methods, and as an incentive mechanism, it may stimulate unique economic structures, perhaps resulting in a new dynamic among diverse medical partners such as clinicians and consumers. A blockchain-enabled shared confidence and reward system, for example, may allow a patient-centric healthcare paradigm and a global Health Information Exchange. Similarly, blockchain-based shared networks and services in healthcare mitigate the chance of provider lock-in. In this chapter, the main goal to use blockchain technology for telemedicine networks by addressing its core features for providing tamper-proof, decentralized, irreversible, traceable, stable, and auditable remote healthcare services is discussed in detail. In addition, the chapter addressed the possible benefits of blockchain technologies for telemedicine applications. A new remote health management system built on blockchain is also proposed, as well as a discussion of the current blockchain-based programmes that doctors are using to provide healthcare services remotely is included. The chapter concludes with a list of issues that need to be addressed in order to improve telemedicine applications by extending the functionality of emerging blockchain-based networks.

References

1. Kirsh S, Su GL, Sales A, et al. Access to outpatient specialty care: solutions from an integrated health care system. Am J Med Qual. 2015;30:88–90.
2. Serper M, Volk ML. Current and future applications of telemedicine to optimize the delivery of care in chronic liver disease. Clin Gastroenterol Hepatol. 2018;16(2):157–161.e8. https://doi.org/10.1016/j.cgh.2017.10.004.
3. Branagan L, Chase LL. Organizational implementation of telemedicine technology methodology and field experience. In: IEEE Global Humanitarian Technology Conference. IEEE; 2012. p. 271–6.
4. Katal A, Sethi V, Lamba S. Blockchain consensus algorithms: study and challenges. In: Choudhury T, Khanna A, Toe TT, Khurana M, Gia NN, editors. Blockchain applications in IoT ecosystem. Cham: EAI/Springer innovations in communication and computing, Springer; 2021.
5. Wood G. Ethereum: a secure decentralised generalised transaction ledger. Ethereum Project Yellow Paper. 2014;151:1–32.
6. Colin LeMahieu. NEM—Distributed Ledger Technology, 2018 (accessed November10, 2018). https://nem.io/.
7. Androulaki E, Barger A, Bortnikov V, Cachin C, Christidis K, De Caro A, Enyeart D, Ferris C, Laventman G, Manevich Y, et al. Hyperledger fabric: a distributed operating system for permissioned blockchains. In: Proceedings of the Thirteenth EuroSys Conference. ACM; 2018. p. 30.
8. Iris. Develop the world's new financial system, 2018 (accessed Nov15, 2018). https://www.stellar.org/.
9. Neo-project. NEO. https://neo.org/.
10. Benet J. IPFS—Content addressed, versioned, p2p file system (draft 3), 2014.
11. https://searchhealthit.techtarget.com/definition/telemedicine. Accessed on 01 March 2021.
12. Tang PC, Ash JS, Bates DW, Overhage JM, Sands DZ. Personal health records: definitions, benefits, and strategies for Overcoming barriers to adoption. J Am Med Inform Assoc. 2006;13(2):121–6. https://doi.org/10.1197/jamia.m2025.
13. https://www.statnews.com/2016/10/06/immunotherapy-cancer-clinical-trials/
14. Parkin DM. The evolution of the population-based cancer registry. Nat Rev Cancer. 2006;6(8):603–12. https://doi.org/10.1038/nrc1948.
15. Swan M. Blockchain thinking: the brain as a decentralized autonomous corporation. IEEE Technol Soc Mag. 2015;34:41–52.
16. Genestier P, Zouarhi S, Limeux P, Excoffier D, Prola A, Sandon S, Temerson J-M. Blockchain for consent management in the eHealth environment: a nugget for privacy and security challenges. J Int Soc Telemed E-Health. 2017;5(1–4):e24. Retrieved from https://journals.ukzn.ac.za/index.php/JISfTeH/article/view/269
17. Prokofieva M, Miah SJ. Blockchain in healthcare. Aust J Inform Syst. 2019;23 https://doi.org/10.3127/ajis.v23i0.2203.

18. Kazmi HSZ, Nazeer F, Mubarak S, Hameed S, Basharat A, Javaid N. Trusted remote patient monitoring using blockchain-based smart contracts. In: Barolli L, Hellinckx P, Enokido T, editors. Advances on broad-band wireless computing, communication and applications. BWCCA 2019, Lecture notes in networks and systems, vol. 97. Cham: Springer; 2020.
19. El-Miedany Y. Telehealth and telemedicine: how the digital era is changing standard health care. Smart Homecare Technol TeleHealth. 2017;4:43–51. https://doi.org/10.2147/shtt.s116009.
20. Griggs KN, Ossipova O, Kohlios CP, Baccarini AN, Howson EA, Hayajneh T. Healthcare blockchain system using smart contracts for secure automated REMOTE patient monitoring. J Med Syst. 2018;42(7)
21. Pham HL, Tran TH, Nakashima Y. A secure remote healthcare system for hospital using blockchain smart contract. In: 2018 IEEE Globecom Workshops (GC Wkshps); 2018. https://doi.org/10.1109/glocomw.2018.8644164.
22. https://medicalchain.com/en/. Accessed on 01 March, 2021.
23. https://healpoint.io/. Accessed on 02 March, 2021.

Security and Privacy issue in Telemedicine: Issues, Solutions, and Standards

11

Hitesh Kumar Sharma, Tanupriya Choudhury, Avita Katal, and Jung-Sup Um

11.1 Introduction

In the twenty-first century, technology made it possible to provide healthcare treatment from remote location. The advancement in technologies like IoT [1], cloud computing, network security, etc. provides a strong support to telecare medicine information systems (TMISs) for remote healthcare [2, 3]. TIMS are intelligent systems which help doctors to provide treatment remotely to their patient who are in rural areas and unable to visit hospitals. The patients store their medical reports and their treatments in TIMS repository and the doctor can access this repository to check the medical history of the patient. It helps the patient to reduce hospital visit expense and saves time. It also reduces overhead to the doctor and hospital to attend patient physically. Whenever a patient needs medical treatment, he/she needs to authenticate himself/herself and provide his/her smart card details to a smart device. After authentication, the patient needs to send his/her information to a medical server via a free network channel. Since patients are sharing their medical information to the server using a common network channel and these medical information are very critical information from their personal perspective. The basic diagram of a TMIS system is shown in Fig. 11.1. The integration and accessibility of various

Hitesh Kumar Sharma, Tanupriya Choudhury, Avita Katal and Jung-Sup Um contributed equally to this work.

H. K. Sharma (✉)
School of Computer Science, University of Petroleum & Energy Studies (UPES),
Energy Acres, Bidholi, Dehradun, Uttarakhand, India

T. Choudhury (✉) · A. Katal (✉)
School of Computer Science, University of Petroleum and Energy Studies (UPES),
Dehradun, Uttarakhand, India
e-mail: tanupriya@ddn.upes.ac.in; akatal@ddn.upes.ac.in

J.-S. Um
Department of Geography, College of Social Sciences, Kyungpook National University,
Daegu, South Korea

© The Author(s), under exclusive license to Springer Nature
Switzerland AG 2022
T. Choudhury et al. (eds.), *Telemedicine: The Computer Transformation of
Healthcare*, TELe-Health, https://doi.org/10.1007/978-3-030-99457-0_11

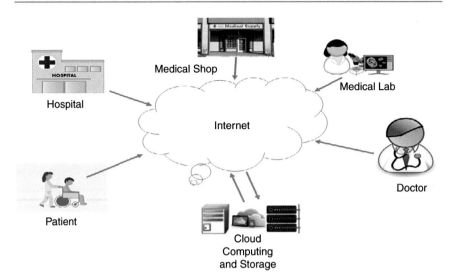

Fig. 11.1 Telemedicine system (Basic Model)

stakeholders is shown in the diagram. In this case, privacy, security, confidentiality, and integrity of their record are important for them. Since all these medical information are floating through a network and stored in a cloud sever, the chance of network attack is highly possible by an attacker to theft these medical records. Attackers can also take control over the medical server and provide wrong treatment to the patient, which can cause a severe medical problem with the patient. Health is the most critical concern and security of such systems involved in remote medical treatment is a major concern. In this view, so many authentication systems were proposed for TIMS. However, these authentication systems were having some security issues and network attacks are possible on them.

The necessity of various advance technologies like cloud computing and machine learning has been described in the following sub-sections.

11.1.1 Cloud Computing Is Backbone for Telehealthcare System

The first technology which comes in the role while making this service for helping doctors and patients is cloud computing. Cloud computing is the platform which is the backbone of proposed telecare health service where our doctors and patients can share medical reports, share updated reports whenever doctors will receive patient's previous report. The proposed telecare service will also provide the prescription prescribed by the doctor. This cloud is a backhand service of this telecare health services and from there only patients and doctors can easily communicate and share their reports. Cloud also ensures the confidentiality, availability, and integrity of data to patients and doctors; this helps them to communicate easily and also make the data as it is, not someone will misinterpret the patient's data. With the help of cloud-based services, if there will be a case when demand for this telecare server will suddenly arise, then in this case also, the cloud can scale their services where this server is running, and also whenever demand goes down, it can scale down the services [4]. It will help us to maintain the cost of our telecare health server. Cloud computing, with its on-demand availability, helped us to reach out to customers easily [5] as shown in Fig. 11.1.

11.1.2 Machine Learning in Healthcare

The second vastly known technology which comes in the role of making the telecare health services the most efficient is machine learning [6, 7]. Here, we have one issue like some of the diseases are common to some of the patients, so that's the waste of time of us and doctors also to come to reach out to the patient and treat them. So, we have some machine learning algorithms by which we can make our machine intelligent so that our machine will detect that the newer patients have similar symptoms of some disease and treat them with the previous treatment given to the patients having the similar disease. It helps us to save our and doctor's time because now there is no need to treat the patients with similar problems. It also makes the whole system more efficient. Machine learning algorithms are used for diagnosis and prescribed treatment in much better way because of the ability to maintain huge datasets and afterwards filtering that dataset for the patient's use according to the requirement [8]. This ultimately led to the lower cost and making the whole system powerful. Patient satisfaction is also the prime concern for telecare health services, but because of machine learning algorithms, we are ready to provide that to patients also [9]. So, this is how the telecare health services play an important role in providing the better services to us without even having fear of going out of our homes.

In the following figure (Fig. 11.2), we have shown a basic comparison of artificial and natural brain.

In this post COVID-19 situation, we don't now need to move here and there for our treatments as we can see there is so much hustle in hospitals for treatment, so we will be safeguarded by this telecare server as we don't need to go outside and can get proper treatment on the cloud.

11.2   Literature Review

In 1981, Lamport for the first time introduced an authentication algorithm for accessing remote system. In 2000, Hwang and Li [10] suggested a system as user authentication exercising the ElGamals public key cryptosystem. Sun (2000) [11] defined a smart card-based advanced scheme for user authentication scheme with more benefits over authentication system proposed by Hwang and Li (2000) [10] in their scheme. In 2003, Wu and Chieu proposed more user-friendly authentication model based on smart card for remote users. The shortcoming of Sun's (2000) [11] smart card-based model was resolved by Wu and Chieu in their model. Lee and Chiu reviewed the Mu and Chieu model and identified a forgery attack in their authentication system and they proposed an improved model after fixing all security

Machine Learning is
basically making the
machine so intelligent
that it can have ability to
learn (6).

Machine Learning simply
implies learing from
previous analyzed data so
that it can further be
used (7).

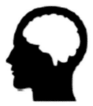

=

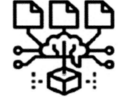

Human Brain

Machine Learning is nothing
less than human brain.

Fig. 11.2 Machine learning in telemedicine system

flaws and possible attacks. In 2006 Liao [12] came up with a one-factor authentication system using the Diffie Hellman key exchange theory and they used one-way hash function to secure unsafe networks and provide security for some general network attacks like stolen-verifier attack, replay attack, guessing attack, and modification attack.

In 2011, Wang et al. declared a secure and efficient authentication system with some unique features. It includes no need to maintain password documentation and no need to update master key every time a new service provider joins to the system. Pu et al. in 2012 found some security problems regarding forward secrecy in authentication model of Wang et al. and then they proposed a new authentication model with better scheme to improve security features. In 2012, Wu et al. [13] proposed a new model in which they have reduced some exponential operators to minimize computing time and they have also claimed that with reducing computing time their model is more effectively secure for any kind of network attack. After Wu et al.'s work, [13] Debiao et al. [14] in the same year 2012 reviewed Wu et al' s [13] model and found vulnerabilities like an insider attack and an impersonation attack. To overcome these two major attacks in Wu et al.' s scheme, they proposed their own model. Wei et al. in 2012 [13] analysed both models, Wu et al. (2012) [13] and Debiao et al. (2012), [14] and they identified an offline password guessing attack is possible in both the authentication schemes. Wei et al. in 2012 proposed a new model to remove mainly these security issues. In 2013, Khan and Kumari [15] identified that Zhu's 2012 [16] as well as Wei et al.'s 2012 authentication models were weak to the stolen/lost smart card, offline password guessing, and denial-of-service attacks. At the same time, Lee and Liu (2013) found session key agreement attack in Zhu 2012 scheme [16]. To remove these flaws in previous authentication schemes, they introduced a new scheme to defeat the security attacks like facing session key disclosure, password guessing, and parallel session.

In 2013, Awasthi and Srivastava introduced a three-factor authentication system for TMIS using biometric system and random numbers. Analysing their schemes, Tan in 2014 caught an issue of user anonymity and a reflection attack in their work. Arshad and Nikooghadam in 2014 identified replay attacks and denial-of-service in Tan's scheme. In 2015, Giri et al. [17] reviewed Lee and Liu's (2013) user authentication scheme for TMIS and found an offline password guessing attack vulnerability. In same year, Amin and Biswas (2015) [18] identified some flaws in authentication schemes of Giri et al.'s (2015) [17]. These flaws or weaknesses are: offline password guessing, lack of user anonymity, and insider attacks, and they proposed a new RSA-based scheme.

In continuous effort, to enhance the security in previous schemes, Bin Muhaya in 2014 introduced an enhanced authentication and key agreement scheme for TMISs. However, it was proved that Bin Muhaya's scheme also has a weakness for offline password guessing attacks and it is not able to perfect forward secrecy. To remove the security weaknesses of authentication scheme of Bin Muhaya, Arshad et al. in 2015 proposed a new two-factor key agreement scheme and user anonymity preserving authentication for TMISs. Limbasiya et al. (2017) [19] analysed Arshad et al.'s [20] authentication schemes mathematically with the help of irreversible hash function, concatenation, and exclusive-or operations and identified some vulnerabilities. Then, they introduced a new authentication scheme to overcome the issues in the previous schemes.

11.3 Network Security Attacks

Network security attacks are mainly classified into two main categories.

- Passive attack
- Active attack

In passive attack, the attacker only captures data packets sent from sender to the receiver and understands the information passed through these data packets but the attacker does not modify the data packets that flow into the network [10]. But in active attack the attacker captures the data packets and also modifies these data packets and sends the modified data packet to receiver on behalf of actual sender. As shown in the following figure, the middle attacker is capturing sender's data. In the following figures (Figs. 11.3 and 11.4), we have shown the presence of an attacker in network.

As shown in the following figure, the attacker is capturing the data packets and modifying captured data as well.

In active attack, the attacker sends his modified packet on behalf of sender. The receiver thinks that the data packet is actual data packet which was initially sent by actual sender.

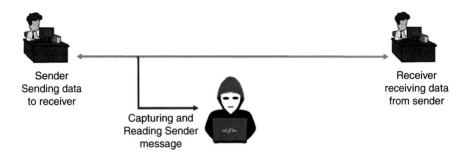

Fig. 11.3 Passive attack

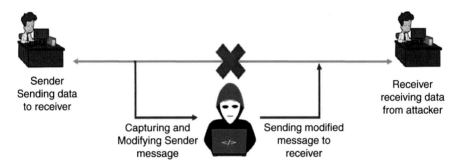

Fig. 11.4 Active attack

11.4   Telemedicine Security Services and Their Application

There are some major services that need to be provided by TMIS systems. These security services are mandatory to be taken care by TMIS systems for the patients and doctors.

Security service	Description
Confidentiality	TMIS system should be accessible by the authenticated users. Information should be encrypted. Individual user should access to his/her records only.
Availability	It should be available 24 × 7. It should be accessible from anywhere. It should be fast performing. Stored HER should be easily available for authenticated user.
Integrity	EHR records or other critical information should be the same at all servers. It should be digital format. It should be encrypted so that unwanted changes can be avoided.

The common network threats are interruption, interception, modification, fabrication, etc. These security threats are possible in network-based systems. In normal information flow, there is no threat active on system, but in interruption, the information flow will be blocked by the threat and normal flow will not be possible. In interception, the normal flow will continue in sender and receiver but the same information will also be read by the attacker. In modification, the attacker will capture sender packet and modify it and send to the receiver after modification. In fabrication, the information received by the receiver is actually transmitted by attacker but receiver thinks that the information is coming from actual sender. All these threats are very harmful in network-based systems, specially in TMIS. So there should be more focus given on these security attacks and security threats to provide a reliable platform in healthcare [21].

11.5 Two-Factor Authentication Scheme for Telemedicine Systems

The detailed authentication process is described in next sections of this paper. There are three main blocks for TIMS, patient, doctor, and telecare server. In Fig. 11.5, we have explained the basic authentication mechanism of TIMS.

Many authentication schemes have been proposed for secured access to telemedicine systems. One popular scheme has been defined in the following section.

11.5.1 Limbasiya et al.'s (2017) Authentication Scheme

Limbasiya et al. (2017) introduced some security attack issues, named as session key disclosure and user impersonation in Arshad et al.'s [22] system. Then, they have proposed an improved two-factor authentication scheme after eliminating all security issues found in Arshad et al. [22]. Proposed authentication system is having three phases. First is registration phase, second is authentication phase, and third is password update phase. The notations used in this scheme have been specified in Table 11.1. The step-by-step procedure of all three phases has been described in the following section.

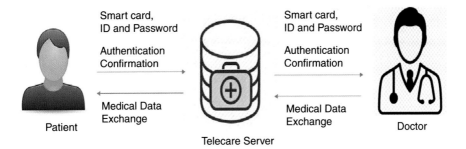

Fig. 11.5 Telecare medical information system block diagram for user authentication

Table 11.1 Symbols and notation used in Limbasiya et al.'s (2017) system

Symbol	Definition
IDi	Identity of user
PWi	Password of user
NU	A randomly generated number chosen by user
NS	A randomly generated number chosen by Server
xi	Secret key per-user by server
Yi	User's key for sever
MIDi	Masked Identity for user
T2, T3	Time measures at receiver end
T1, T4	Time measures at sender end
ΔT	The maximum delay allowed for transmission
SK	A session key with mutual agreement
$\parallel$	Operation for concatenation
$\oplus$	Operation for XOR
S	Server notation
Ui	User notation
SCi	Smart card for user
$h(\cdot)$	hash function used for one-way

11.5.1.1   Registration Phase

Registration phase consists of mainly four steps. The flow of these four steps with mathematical formulas has been given in Table 11.2. It will be processed only once for each user. A new user can register directly to the system without intervention of an intermediate authentication system. Using a private communication channel, a new user can register to the health server after performing the following steps.

Step 1 Ui: user picks IDi, PWi, and random number NU. Calculates $Mi = h(PWi \parallel NU)$ and sends a registration appeal message {IDi, Mi} to the server via a private medium.

Step 2 S: selects NS and calculates $MIDi = h(IDi \parallel NS)$, $Ai = h(IDi \parallel Yi \parallel MIDi)$, $Pi = Ai \oplus Yi$, $Ni = Mi \oplus xi$.

Step 3 S: in this step server will store IDi and MIDi in its data centre, and {Ai, MIDi, Pi, Ni, $h(\cdot)$} in SCi and provide the SCi information to the new user.

Step 4 Ui: calculates $Bi = Ai \oplus h(IDi \parallel PWi)$ and replaces Ai with Bi in the smart card: $SCi = \{Bi, MIDi, Pi, Ni, h(\cdot)\}$.

11.5.1.2   Authentication Phase

The steps with calculation have been described in Table 11.3. All these steps will be executed routinely and respective measurements are evaluated using free channel.

Step 1 Ui: the user inserts his/her card SCi into the smart card reader and inputs their IDi and PWi. Then,

Table 11.2 Registration phase of Limbasiya et al.'s (2017) scheme

User		Medical server
Chooses IDi, PWi and NU Computes Mi = h(PWi ǁ NU)		
	{IDi, Mi} ————————▶ Secure Channel	
		Chooses NS Computes… MIDi = h(IDi ǁ NS) Ai = h(IDi ǁ Yi ǁ MIDi) Pi = Ai ⊕ Yi Ni = Mi ⊕ xi SCi = {Ai, MIDi, Pi, Ni, h(·)} Stores IDi and MIDi in the database
	{SCi} ◀———————— Secure Channel	
Computes Bi = Ai ⊕ h(IDi ǁ PWi) Replace Ai and Bi in SCi SCi = {Bi, MIDi, Pi, Ni, h(·)}		

Calculates Ai = Bi ⊕ h(IDi ǁ PWi) where Ai = h(IDi ǁ Yi ǁ MIDi), Yi = Ai ⊕ Pi, xi = Pi ⊕ Ni. A random number dC is generated and QC = dCYi, V1 = h(IDi ǁ Ai ǁ QC ǁ T1), K1 = dCxi, V1′ = V1 ⊕ (K1 ǁ T1), MIDi′ = MIDi ⊕h(K1) are evaluated. A request for login {MIDi′,V1′, QC, T1} is given to the server.

Step 2 S: after getting {MIDi′,V1, QC, T1}, the server checks T2 – T1 ≤ ΔT. The server then calculates

$$K_1^* = dC\ xi = \frac{QCxi}{Yi} \quad V_1 = V_1' \oplus h\left(K_1^* \quad T_1\right), \text{ MIDi = MIDi′} \oplus h(K1^*) \text{ and checks}$$
for

h(IDi ǁ h(IDi ǁ Yi ǁ MIDi) ǁ QC ǁ T1) =?V1. Then, the server generates a number randomly dS, and calculates QS = dSYi, K2 = h(dSQCT3) = h(dSdCYiT3), where T3 is the measured time at server end when K2 is calculated and V2 = h(QS ǁ V2 ǁ K2). Finally, the server generates its session key SKS = h(IDi ǁ K2) and sends back a challenge message to user{QS, V2, T3}.

Step 3 Ui: after receiving the challenge message from server S, the Ui checks T4 – T3 ≤ ΔT. The user then calculates

the values dS = QSYi, K2* = h(dCQS) = h(dSdCYiT3) and checks * h(QS ǁV1 ǁ K2*) =? V2. Then, the user side session key SKU = h(IDi ǁ K2*) is calculated. Finally, the SKU =?SKS is compared, and if it is equal, then sever authenticates the session; If it is not found equal, server will terminate the session forcefully.

Table 11.3 Authentication phase of Limbasiya et al.'s (2017) scheme

User		Medical server
Inserts smart card into card reader Enters IDi and PWi SCi = {Bi, MIDi, Pi, Ni, h(·)}. Computes… Ai = Bi ⊕ h(IDi ‖ PWi) Where Ai = h(IDi ‖ Yi ‖ MIDi) Computes… Yi = Ai ⊕ Pi xi = Pi ⊕ Ni Generates a random number dC Computes… QS = dCYi V1 = h(IDi ‖ Ai ‖ QC ‖ T1) K1 = dCxi $V_1' = V_1 \oplus h(K_1 \quad T_1)$ MIDi' = MIDi ⊕h(K1)		
	$\{MIDi,\ V_1', Qc, Ti\}$ $\longrightarrow$	
		Checks T2 – T1 ≤ ΔT Computes… $K_1^* = dC\ xi = \dfrac{QCxi}{Yi}$ $V_1' = V_1 \oplus h(K_1 \quad T_1)$ MIDi = MIDi' ⊕h(K1*) Checks… h(IDi ‖ h(IDi ‖ Yi ‖ MIDi) ‖ QC ‖ T1 =? V1 Generates random number dS Computes… QS = dSYi K2 = h(dSQCT3) = h(dSdCYiT3) V2 = h(QS ‖ V1 ‖ K2) SKS = h(IDi ‖ K2)
	{Qs, V2, T3} $\longleftarrow$	
Checks T4 – T3 ≤ ΔT dS = QSYi K2* = h(dCQS) = h(dCdSYiT3) Checks h(QS ‖V1 ‖ K2*) =? V2 Computes * SKU = h(IDi ‖ K2*)	Checks SKU =? SKS	

11.5.1.3 Password Update

If a user wants to update his/her password for any reason, then the third phase will be used and the steps defined for updating password will be processed.

- Step 1 Refer to Step 1 of Sect. 2.2, authentication phase.
- Step 2 Refer to Step 2 of Sect. 2.2, authentication phase.
- Step 3 Upon acquiring the challenge $\{Q_S, V_2, T_3\}$ from the server, the user calculates $K_2{}^* = h(d_C Q_S) = h(d_C d_S Y i T_3)$ and verifies whether $h(Q_S \| V_1 \| K_2{}^*)$ matches the received V_2 or not. If they do not match, the process is terminated. If they do match, the smart card calculates $B_i^{new} = Ai \oplus h (IDi \| PWi^{new})$. Then, it updates Bi with B_i^{new} in SC_i.

11.6 Conclusion

In this chapter, the proposed approach provides a patient an easy access to healthcare services without being physically present at hospitals. This approach is suitable for remote patients, a patient can easily login and submit their symptoms to a cloud-based TMIS server through this portal. Patients do not have to search for a doctor or visit hospitals. After receiving patient's data, the telecare server, which has suitable ML models deployed, performs the task of predicting disease, giving prescriptions, filtering patients, and sending data to telehealth service providers (or doctors). This approach is favourable for patients as well as doctors. The task of doctors becomes comparatively easy, since at initial level, disease is predicted and sorting of patients is done by server, based on severity of disease. In this approach, health services are provided over network, so it does have data security vulnerabilities and there may be chances of wrong prediction by ML model; we can try to overcome these problems by using efficient security protocols for all the tasks (authentication, data transfer, data access) and training ML model with large, authentic data set; applying continual learning to ML model may also help.

References

1. Krishnan DSR, et al. An IoT based patient health monitoring system. In: 2018 International Conference on Advances in Computing and Communication Engineering (ICACCE). IEEE; 2018. p. 1–7.
2. Chauhan A, et al. Healthcare information management system using android OS. In: Proceedings—2017 International Conference on Computational Intelligence and Networks CINE 2017; 2018.
3. Sinha H, et al. Effective E-Healthcare system: cache invalidation mechanisms for wireless data access in mobile cloud computing. Int J Big Data Anal Healthcare (IJBDAH). 3(2) https://doi.org/10.4018/IJBDAH.2018070102.
4. Pramanik PKD, Pal S, Mukhopadhyay M. Healthcare big data: a comprehensive overview. In: Bouchemal N, editor. Research anthology on big data analytics, architectures, and applications; 2022. p. 119–47.

5. Sharma HK, Patni JC. Pandemic diagnosis and analysis using clinical decision support systems. J Crit Rev. 2020;

6. Gupta S, Sharma HK. User anonymity based secure authentication protocol for telemedical server systems. Int J Inform Comput Security. 2021;

7. Shailender SHK. Digital cancer diagnosis with counts of adenoma and luminal cells in plemorphic adenoma immunastained healthcare system. IJRAR. 2018;5(12)

8. Patni JC, Ahlawat P, Biswas SS. Sensors based smart healthcare framework using internet of things (IoT). Int J Sci Technol Res. 2020;9(2):1228–34.

9. Taneja S, Ahmed E, Patni JC. I-Doctor: an IoT based self patient's health monitoring system. In: 2019 International Conference on Innovative Sustainable Computational Technologies, CISCT 2019; 2019.

10. Hwang MS, Li LH. 'A new remote user authentication scheme using smart cards', IEEE Transactions on Consumer Electronics, 2000;46(1):28–30.

11. Sun HM. 'An efficient remote use authentication scheme using smart cards', IEEE Transactions on Consumer Electronics, 2000;46(4):958–61.

12. Liao IE, Lee CC, and Hwang MS. 'A password authentication scheme over insecure networks', J Comput Syst Sci. 2006;72(4):727–40.

13. Wu ZY, et al. 'A secure authentication scheme for telecare medicine information systems', J Med Syst. 2012;36(3):1529–35.

14. Debiao H, Jianhua C, and Rui Z. 'A more secure authentication scheme for telecare medicine information systems', J Med Syst. 2012;36(3);1989–95.

15. Aji A, et al. Hadoop-GIS: A high performance spatial data warehousing system over MapReduce. In Proceedings of the VLDB Endowment International Conference on Very Large Data Bases 2013;6(11). NIH Public Access.

16. Zhu, Z. 'An efficient authentication scheme for telecare medicine information systems', J Med Syst. 2012;36(6):3833–38.

17. Giri D, Maitra T, Amin R, and Srivastava PD, 'An efficient and robust rsa-based remote user authentication for telecare medical information systems', J Med Syst. 2015;39(1):1–9.

18. Amin R, Biswas GP. 'An improved rsa based user authentication and session key agreement protocol usable in tmis', J Med Syst. 2015;39(8):1–14.

19. Trupil Limbasiya, Sachit Shivam. "A two-factor key verification system focused on remote user for medical applications, Int J Critical infrastructures. 2017;13(2/3).

20. Arshad H, Nikooghadam M. 'Three-factor anonymous authentication and key agreement scheme for telecare medicine information systems', J Med Syst. 2014;38(12):1–12.

21. Arshad H, Teymoori V, Nikooghadam M, Abbassi H. On the security of a two-factor authentication and key agreement scheme for telecare medicine information systems. J Med Syst. 2015;

22. Joshi A, et al. Data mining in healthcare and predicting obesity. In: Proceedings of the Third International Conference on Computational Intelligence and Informatics, Hyderabad, India; 2020. p. 877–88.

Virtual Diet Counseling as an Integral Part of Telemedicine in COVID-19 Phases

12

Swapan Banerjee, Bhaswati Samaddar, Corinna van der Eerden, Tanupriya Choudhury, and Manish Taywade

12.1 Introduction

12.1.1 Telehealth

It signifies delivery and facilitation of healthcare services: consultation, education, and information via remote technologies, i.e., telecommunication and digital communication technologies. Telehealth can be done by live videoconferences where medical facilities and the patient party can sit on either side and consult over videoconferences or mobile health apps. According to the WHO, telemedicine is defined as providing healthcare services to all possible areas using electronic media. In

S. Banerjee (✉)
Department of Nutrition, Seacom Skills University, Kendradangal,
Birbhum, West Bengal, India

B. Samaddar
Dietetics and Food Service Management, Indira Gandhi National Open University,
New Delhi, India

C. van der Eerden
Family Food Coach and Functional Medicine Certified Health Coach,
Bernkastel-Kues, Germany

T. Choudhury (✉)
School of Computer Science, University of Petroleum and Energy Studies (UPES),
Dehradun, Uttarakhand, India

M. Taywade
Department of Community Medicine & Family Medicine, All India Institute of Medical
Sciences Bhubaneswar, Sijua, Patrapada, Bhubaneswar, Odisha, India

© The Author(s), under exclusive license to Springer Nature
Switzerland AG 2022
T. Choudhury et al. (eds.), *Telemedicine: The Computer Transformation of
Healthcare*, TELe-Health, https://doi.org/10.1007/978-3-030-99457-0_12

1960, telemedicine was remotely used with wireless broadband technology in the military and space. Still, slowly with due course of time, it is widely used among other fields also [1, 2].

12.1.2 Telemedicine

This technology allows medical professionals to evaluate, diagnose, and treat patients at a distance using telecommunication technology. This telemedicine technology is frequently used for follow-up visits, chronic conditions management, medication management, and consulting specialists [2]. Modern-day telemedicines partially originated in Europe in the ancient ages and has been continuously rising. Dutch physician Willem Einthoven used this technology in 1905 for electrocardiograms that were the first clinical application of telemedicine. In 1920, radio consultation started for patients aboard ships at sea and remote islands like France, Italy, Norway. The internet age brought this profound change in health practice. This history of telemedicine is closely parallel to communication and information technology [3].

12.1.3 COVID-19 and Economic Crisis

Coronavirus or COVID-19, a global pandemic that the world is facing after World War II, an outbreak from China, has eventually gone everywhere in the last few months. According to WHO data, as of 15 June 2021, more than one hundred seventy-six million people have already been affected, and three million people have died worldwide. Similarly, above twenty-nine million confirmed cases and three lakhs eighty-two thousand deaths were also reported in India [4]. In this situation, the world economy is showing significant risks that may induce hyper-globalization or a start of deglobalization. Moreover, the world will face a recession and a global economic crisis. From the Indian perspective, the country faces a similar financial crisis; millions of people are losing their jobs. In addition, the gross domestic product (GDP) level is coming down daily, affecting poor and middle-class people [4, 5].

12.1.4 Lockdown Phases

Telehealth was already there before lockdown, but this technology was less as people are skeptical regarding online services for a health issue. From the beginning of 2020 till ongoing 2021, people started using telehealth services in lockdown and unlock stages only because there is no other best option to reach a consultant; however, people understood the benefits of this system [5]. According to the WHO mental health department, isolation, fear of life uncertainty, depression, and economic turmoil could lead to psychological distress. Psychologists said that children face severe depression as they are entirely isolated from the outside world, sitting at home [6].

12.1.5 Health Crisis due to COVID-19 in India

Millions of people have lost employment globally, and the health fraternity warns that this anxiety, continuous isolation, and depression may lead to severe mental crises. This nationwide shutdown disrupted the lives of millions of people, which resulted in mass unemployment. In addition, recent research conducted by the Indian Psychiatry Society found that mental illness conditions increased by 20%. Some psychiatrists also suggested that children are at greater risk because of this lockdown, economic turmoil, and family violence. According to the survey, since March 2020, almost 343 people have committed suicide; among them, nearly 125 people have committed suicide due to fear of getting an infection or loneliness [7].

12.2   Methodology

Our paper highlighted the importance of a balanced diet by proper nutrition for all COVID phases. The study was prepared by online available open-access literature search through reliable and high-quality databases. The phrases and keywords applied during database searches were "telemedicine during COVID phases," "diet consultation in the COVID pandemic," "diet consultation, a part of telemedicine," "teleconsultation in the COVID pandemic," etc. All searches were considered both global cum Indian level and emphasized to cite the quality articles. The Boolean keywords were also added to online searches to sort and select the most relevant articles as per the study concept.

12.3   Discussion

12.3.1 Role of Telehealth and Telemedicine in COVID-19 Outbreak in Indian Perspective

Telehealth and telemedicine are based on modern technologies by which health-related services and information get commuted through electronic media. Moreover, these technologies are proven a boon because people can access medical assistance with proper social distancing norms. Technology provides service seekers a digital platform that eases the clinical problem from a distance, especially in semi-urban and rural distance areas. The technology-driven applications can enable patients to avail themselves of medical assistance sitting at home only. The easily downloadable applications from the Google play store can efficiently help people save time by consulting their doctors. Some studies showed that the Indian telemedicine market spiked growth during this pandemic COVID-19 situation. People prefer telemedicine to keep themselves safe and at home, monitoring their health well [8].

12.3.2 Importance of Diet in COVID-19 Pandemic

A balanced diet can assure better prevention against all diseases, including the COVID-19 virus. A proportional amount of protein is required, that is, 1 gram per kg body weight for adults. In addition, the right proportion of water-soluble vitamins (vitamin C and B vitamins) and all essential minerals is also required. All the nutrients can help prepare a properly balanced diet for an individual [9]. Low carbohydrate and edible fat in the diet but plenty of green vegetables and fruits are always helpful for everyone. Undoubtedly, fruits and vegetables supply polyphenols and other bioactive compounds, potent antioxidants, and natural anti-inflammatory agents. Many studies showed that some herbs and spices provide immunity-boosting and different therapeutic roles in Ayurveda and nutritional science. Raw turmeric, coriander leaves and seeds, cumin, cinnamon, garlic ginger, cloves, black pepper, cardamom, and fenugreek seeds cum leaves are the best examples. Egg, fish, and chicken are the best animal protein sources whereas soybean, pulses, beans, milk, and milk products are the best protein sources available and affordable almost in all countries. Around 50–55% of carbohydrate, 15–20% of protein or 1 g/kg body weight, and 20% approx edible fat are significant nutrients in an average balanced diet.

Moreover, 10–12 glasses of water should be consumed daily as an essential component to maintaining hydration [10]. Apart from diet, exercises must be practiced at home during the COVID pandemic. Early morning yoga, some amount of freestyle, and maximum walking, if possible, should be within the exercise regimen, although home-based physical activities are also an alternative. In addition, a minimum of 7 hrs sleep must be there for everyone, whether leading sedentary or mild to moderate activities. However, diet, exercise, and drinking water should be planned by a dietitian and fitness trainer considering an individual's lifestyle, existing diseases, comorbidities, and medications (if any) [11].

12.3.3 Initiatives by the Government of India on Telemedicine and Nutritional Awareness

Telemedicine marks a very positive contribution towards health in this pandemic. It acts as a bridge between people and the health system because it helps people get their medical facility staying at home. Even the Indian government has introduced the Ayushman Bharat scheme, one of the biggest health financing schemes that facilitate and develop ideology [12, 13]. In diet selection, intermitted fasting diet, ketogenic diet, and other fad diets should be avoided during this time. Apart from proteins, minerals, and vitamins, some value-added foods like probiotics, prebiotics, and omega-3,6,9 polyunsaturated fatty acids can be very much helpful to prevent COVID virus at home level [14].

12.3.4 Telemedicine Management in International Perspectives

Telemedicine is now a global concept for the benefit of international people. Many countries have had already imposed specific regulations under their countries' laws system. Europe and American countries are always one step ahead despite many challenges in telemedicine. There was a rapid change in legislative circumstances around telemedicine and acceptance of this kind of support from patients and customers in Germany. It is a very tech-averse country where patients are actively seeking telemedicine opportunities, mainly in video consultations. Health insurance companies quickly adjust their billing methods per reimbursement policy, integrating telemedicine into their portfolio [15].

The German Federal Ministry of Health has communicated its goal on telemedicine with the initiative "Digital Health 2025": The initiative aims to improve healthcare in Germany. It includes various activities, including introducing electronic patient records, prescriptions, digital health applications ("App on prescription"), telemedicine advancements, and establishing a data center for research. Additionally, the Federal Ministry has set up an initiative to bring digital solutions into more practical applications and learn about their use. The German Federal Ministry of Health claims that it is necessary to make high-quality digital services available to patients with prompt services such as video consultations, electronic prescriptions, and electronic patient files that should become a natural part of everyday care. However, Germany is still facing some challenges and lacks various aspects. Some reports show that despite the growth of the telemedicine market, there are some challenges usually faced by the people of low- and middle-level economic countries. Most of the issues are lack of nationwide broadband expansion, insufficient training of medical specialists, and reimbursement issues for many services by health insurance companies [16]. Other European countries have already developed patient-friendly solutions: the Netherland, one of the most progressive countries where telemedicine services are integral parts of routine healthcare. Every hospital and doctor's office uses a portfolio (e.g., remote monitoring or teleradiology) of services and mobile applications for patients. In Sweden, the state finances its e-health authority through a separate budget. In general, digital services are reimbursed as conventional services by health insurance [17].

Almost 75% of adults in the United States have been using broadband internet service at their homes located in the metro or major cities. On the other end, older adults, racial minorities, rural people, low education, and low income are deprived somehow or yet to receive the services. Therefore, it is essential to have a uniform distribution of minimum technologies for teleconsultations even in the most advanced countries in the world [18]. In this context, there is a small percentage of patients who are availing the virtual diet consultations for the health issues like obesity, diabetes, and chronic kidney disorders as common lifestyles disorders.

In the South Asian zone, some countries have already developed telemedicine laws following international guidelines. Singapore is the example, but Indonesia and Vietnam remain with older technologies. However, their government has

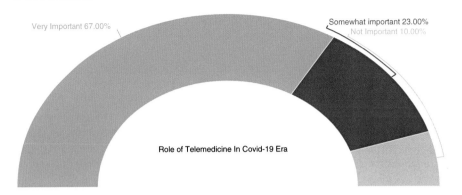

Very Important 67.00%   Somewhat important 23.00%
                                          Not Important 10.00%

Role of Telemedicine In Covid-19 Era

Fig. 12.1 Role of telemedicine in COVID-19 era

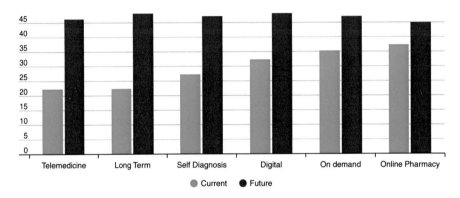

Telemedicine   Long Term   Self Diagnosis   Digital   On demand   Online Pharmacy

● Current   ● Future

Fig. 12.2 Adoption of telemedicine globally: current vs. future (in percentage)

provided some provisions for patients to go and get medical facilities from advanced countries [19]. As far as diet is concerned in telemedicine practices, many patients are usually referred by consultant physicians or specialist doctors to recover from the overweight, poor dietary and lifestyles.

The above Fig. 12.1 shows the response of the global population towards telemedicine in the COVID-19 era. In this figure, 67% responded favoring telemedicine, 23% reacted somewhat necessary, and 10% found it unnecessary.

Due to various factors, some countries are still struggling with telecommunications technologies. Therefore, we have insufficient data based on every nation; hence we have tried as best as possible to show the importance and non-importance percentages. Due to post-pandemic circumstances, authors and telemedicine researchers expect more relevant data in the coming days. In the last few years, there has been significant growth in the telemedicine industry, but the scenario is more prominent since 2020.

The above Fig. 12.2 shows the acceleration of the adoption of telemedicine in the current time vs. the future (in percentage: 0–45%) by different healthcare departments based on the global population. Table 12.1 shows the various applications and tools used in the telemedicine fields.

Table 12.1 Various tools for telemedicine [17–19]

Various Applications	Tools	Tools used in telemedicine
Patient and telecoms health service	Health apps	These are used for physical fitness
Medical practitioners	Video call, telecommunication, e-mail, WhatsApp.	1. Chronic illness conditions, 2. Various medical counseling 3. Routine checkup for various diseases
Medical practitioner to medical practitioners	E-mail, video call	Dermatology, Radiology, Surgical topics, or related issues as case studies
Dietitians: referred by the doctor	E-mail, video, phone	Customized application for the dietitian to write diet advice and attachment of diet prescriptions

12.3.5 Teleconsultation and Diet Consultation [19, 20]

Teleconsultation is termed synchronous and asynchronous consultation performed using various communication technologies. It is helpful regarding omitting the geographical and functional distance between two parties. Examples are as follows:

(1) Physicians and patients can directly show reports for a health-related problem for consultation.
(2) Dietitians and patients can directly communicate with their dietitians and seek health tips.

There is another term, remote consultation that means consultation done by remote telecommunication. Generally, it is used for diagnosis or treatment purpose of the patient at a remote site from doctors/physicians.

12.3.6 The Basic Process for Telecommunication [21]

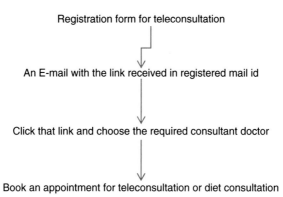

Registration form for teleconsultation

An E-mail with the link received in registered mail id

Click that link and choose the required consultant doctor

Book an appointment for teleconsultation or diet consultation

12.3.7 Web-Based Appointments

Age-year-old practice regarding appointment was to book appointment slot by calling up doctor's assistant. This type of booking system involves verbal communication with real people. However, this is troublesome as getting a timely appointment depends on the scheduler's availability near the telephone. After finding flaws in this technique, a new approach evolves that is web-based appointment booking or E-appointment. Nowadays, various apps are available like Practo, Lybrate, etc., in India. People can read the doctor's medical background and book a slot for appointments per their medical requirements. Patients or patients' parties can choose an appointment as per their convenient date and time; however, an appointment is subject to the availability of a doctor or dietitian in a private clinic or institute setting [22].

There are two types of web-based medical appointment services:

(1) Medical scheduling software as service: This appointment system is not built up by medical practitioners themselves; instead, it is provided and maintained by health IT Companies such as Zocdoc and InQuicker (paid or subscription-based). The health professional owns this management system that can assess cloud-based services.
(2) Proprietary appointment system: The system is integrated into the patient portal on the service provider's website. A patient can directly communicate with their healthcare provider at any time.

Two modes of web-based appointment system are:

(1) Asynchronous: The appointment is initiated using electronic media, either mail or app-based.
(2) Real-time mode: The patients can now interact with the service provider and schedule their appointment.

Physician and patient trust on teleconsultation during COVID-19 particularly. All doctors, dietitians, and other health practitioners enroll under various online medical portals. They provide medical health assistance to their patients through these online platforms due to COVID-19 situations where people are badly stuck. Altogether, telemedicine technology has proved a boon [23].

12.3.8 E-pharmacy

E-pharmacy or electronic pharmacy, or online pharmacy, is the same and operated by the pharmaceutical industry. However, many app-based pharmacies are now available to access all services efficiently, e.g., PharmEasy, Medlife, 1 mg, Netmeds, Apollo, and MedPlus.

12.3.9 There Are a few Drawbacks of Internet Pharmacy [24]

(1) The Pharmacy's web pages sometimes contain improper information about its parent country, procedure, certification, pricing, and authentication. This type of pharmacy occasionally even sells short expiry medicine.
(2) Medicine packing techniques to be checked whether meeting quality or not.
(3) Order controlled substances without proper parental guidance.

12.3.10 Role of Virtual Laboratory (E-Lab)

Lab testing is the most critical clinical act through screening, diagnosis management, and monitoring disease or therapies. Comprehensive lab software generates laboratory reports and does accounting jobs much more straightforward, quicker way as affordable as possible. The laboratories also offer many packages of various tests and simultaneously customized or on-demand tests. Hence, no need to wander but get all test reports within a day or two. In the E-lab context, LIS (laboratory information system) records, manages, and stores data associated with the clinical laboratory [24, 25]. However, dietitians are dependent on the tests, doctors' prescriptions, and other medical reports to analyze and plan a diet for a particular patient. Therefore, the laboratories industry follows doctors' prescriptions and helps them confirm the diagnosis and subsequent treatment process. A laboratory information management system (LIMS) effectively manages samples and other related information to improve the Lab's efficiency. The system includes all the tests conducted under a particular facility. Cloud storage is helping widely in LIMS because it can store large files, but it does not have a specified storage capacity. Patient accessibility: The interconnection of LIMS software helps patients access internal lab information; they can easily track their records [25].

Benefits of Using LIMS in the Lab as Follows [24, 25]
(1) Workflow automation.
(2) Integrated instruments.
(3) Data can be accessed by centralizing.
(4) Data tracking facility.

12.3.11   Flow Chart of LIMS Technique

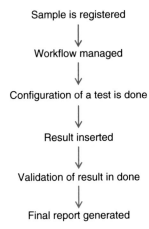

One of the highly used LIMS software is MocDoc, endorsed by many doctors and patients most inclined towards teleconsultation.

It is necessary in the paperless healthcare industry because we all know the world is going through a pandemic condition where going outside is restricted. Hence, in this condition, a paperless hospital is a boon service.

12.3.12   International Telemedicine Companies and their Business/Sales [26]

(1) MD. Live (USA): MDLive provides extensive access to registered therapists, dietitians, pediatricians, and doctors. It is affordable and convenient to use, having more than 45 global members.
(2) iCliniq (India): One of the best telemedicine portals since 2010 offering virtual consultation located at Tamil Nadu (India) headquarter. It has a very high volume of contacts of both medical professionals and patients looking for second medical opinion sitting at home.
(3) Sermo (USA): A social platform opened for licensed MDS and DOS of the USA, Europe, North and South America, etc. It was established by a physician named Daniel Palestrant in 2005, and then after the year 2012, this entity was acquired by the world.
(4) AMD Global Telemedicine (USA): Since 1991, it has been the complete platform from medical, where presently seven categories are there, i.e., emotional, environmental, intellectual, occupational, physical, social, and spiritual. Doctors treat people under these categories.
(5) Trihealth services (Ohio): It was established in 1995, operated from Cincinnati, Ohio. It is the first fitness facility recognized by MFA. It works with profession-

als from Bethesda and good Samaritan hospitals. People have to purchase membership plans, and they even provide internship facilities.

(6) Teladoc Health (USA): Teladoc Health is one of the leading players in telemedicine, having over 125 countries globally. The company is applying the latest technologies, including artificial intelligence-based telemedicine. In 2018, the company showed 2.5 million telehealth visits across the globe. The renowned brands are "healthiest you" and "better help" from the company.

12.3.13   Indian Telemedicines Companies and Their Business [27]

(1) Practo: It was established in the year 2008 in May month. The Health Insurance Portability and Accountability Act (HIPAA) is a gateway for doctors and hospitals to book medical appointments or consultation appointments. This app can also get insurance, store their health record and medical deliveries. Unique selling points (USP) of Practo is that they check it rigorously to build up trust factors with a customer before feeding any pieces of information. Furthermore, Practo follows the compliance activities to maintain patient privacy. They are also running a vast online city-wise network on virtual diet consultation through India's best dietitians empaneled since 2012. They also have good teleconsultations coverage even in Singapore, Indonesia, and the Philippines.

(2) 1 mg: The organization was established in 2015; through this app, medicines are delivered all over India from licensed and verified pharmacies. An unlimited free consultation can be done within 30mins. 1 mg is very popular in offering customized diet plans through their city-wise enlisted dietitians paid satisfactory fees in a systematic reimbursement process.

(3) Lybrate: It was established in 2013, and it is India's first mobile healthcare, communication, and delivery platform. It helps patients to undergo one-one consultations with doctors.

(4) Medlife: It was founded in 2014; the main aim is to make healthcare accessible and affordable for all people. Medical consultation can be done through this app, medicine delivery, lab test, etc. They also tied up with online digital payment portals like MobiKwik, free charge, etc.

(5) Portea Medical: Portea as a portal was established in 2013, which provides healthcare services that include primary care, chronic care of diseases, and physiotherapy. Various doctors and nurses enlisted their names here because of multiple benefits, including home care services.

(6) Truworth wellness: The company was established in the year 2014. They tie up with IT professionals, banking sectors, insurance, retail, pharma, etc., for a medical checkup. Overall, this app provides a customized health plan and many social projects.

12.3.14   Quality Assurance of Teleconsultation of Following Parameters [21, 28]

12.3.14.1   Operational Management

- Online Management team: It is teamwork through an online management team that looks into the workflow's total operation and smooth functioning. This team includes a software engineer, virtual voice assistant, and virtual help desk.
- App management: It is critical management when an app launches in the telemedicine market; a team works behind it and manages the 24/7 smooth functioning of the app.
- Data security: In telemedicine, patients feed their information during consultation, and it is essential to keep that information secure as the doctors check patients.
- Payment gateway and payment releases are the pathways through which payment is made. The different app uses different payment systems and gateways. The popular uses are Unified Payment Interface (UPI) mode like Paytm, BHIM app, and credit card, debit cards of all banks duly tied up with them.
- Doctors and medical professionals online verification: Doctors, dietitians, and other medical practitioners get enlisted in the respective app by self-uploading educational and other supporting documents. The visibility of their profile can easily fetch regular leads and other assignments along with existing follow-up; however, the overall return is subject to a free or paid subscription.
- Special department-wise COVID awareness (free or paid): In this COVID pandemic situation, every app has a unique COVID care facility where patients can feed up their symptoms regarding COVID and get proper guidance.

12.3.14.2   Role of Doctors and Dietitians in COVID-19 Phases [29, 30]

- Numbers of doctors and qualifications: 10–12 specialist doctors are always on-job in their respective departments: nephrology, urology, gynecology, gastrology, diabetology, cardio, etc. Additionally, another general medicine is ready to provide COVID care and other medical services following COVID safety protocol.
- Each consultation timing and duration: General office hours from 10 am till 8 pm for total timing of any institution and period for each consultation is average 15–30 min or variable as per the company.
- Doctors' involvement in maintaining records of prescriptions: The patient has to feed up their report beforehand to consult and prescribe medicine. The virtual consultation modes are usually mail prescriptions or WhatsApp.
- Special COVID team of doctors for awareness: In this pandemic situation, every app has an impressive COVID care facility where patients can feed up their symptoms regarding COVID and get proper guidance. In addition, dietitians and nutritionists contribute by sharing their nutritional knowledge with patients and society.
- Home visits/emergency visits at home - In emergency or elderly cases, home visits are offered special facilities. In 2020, their elder groups were identified as the most vulnerable section to COVID-19. Dietitians took significant roles, start-

ing from the intensive care unit to private clinic by advising an immunity-boosting diet.

- Feedback system: In every institution, a nodal department is assigned to check the feedback and patients' compliance with the institution's services. Whether the establishments are private or government, feedback or comment system must have been there. However, some advanced countries can manage this quality management system as best as possible despite several challenges. Still, countries like India, Bangladesh, and other low-economic high population countries have already faced much trouble due to the faster rate of infections.

12.3.14.3 Role of Nurses

Nurses are the backbone of the medical and healthcare industry. They are just like a mother cares for a baby constantly. They cooperate and work in nursing homes or hospitals with the doctors. From the COVID outbreak in February 2020 till ongoing 2021, their roles in every ward are indispensable. During COVID lockdown and emergency, they tirelessly work more than 12 h a day [31].

12.3.14.4 Role of Functional Medicine Coach and Practitioners

In the phases of lockdown and post lockdown in 2020, there were many micro-level health interventions where functional medicine coaches played essential roles. Functional medicine coaches and practitioners are highly skilled with versatile expertise in health, hygiene, and essential nutrition. They have had such capacity to move for the suffering people within their zone and provided knowledge of COVID safety measures. As per data, many practitioners (FMP) attended to the COVID-positive patients for their vital health and psychological counseling. Additionally, they provided instant cum helpful suggestions on good functional foods virtually through video calls. That effort was indeed beneficial in preventing COVID infections primarily for their neighbors and friends' circles available on social media [32].

12.3.14.5 Patients Records and Feedbacks [33]

- Patient data and records are stored in-app memory. Different apps have different systems, like in some app, patients can open their profile to feed their data, which they can themselves track; this is useful in weight management cases.
- Outdoor/start-up consultation and follow-up consultation department wise.
- COVID patients and recovery data.
- Online COVID patients status assessments (city wise) and hospital admissions.
- Emergency services for COVID and other patients.
- Satisfactions assessments by feedbacks.
- Repeat visits online and overall reputation by Google/other search engines.

12.3.14.6 Continuum Care

Continuum care is an integrated system that systematically guides and tracks a patient under the comprehensive array of health services. It consists of caring for pregnant ladies from pre-delivery to postnatal care and continuous follow-ups. It also works with chronic patients. Continuum care is moreover essential for older adults [34].

12.3.14.7 Growing Demand of Virtual Diet Consultation: A Clinical Evidence

One of our authors is a practicing dietitian in Kolkata who contributed data from his database to compare the five-year status of virtual diet patients. The graph (Fig. 12.3) shows a significant hike in percentage in 2020 due to the COVID pandemic. People preferred to take consultations only on virtual modes. The graph shows nearly 90% of patients attended online for a virtual consultation in 2020, whereas 10–30% of patients consulted from 2016 to 2019.

The same author, one of the best practicing dietitians, got virtual diet consultations and identified the health issues shown in the graph (Fig. 12.4). Obesity among all lifestyles disorders was highest in December 2020 from April 2020 to March 2021.

12.3.15 Significant Challenges in Telemedicine and Diet Consultations

In the urban areas, telehealth and telemedicine have already got popularity due to instant access to all medical services. In the rural sections, people worldwide are facing challenges. There are issues like the broadband network not being available in the rural and some micro areas almost in every country. Low-economic countries face more issues with these services due to installation problems and financial returns from the villagers. India and other South Asian countries have more than 50% of people living below the poverty line who struggle with food, clothes, and shelter as basic needs. Most African countries are also deprived of internet and telecommunications facilities like India and Bangladesh. However, the respective

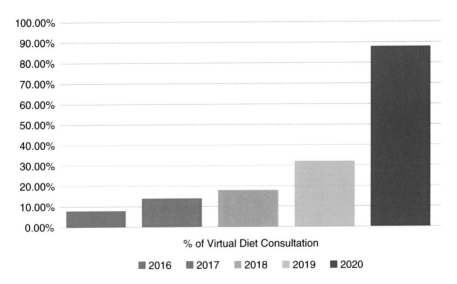

Fig. 12.3 Five years (2016–2020) virtual diet consultation by a leading dietitian located in a metro city

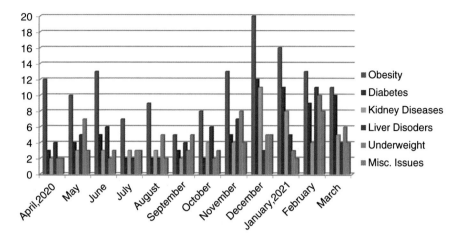

Fig. 12.4 Health issues identified through the virtual diet consultation from April 2020 to March 2021

governments adopt various easy regulations cum policies to reach modern digital services everywhere [35].

Diet consultations through telemedicine have been growing and getting popular over the decades in India and other countries. American, European, and Asian countries are significantly progressing with on-demand diet consultation through various popular teleconsultations portals where they generate revenues. However, there are some primary challenges on diet parts also. Diet and nutritional counseling are still not reachable in rural areas due to a lack of awareness and financial issues despite the internet. The perceptions of ordinary people are not updated and upgraded even in the urban areas. Diet consultations are limited to weight management, particularly obesity, diabetes, and other lifestyle disorders, but it has a wide practicing area [36]. A well-planned (customized) diet prepared duly with affordable and available food can help many diseases and conditions. Physicians and specialists refer the patients to dietitians for primary consultations and counseling to get rid of weight, sugar control, and other health issues. Therefore, diet consultations and basic nutritional counseling have been the sub-domains of telehealth in almost all countries for the last few years. Some key points to overcome challenges are nutrition education, care plan development, counseling, screening, assessments, and discharge planning in institutional and private settings. We are hopeful about the coming days that people will be more aware and concerned about diet consolations because food as medicine believed since old age.

12.4   Conclusion

In the COVID-19 phases, it has become of utmost concern to follow safety measures to avoid virus transmission in patients and healthcare professionals. Doctors, dietitians, and functional medicine coaches must attend to patients on general health issues or COVID infections. Our study significantly focussed on the roles of diet and dietitians during the COVID pandemic, which is still ongoing. A healthy lifestyle is essential to prevent any virus, including COVID-19, primarily through a balanced diet, minimum level of exercise, and a positive mind. Food as medicine is considered because food can only protect a human body from any pathogen by solid immunity. Therefore, effective and customized diet planning based on available and affordable food has become an integral part of telemedicine services during the COVID era.

References

1. Kichloo A, Albosta M, Dettloff K, et al. telemedicine, the current COVID-19 pandemic, and the future: a narrative review and perspectives moving forward in the USA. Fam Med Commun Health. 2020;8:e000530. https://doi.org/10.1136/fmch-2020-000530.
2. Dasgupta A, Deb S. Telemedicine: a new horizon in public health in India. Indian J Commun Med. 2008;33:3–8. https://doi.org/10.4103/0970-0218.39234.
3. Ryu S. History of telemedicine: evolution, context, and transformation. Health Inform Res. 2010;16:65–6. https://doi.org/10.4258/hir.2010.16.1.6.
4. COVID situation. Source: World Health Organization. https://covid19.who.int/region/searo/country/in. Accessed on 10th May 2021.
5. Serper M, Volk ML. Current and future applications of telemedicine to optimize the delivery of care in chronic liver disease. Clin Gastroenterol Hepatol. 2018;16:157–161.e8. https://doi.org/10.1016/j.cgh.2017.10.004.
6. Rodríguez-Rey R, Garrido-Hernansaiz H, Collado S. psychological impact and associated factors during the initial stage of the Coronavirus (COVID-19) pandemic among the general population in Spain. Front Psychol. 2020;11:1540. Available from: https://www.frontiersin.org/article/10.3389/fpsyg.2020.01540
7. Roy A, Singh AK, Mishra S, Chinnadurai A, Mitra A, Bakshi O. Mental health implications of COVID-19 pandemic and its response in India. Int J Soc Psychiatry. 2021;67(5):587–600. https://doi.org/10.1177/0020764020950769.
8. Dash S, Aarthy R, Mohan V. Telemedicine during COVID-19 in India—a new policy and its challenges. J Public Health Policy. 2021; https://doi.org/10.1057/s41271-021-00287-w. Accessed on 25th May 2021
9. Aman F, Masood S. How nutrition can help to fight against COVID-19 Pandemic. Pak J Med Sci. 2020;36:S121–3. https://doi.org/10.12669/pjms.36.COVID19-S4.2776.
10. Banerjee S, Srivastava S, Giri AK. Possible nutritional approach to cope up COVID-19 in Indian perspective. Adv Res J Med Clin Sci. 2020;06:207–19.
11. Banerjee S. The essence of Indian indigenous knowledge in the perspective of Ayurveda, Nutrition, and Yoga. Res Rev Biotechnol Biosci. 2020;7:20–7.
12. Kotecha R. The journey with COVID-19: initiatives by Ministry of AYUSH. J Ayurveda Integr Med. 2021;12:1–3. https://doi.org/10.1016/j.jaim.2021.03.009.
13. Paper W, Kumar P, Thakker D, Arora L. Assessing impact of COVID-19 on AB-PMJAY. Available at: www.pmjay.gov.in. Accessed on 10th May 2021.
14. Diabetes (India), National Diabetes Obesity and Cholesterol Foundation (NDOC), and Nutrition Expert Group, India. Balanced nutrition is needed in times of COVID19 epidemic in India: a call for action for all nutritionists and physicians. Diabetes Metab Syndr. 2020;14:1747–50. https://doi.org/10.1016/j.dsx.2020.08.030.
15. Margarethe Urbanek. Is the corona crisis pushing telemedicine? Published on 19th May 2020. Available at: https://www.aerztezeitung.de/Podcasts/Pusht-die-Corona-Krise-die-Telemedizin-409613.html. Accessed on 15th May 2021.

16. E-Health—Digitization in Health Care. May 26.2021. https://www.bundesgesundheitsminis-terium.de/e-health-initiative.html. Accessed on 5th June 2021.
17. Cioti A, Stănescu A, Grăjdeanu I, et al. Telemedicine in Europe: current status and future perspectives. Mod Med. 2019;26:165–8. https://doi.org/10.31689/rmm.2019.26.4.165.
18. Almathami HKY, Win KT, Vlahu-Gjorgievska E. Barriers and facilitators that influence telemedicine-based, real-time, online consultation at patients' homes: systematic literature review. J Med Internet Res. 2020;22:e16407. https://doi.org/10.2196/16407.
19. Intan Sabrina M, Defi IR. Telemedicine guidelines in South East Asia: a scoping review. Front Neurol. 2021;11:1760. https://doi.org/10.3389/fneur.2020.581649.
20. Mehta P, Stahl MG, Germone MM, et al. Telehealth and nutrition support during the COVID-19 pandemic. J Acad Nutr Diet. 2020;120:1953–7. https://doi.org/10.1016/j.jand.2020.07.013.
21. Deldar K, Bahaadinbeigy K, Tara SM. Teleconsultation and clinical decision making: a systematic review. Acta Inform Med. 2016;24:286–92. https://doi.org/10.5455/aim.2016.24.286-292.
22. Zhao P, Yoo I, Lavoie J, Lavoie BJ, Simoes E. Web-based medical appointment systems: a systematic review. J Med Internet Res. 2017;19:e134. https://doi.org/10.2196/jmir.6747.
23. Kogan S, Zeng Q, Ash N, Greenes RA. Problems and challenges in patient information retrieval: a descriptive study. Proc AMIA Symp. 2001;329-333
24. Chordiya SV, Garge BM. E-pharmacy vs. conventional pharmacy. IP Int J Compr Adv Pharmacol. 2020;3:121–3. https://doi.org/10.18231/2456-9542.2018.0027.
25. Kapilan N, Vidhya P, Gao X-Z. Virtual laboratory: a boon to the mechanical engineering education during Covid-19 Pandemic. Higher Educ Future. 2021;8:31–46.
26. Top 10 Telemedicine Companies in the World, 2020. Available at: https://www.fortunebusinessinsights.com/blog/top-10-telemedicine-companies-2020-10077. Accessed on 25th May 2021.
27. Eight Indian digital health companies received $40 million in VC funds in Q3 2020. Available at: https://www.expresshealthcare.in/news/eight-indian-digital-health-companies-received-40-million-in-vc-funds-in-q3-2020/425334. Accessed on 25th May 2021.
28. Wootton R, Liu J, Bonnardot L. Quality assurance of teleconsultations in a store-and-forward telemedicine network – obtaining patient follow-up data and user feedback. Front public Heal. 2014;2:247. https://doi.org/10.3389/fpubh.2014.00247.
29. Brugliera, L., Spina, A., Castellazzi, P., et al. Nutritional management of COVID-19 patients in a rehabilitation unit. Eur J Clin Nutr, 2020; 860–863. https://doi.org/10.1038/s41430-020-0664-x
30. Monaghesh, E., Hajizadeh, A. The role of telehealth during COVID-19 outbreak: a systematic review based on current evidence. BMC Public Health 2020; 1193. https://doi.org/10.1186/s12889-020-09301-4.
31. Fawaz M, Anshasi H, Samaha A. Nurses at the front line of COVID-19: roles, responsibilities, risks, and rights. Am J Trop Med Hyg. 2020;103:1341–2. https://doi.org/10.4269/ajtmh.20-0650.
32. Evans JM, Luby R, Lukaczer D, et al. The functional medicine approach to COVID-19: virus-specific nutraceutical and botanical agents. Integr Med (Encinitas). 2020;19:34–42.
33. Wali RM, Alqahtani RM, Alharazi SK, Bukhari SA, Quqandi SM. Patient satisfaction with the implementation of electronic medical records in the Western Region, Saudi Arabia, 2018. BMC Fam Pract. 2020;21:37. https://doi.org/10.1186/s12875-020-1099-0.
34. De Regge M, De Pourcq K, Meijboom B, Trybou J, Mortier E, Eeckloo K. The role of hospitals in bridging the care continuum: a systematic review of coordination of care and follow-up for adults with chronic conditions: a BMC Health Serv Res. 2017;17:550. https://doi.org/10.1186/s12913-017-2500-0.
35. Board on Health Care Services; Institute of Medicine. The Role of Telehealth in an Evolving Health Care Environment: Workshop Summary. Washington (DC): National Academies Press (US); 2012 Nov 20. 4, Challenges in Telehealth. Available at: https://www.ncbi.nlm.nih.gov/books/NBK207146/. Accessed on 29th May 2021.
36. Brunton C, Arensberg MB, Drawert S, Badaracco C, Everett W, McCauley SM. Perspectives of registered dietitian nutritionists on adoption of telehealth for nutrition care during the COVID-19 pandemic. Healthcare (Basel). 2021;9:235. https://doi.org/10.3390/healthcare9020235.

Telemedicine and Healthcare Ecosystem in India: A Review, Critique and Research Agenda

13

Parag Sunil Shukla and Sofia Devi Shamurailatpam

13.1 Introduction

Over the decades, the information and communication technology has revolutionized how individuals across the globe connected, seek for exchange of resources and play a significant potential to help and address contemporary health problems. This makes us redesign the form of telemedicine which has a broader applicability resulting into the use of ICT in order to improve the health of the patients. The concept of telemedicine signifies an important position in the distribution and allocation of healthcare services with an aim to reduce the distances and expansion of outreach particularly in remote and underserved regions for diagnosis, treatment as well as prevention of life-threatening diseases [1]. The main objectives of adoption of the ICT in the healthcare sector is to improve health outcomes of the patients through clinical support, overcoming the geographical boundaries/barriers provided the availability of various forms of ICT across the regions and places of corners of the country. The concept of telemedicine is a major development in the healthcare sector and its demand is expected to increase over the years to come. However, there are constraints in such adoption of technology-based platform in healthcare setting where personal interaction is preferred and patients are reluctant to adapt to newer formats of medical consultation. In other words, how technology can intervene in such a way to capitalize on the advantages of telemedicine so as to produce robust system that will deliver an acceptable, affordable services with suitable prices for

P. S. Shukla (✉)
Department of Commerce and Business Management, Faculty of Commerce, The Maharaja Sayajirao University of Baroda, Vadodara, Gujarat, India

S. D. Shamurailatpam
Department of Banking and Insurance, Faculty of Commerce, The Maharaja Sayajirao University of Baroda, Vadodara, Gujarat, India
e-mail: sofia.devi-bi@msubaroda.ac.in

the masses. With this backdrop, this research study aims to present a conceptual framework with regard to technology in healthcare system and throw light on the research gaps in the extant literature that can be furthered upon for enhancing the service delivery of healthcare system using digital technology. This chapter highlights the significance of telemedicine, the scope and availability in the healthcare delivery system and also the critical aspects to address for optimal healthcare system given the institutional, economic, political and regulatory framework.

The market for telemedicine has grown significantly in the recent years, preferably after the onset of COVID-19 pandemic. According to the recent data of WHO, telemedicine at the global market value is placed at around 50 billion US dollars and the forecast value is projected to nearly 460 billion US dollars by the year 2030. This rise in the market segment of telemedicine in the near future is a key driver for use of digital health tools and infusion of new investment funding in the digital health industry.

As against the investment in digital health industry to around one billion US dollars in 2010, it soared up to over 21 billion US dollars in 2020. One of the significant contributions of telemedicine is increase in access to healthcare services particularly to underserved segments of population, whereby impacting positively for health services enabling them to seek treatment and improving the quality of life.

Economic infrastructure in most of the developing countries is poor and inadequate, along with limited financial resources, posing limitations on where telemedicine can be implemented. According to the WHO (2010), provision of telemedicine is much progressed in high-income countries than other classifications of global population group as per the World Bank database, with African and Eastern Mediterranean regions having the least coverage. The economically developed nations have a sufficient level of information technology which is a foundation for telemedicine which is vice versa with emerging economies. The chapter contains eight different sections. The next section gives a blueprint of adoption of telemedicine across countries over a period of time. Section 13.3 gives the rationale of the study. The next section addresses about the objectives of the study, data and methodology. Section 13.5 gives a summary of the review of literature collected based on diverse aspects of telemedicine. Sections 13.6 and 13.7 gives strategic implications and policy imperatives, respectively, followed by concluding remarks.

13.2 A Blueprint of Telemedicine Adoption

In this section, we put forward different dimensions of adoption of telemedicine under given phases of gradual development. The first figure gives the strategy of telemedicine under three different phases as shown (Fig. 13.1). Generally, telemedicine can be used as a strategy to reach out the masses through various phases. In other words, telemedicine services are approved or sanctioned through a proper regulatory mechanism to reach the markets.

As discussed in Fig. 13.1, the authors have explained the telemedicine strategy which has evolved over a period of time. Phase I relates to targeting the prioritized

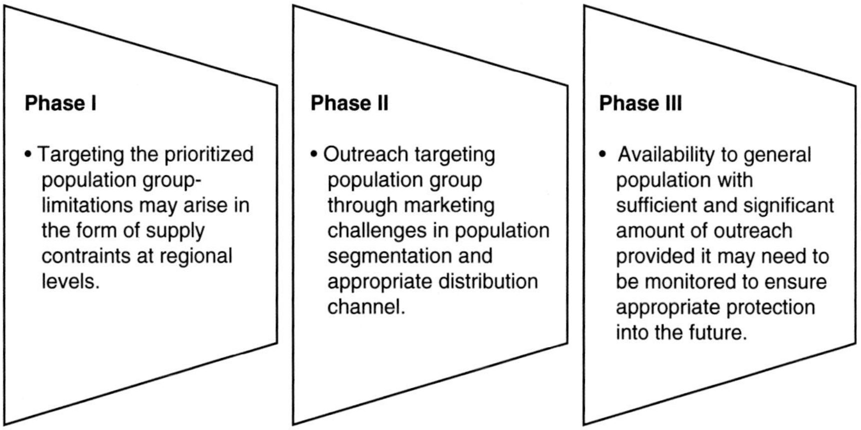

Phase I

- Targeting the prioritized population group-limitations may arise in the form of supply contraints at regional levels.

Phase II

- Outreach targeting population group through marketing challenges in population segmentation and appropriate distribution channel.

Phase III

- Availability to general population with sufficient and significant amount of outreach provided it may need to be monitored to ensure appropriate protection into the future.

Fig. 13.1 Telemedicine strategy: a phased approach
Source: Prepared by Authors

population group particularly the remote and rural areas with poor health infrastructures, provided proper necessary framework of connectivity for performing services of telemedicine.

In Phase II, the outreach is expanded to cover the other population group through marketing with population segmentation and appropriate instruments. In the Phase III, the general population be targeted with full fledge marketing and coverage with monitoring and appropriate facilities.

There are certain parameters that determine the adoption of telemedicine across different segments of population, particularly from the perspectives of the developing countries especially India. To put together, adoption and implementation of technology is contingent on institutional arrangements and economic infrastructures facilitated in terms of six A's– availability, administrations, accessibility, acceptability and affordability as well as accountability [2].

Exhibit 13.1 explains the key parameters of telemedicine adoption under 6As, namely availability, administrable, accessible, acceptable, affordability and accountability aspects. Each of the attributes has significant impact in the adoption and implementation of telemedicine across time and space, and a detailed aspect under each of the A's is highlighted in the Box which is self-explanatory

The model exhibited in Fig. 13.2 elucidates the concept of telemedicine and depicts how various ingredients, viz. telementoring, telemonitoring and teleconsulting, are affected by the enablers; for example, improving accuracy, effective diagnosis, remote treatment and the advances in human intelligence are acting as drivers of growth for telemedicine. The aspects of AI, ML, VR and sensor technologies are taking telemedicine to greater heights. On the other hand, there are some forces that restrain the growth of telemedicine, viz. lack of connectivity, infrastructure bottlenecks, lack of digital awareness, regulatory mechanisms, inadequate training,

Exhibit 13.1 Key parameters of telemedicine adoption: a continuum

Availability	• Availability of adequate information technology (IT) infrastructure for delivery of the services • Services are available through a proper regulatory mechanism to reach to the markets • Upstream/downstream sources of telemedicine services and significance of public policy planning • Telemedicine be available as a public good with all its characteristics of non-rivalry and non-excludability
Administrable	• End-to-end services be administered at regular intervals • Administering the population segment particularly rural and hinterland areas • Centre to administer for handling technology discrepancy in the delivery of services
Accessible	• Easy and comfort applications preferably in local languages and simple steps so as to understand easily and get access • Infrastructure to access the services from different locations and for ordering/purchasing of the products • Accessibility to internet services
Acceptable	• Consumers have accurate information and develop trust, and they choose to adapt telemedicine services • Better information and awareness campaign to bring trust and confidence towards the people
Affordability	• Costs of such services/products available are amenable to both the parties—the suppliers including government and the private bodies on the one side and the consumers/patients on the other side for proper diagnosis and treatment • Funding and financing facilities to make operational at efficacy • Concession rates or lower fees structure for underprivileged groups and weaker sections of the society living in rural and remote areas
Accountability	• Patients receive full course of treatment and monitoring after the implementation of such strategy at mass level • Role of information technology (IT) infrastructure and interoperability • Ongoing monitoring and reporting mechanism and disclosure practices

Source: Prepared by authors

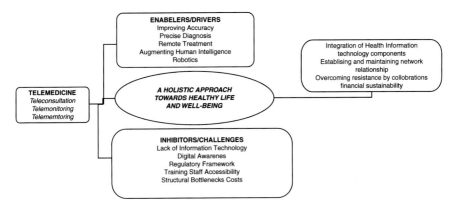

Fig. 13.2 A conceptual model of telemedicine—an integrative approach

problem of accountability, and costs. The authors in this research paper have identi-fied key result areas to mitigate the ill effects caused by the challenges and restrain-ing forces and have identified some critical factors, viz. integration of health information and technology-based components. This can be better achieved by establishing and maintaining network of relationships between the service provider and beneficiaries of telemedicine. Further, to overcome the resistance in terms of outlay costs and financial implications, there is a need for a collaborative approach for shared sense of purpose.

13.3   Rationale and Significance of the Study

According to a forecast by international consultancy Price Waterhouse Coopers, it is estimated that India would be among the top 10 global growth markets for health-care and nutrition. The significance of telemedicine and telehealthcare services stands substantial in the optimal healthcare system in India in the years ahead. To say, India's healthcare sector was expected to grow by threefold between the years 2016 and 2022 to reach US dollar 372 billion [3]. The painstaking efforts of the Indian government have resulted into Ayushman Bharat initiative for healthcare and Unnat Bharat Initiative [UBA] to offer services to the rural hinterlands that survive with vulnerability. The concept of telemedicine is a major development in the healthcare sector and its demand is expected to increase over the years to come. However, there are constraints in such adoption of technology-based platform in healthcare in that the conventional form of healthcare delivery system with face-to-face interaction stands essential to the processes of optimal healthcare system and such mechanisms could not replace the real thing experienced through physical way of consultation. In other words, how technology can intervene in such a way to capi-talize on the advantages of telemedicine so as to produce robust system that will deliver an acceptable, affordable services with suitable prices for the masses. With this backdrop, this chapter attempts to present a conceptual framework with regard to technology in healthcare system and throw light on the research gaps in the extant literature that can be furthered upon for enhancing the service delivery of healthcare system using digital technology.

13.4   Objectives, Data and Methodology

In this chapter the researcher proposition is to provide a firm theoretical perspective with regard to telemedicine that is at the nascent stage particularly when it comes to penetration of services to the masses. Further, the researchers also proposed a con-ceptual model in which there is interplay of enablers/drivers of telemedicine along with the inhibitors and challenges. This dynamism can be managed with the judi-cious use of technology by seamless integration of health technology components which ultimately results into a holistic approach towards healthy life and well-being for the masses and not only for the classes.

The study adopts a simple methodology to analyse the various aspects of telemedicine and its significance in the healthcare industry system.

The methodology approach used in this chapter is presented into different forms: (i) databases are distinguished from Science Direct, Web of Science, JSTOR and Google scholar; (ii) in order to collect data, keywords are used in the search standards; (iii) all the collected papers/articles are analysed from key dimensions of telemedicine; (iv) in the next step the studies are grouped based on major issues and themes pertaining to telemedicine; and (v) lastly, the study pattern highlights the research gaps, loopholes and setting up scope for future studies.

The chapter tries to assimilate various research studies that have been conducted with objective with purpose to add on the extant literature. From the various analyses of research papers/articles, huge gap exists between the content of available literatures on the telemedicine and thus this work will prove to be helpful to policy makers, practioners and entrepreneurs to further the scalability of telemedicine.

13.5   Tabular Summary on Telemedicine: Review of literature

This section gives a summary on the aspects of telemedicine based on review of literature of research papers and articles. The rationale behind undertaking this summarization is to pin down the context, type, and the categories of research work undertaken in the domain of telemedicine.

Sr. no.	Author/s	Year	Type of paper/ research	Context	Source
1	Gachabayov et al. [4]	2020	Conceptual	Telemedicine and use of robotic technology in super speciality hospitals and treatment of patients in COVID-19 Pandemic	International Journal of Surgery Protocol
2	Wu et al. [5]	2021	Empirical	Investigating the key facets of adoption of telemedicine by resident doctors and their intentions towards teleconsultation, telemonitoring. The social-cognitive theory was tested with the Cohorts	Health Policy and Technology
3	Verbraecken [6]	2021	Conceptual	Adoption of telemedicine in sleep disordered breathing	Sleep Medicine Clinics
4	Cassar et al. [7]	2021	Empirical	Telemedicine and its use during pandemic for saving people of Malta from the virus attack by rehabilitative care	International Journal of Infectious Diseases

Sr. no.	Author/s	Year	Type of paper/ research	Context	Source
5	Sekhon et al. [8]	2020	Conceptual	Role of telemedicine in monitoring, treatment, and overall well-being of senior citizens and elderly single couples suffering from mental disorders	Maturitas
6	Kruse et al. [9]	2020	Conceptual	Telemedicine and its connotation with healthcare service providers and the claim settlement aspect with mediclaim service provider companies	Health Policy and Technology
7	Corbett et al. [10]	2020	Conceptual	Adoption of telemedicine for treatment of chronic disease	International Journal of Cardiology Hypertension
8	William et al. [11]	2020	Conceptual	Adoption of telemedicine to connect and fill up a gap in current healthcare delivery, particularly remote and rural populations	Fertility and Sterility
9	Breitinger et al. [12]	2020	Conceptual	The use and adoption of telemedicine although in less reach and magnitude has created an impact in the minds of people and now they seek comfort, care and ease of services. The only untapped area is to build applications, software, and low-cost solutions to cultivate resilience and build capacity of existing system	Mayo Clinic Proceedings
10	Kondakov and Kulik [13]	2020	Conceptual	Development of Effective, low-cost technology and laser treatment for psoriasis	Procedia Computer Science
11	Paruthi [14]	2020	Review	Telemedicine can be delivered through many modalities to address the paediatric sleep disorders and can add significant information, saving travel time and costs	Sleep Medicine Clinic
12	Ortega et al. [15]	2020	Review	The critical function relates to government maintaining stricter regimes and rules for the telemedicine to ensure last mile coverage across the weaker and deprived classes	Health Policy and Technology

Sr. no.	Author/s	Year	Type of paper/ research	Context	Source
13	Albahri et al. [16]	2020	Empirical	In-depth study of telemedicine tools, mobile applications and how the service providers are making new infrastructural changes to equip for better services	Journal of Network and Computer Applications
14	Jha et al. [17]	2021	Conceptual	Examination of telemedicine and Community Health Projects in Asia with challenges for financial sustainability, technological infrastructure, integration in the healthcare system towards optimal implementation of telemedicine	Dermatologic Clinics
15	Zobair et al. [18]	2019	Empirical	A study of patient feedback and assessing family relatives sense of worth towards telemedicine	Social Science & Medicine
16	Avanesova, and Shamliyan [19]	2019	Review	The effectiveness of telemedicine is contingent upon the advances in software, international know-how, technical soundness and other macro-economic variables in a given political, social, and economic setting	Health Policy and Technology
17	Suzuki et al. [20]	2020	Empirical	IT penetration in select countries in Asia and Africa and its effects on adoption of telemedicine	Health Policy and Technology
18	Weinstein and Krupinski [21]	2018	Review	Telemedicine is at a preliminary stage and requires alignment with existing frameworks to offer specialized services	Medical Clinics of North America
19	Botrugno [22]	2018	Review	The ushering of telemedicine is changing the rules of the game and not only aims to provide care but also relates with deeper patient insights and control for diseases with wearables that help patients track and monitor their own health	Health Policy and Technology
20	Aaron P Lesher and Shah [23]	2018	Review	Telemedicine as a holistic care model for infant and childcare with reference to gynaecological problems	Seminars in Paediatric Surgery

Sr. no.	Author/s	Year	Type of paper/ research	Context	Source
21	Parimbellia et al. [24]	2018	Review	Governance and legal aspects with reference to patient safety and risk sharing with the use of latest gadgets for surgery	International Journal of Medical Informatics
22	Blue et al. [25]	2020	Review	Telemedicine is a front runner in terms of the advantages and an array of services it provides	World Neurosurgery
23	Abuzeineh et al. [26]	2020	Conceptual	Telemedicine can be effective source for various surgical interventions especially in a COVID-19 induced environment where physical distance is advisable. It gives secured, transparent and effective care	Transplantation Proceedings
24	Yamin and Alyoubi [27]	2020	Empirical	Analysis of individual behaviour towards adoption of telemedicine with Internet of things and health tracking wearables particularly amidst pandemic	Journal of Infection and Public Health
25	Samarraie et al. [28]	2020	Review	Adoption of telemedicine UAE and other nations	International Journal of Medical Informatics
26	Mishra [29]	2020	Empirical	Use of telemedicine for Diabetic patients	Health Policy and Technology
27	Rotker and Velez [30]	2020	Conceptual	The COVID-19 pandemic has led the medical community, its patients, insurance companies, and lawmakers to face the various challenges of telemedicine which stood its stand towards broader adoption	Fertility and Sterility
28	Mouchtouris et al. [31]	2020	Empirical	The study focussed on extent of use of telemedicine for critical surgeries and subsequent monitoring and care	World Neurosurgery
29	Leochico [32]	2020	Conceptual	Adoption of telerehabilitation as an aspect of telemedicine in developing country as a significant dimension of healthcare delivery system	Annals of Physical and Rehabilitation Medicine

Sr. no.	Author/s	Year	Type of paper/ research	Context	Source
30	Miller et al. [33]	2020	Review	Telemedicine is at a burgeoning stage and has a plethora of services ranging from cure, wellness, rehabilitation and continuous care for severe diseases	Journal of Pain and Symptom Management

The summary table shows that in the recent decades the implementation of telemedicine as one of the healthcare system is gradually increased across countries for detection and care of diverse diagnosis and treatment of patients. And in most of the recent studies on telemedicine it is observed that the focused and significance of telemedicine is intense after the pandemic COVID-19. During the post pandemic period, people across the globe with the social distancing norms have options available in the virtual mode as the safe way to deal with all aspects of life, with no exception of healthcare system.

Telehealth and telemedicine has been seen as one the safest way, cost-effective and saving of time to diagnose and undergo processes of curing and treatment for different diseases, detection of symptoms, common diseases, particularly in remote and underserved rural areas of the country. Our present study based on diverse aspects of access to healthcare system through telemedicine demonstrates that during the period from 2018 to 2021 latest studies, people opted for telemedicine as one of the mechanisms of healthcare system.

One significant contribution of this study is that our study is based on the latest studies on aspects of telemedicine adopted for healthcare system across the globe.

13.6 Strategic Implications and Key Discussions

The far-reaching adverse implications of the pandemic are on all the sectors of the economy and the healthcare sector is not an exception to it. Though the government and authorities has provided impetus towards stabilizing the state of the economy, the healthcare sector as a whole had to face crisis to use an access of basic health service. Here, the robust technology of telemedicine can come to rescue as a disruption in technology coupled with strong ties with infrastructure and ubiquitous institutional framework.

The notion of 'Atmanirbhar Bharat' epitomizes reduced dependence on foreign counter parts, thereby taking economy towards ample resources which can have a strong foothold and scope for indigenous telemedicine start-ups that can deliver optimal telehealth services efficiently to populace of India. The entrepreneurial spirit can be leveraged by proactive government actions that can have a positive impending effect on this mushrooming sector.

The Indian healthcare sector occupies a formidable position and has buoyant market in terms of delivery of healthcare service across countries around the world. Therefore, it is imperative for the Government to initiate such mechanisms to incorporate digitization and use of information technology in the healthcare sector which outreaches the rural and underserved areas of the remote areas of India. As a matter of fact, over the last 5 years India has received a significant amount of investment of US Dollar 600 Million out of which Singapore, the United States, and Europe has made significant contribution. The time is ripe for government to rethink and redesign the telemedicine framework with regulatory structure to provide affordable and accessible healthcare services taking into account geographic and demographic profile of the country.

Telemedicine can be enhanced significantly if there is a health worker with the patient when seeking opinion from a specialist. The primary health worker can share the clinical details, relevant past medical records and can also follow-up on the specialists' advice. The primary health worker gives the essential 'human touch' to telemedicine.The primary health worker will also optimize the use of telemedicine. Teleconsultations are manageable for a populous country like India as even the patients can get healthcare advice without putting the doctors at the risk of infection transmission. Teleconsultations works very well with follow-up patients as they already trust the doctor and even the patient's medical history is already known. The problem happens for new patients as the adequate connect have not formed and due to trust issues patients are not comfortable in sharing the images and videos of areas of concern.

Though telemedicine has shown to be very effective in the delivery of non-emergency care, there still does not exist enough awareness and training of doctors to conduct the same. Today telemedicine has become so vast that you cannot learn how to do telemedicine by switching on your video camera. There is a need for formal training and exposure to telehealth. To practice telemedicine, the body language of the doctor is very critical.

The doctor should be able to answer the patients' doubts clearly and make the patients feel that you are empathizing with them. As India battles the third wave of COVID-19, it has become clear that our country must work expeditiously to iron out deficiencies in its vast network of Primary Healthcare Centers. Primary Healthcare Centers (PHCs) are the first and in most cases the only access to medical support in rural and remote areas. The coming together of technology and healthcare over the last decade has changed the face of healthcare, and one outcome has been the empowering of healthcare providers to administer care remotely.

The ongoing transformation of healthcare to a tech-driven digital avatar gained tremendous importance during the past year and a half as it helped to connect patients with doctors even in the face of challenges such as lockdowns and social distancing that impacted access. The adoption has been supported by increased deployment and development of technologies that make digital healthcare convenient and cost-effective. One of the reasons for the rise in the prevalence of such inveterate maladies, viz. diabetes, heart-related ailments and life-threatening diseases like cancer, is due to the increasing stress in the life of people. Digital health has been especially beneficial to patients with non-communicable diseases that require constant monitoring.

In these cases, remote monitoring through m-health technologies and review of data from digital tools and wearables has changed the way chronic diseases can be managed. Connected health has changed the way that patients interact with healthcare and healthcare systems, while also changing the approach from acute and reactive to proactive and preventive.

However, there are challenges to be addressed and overcome in the implementation and integration of digital health by healthcare providers. These include issues of security and interoperability between disparate healthcare organizations, lack of bandwidth leading to low image resolution and video quality that is not adequate for healthcare applications, access to technical support in case of any problems, difficulty in integrating with the organizational culture, and lack of last mile access to providers in remote areas. It is here that technology platforms provide a connected health ecosystem for healthcare providers that address the challenges with regard to digital interfaces and connected devices to facilitate integration. These platforms help healthcare providers desire to take a virtual leap into the digital health space. These platforms also take away the need for healthcare providers to set up IT systems with servers/data centres and IT professionals. Using cloud and mobile-based technology, these technology platforms are helping providers to adopt a new digital health model, overcoming challenges of integration and interoperability.

13.7 Policy Imperatives

Telemedicine has a broad spectrum as it serves to give a patient focused protection and also gives a live expert care to the patients who do not require hospitalization. It also entails patient well-being and information security and offers plethora of rehabilitative services that is focused on preventive care.

Because of its wide range of utility, telemedicine is being taken on by the overall professionals as an enterprising move towards one side while it is likewise being consolidated in well-being arrangements by the legislatures for money saving advantages and to fortify the existing healthcare setting.

Arogya Setu Mobile Application is one such example that epitomizes the ability of technology to trace, track and monitor health and well-being especially in the pandemic.

A hindrance to the expansion of telemedicine is the immature financial framework, i.e. the cost and investment bottlenecks. The whole scope of the convenience of telemedicine is expansive in India.

While the doctors are consolidating the telemedicine devices into their medical practice to offer holistic and continuous care, on the other end the tertiary care centres are connected to those patients and outpatient individuals who seek consultations and medicines/drugs at their place of residence. This is having a positive impact as there is a lesser burden on the hospitalization, saving the tertiary care clinics and hospitals for the sick and patients who need life-saving support systems. As in this digitized modern economy, telemedicine has a significant scope in the efficient delivery of healthcare services though it has constraints in terms of costs and operation, hence a question of affordability and adaptability among the people. For equitable and affordable services across the patients, the role of the tertiary care hospitals is significant and should incorporate telehealth platforms for efficacy in the healthcare delivery system.

13.8 Concluding Remarks

The telemedicine will probably bring a paradigm shift in the medical care system even after the pandemic ends and it will be an important element for the eventual fate of healthcare service providers. There are many uncertainties concerning the job of healthcare works, and in Indian setting an integrative approach is needed to consolidate telemedicine with in-person care for various conditions of diseases across the geographies. Establishing inclusive care and equality with low-cost affordable telemedicine is only possible with public private partnership [PPP] models that are fostered by collaboration and strong alliance for public good. Telemedicine is at a takeoff platform given the use of (AI) applications, which are quickly advancing for rehabilitative and preventive care. A robust well-being and healthcare structure must be set up to empower the telemedicine frameworks. Rules, authorizing pre-essentials, preparing schedules, conventions and interoperability guidelines must be institutionalized and redefined to implement an effective telemedicine adoption in India. The digitization and use of AI will be the forerunners that will take healthcare to the next level.

The authors in this research study purport that a complicated technology will not solve emblematic healthcare problems of a populous country like India. This scenario was figurative especially when COVID-19 pandemic caused panic, disorder, and anarchy for availability of healthcare amenities. Further, the authors would also emphasize that telemedicine has to evolve as an affordable full-bodied network to resolve crisis situations in healthcare too. Newer forms of embedded technologies need to be used for predictive care which can save people's lives especially at the bottom-of-pyramid markets.

The use of emergent technologies such as two-way videos, easy-to-use applications with multi-lingual support and SOS signalling are still to be probed upon to enhance the reach of telemedicine. There is a need to address 'burning issues' in the context of telecommunications and internet availability in the rural and sub-urban areas of India. The question to be addressed is that how telemedicine can make a difference in the lives of people who cannot afford a smart phone. There is a need for purposive deliberation with regard to the interoperatability of mobile applications and user interface. In conclusion, there is a need to determine all the possibilities technology has to offer with regard to the governance, adoption and implementation of telemedicine given the structural and socio-economic milieu.

References

1. WHO Report. https://www.who.int/publications/i/item/9789241564021. 2010. Accessed 12 Dec 2021
2. Mckinsey and Company Report. Path to the next new normal. 2020. https://www.mckinsey.com/~/media/McKinsey/Featured. Accessed 20 Dec 2021
3. PWC Annual Report. Retrieved from https://www.pwc.nl/nl/onze-organisatie/jaarbericht2020/pdf/pwc-annual-report-2019-2020.pdf. 2019, assessed on May 17, 2021.
4. Gachabayov M, Latifi LA, Parsikia A, Latifi R. Current state and future perspectives of telemedicine use in surgery during the COVID-19 pandemic: a scoping review protocol. Int J Surg Protoc. 2020;24(2020):17–20.
5. Wu D, Gu H, Gu S, You H. Individual motivation and social influence: a study of telemedicine adoption in China based on social cognitive theory. Health Policy Technol. 2021;10(2021):100525. 1–10
6. Verbraecken J. Telemedicine in sleep-disordered breathing. Journal of Sleep and Medicine. 2021;16(3):417–45.
7. Cassar MR, Borg D, Camilleri L, Schembri A, Anastasi EA, Buhagiar K, Callus C, Grech M. A novel use of telemedicine during the COVID-19 pandemic. Int J Infect Dis. 2021;103(2021):182–7.
8. Sekhon H, Sekhon K, Launay C, Afililo M, Innocente N, Vahia I, Rej S, Beauchet O. Telemedicine and the rural dementia population: a systematic review. Maturitas. 2021;143(2021):105–14.
9. Kruse CS, Williams K, Bohls J, Shamsi W. Telemedicine and health policy: a systematic review. Health Policy Technol. 2020; https://doi.org/10.1016/j.hlpt.2020.10.006.
10. Corbett JA, Opladen JM, Bisognano JD. Telemedicine can revolutionize the treatment of chronic disease. Int J Cardiol Hypertens. 2020;7(2020):100051.
11. Williams T, Goldstein M, Alexis, and Zev. Clinical Implications of Telemedicine for providers and patients. Fertil Steril Rev. 2020;114(6):1123–33.
12. Breitinger S, Gentry MT, Hilty DM. Key opportunities for the COVID-19 response to create a path to sustainable telemedicine services. Mayo Clin Proc. 2020; https://doi.org/10.1016/j.mayocp.2020.09.034.
13. Kondakov A, Kulik S. Intelligent information system for telemedicine. Procedia Comput Sci. 2020;169(2020):240–3.
14. Paruthi S. Telemedicine in paediatric sleep. Sleep Med Clin. 2020;15(2020):e1–7. https://doi.org/10.1016/j.jsmc.2020.07.003.
15. Ortega G, Rodriguez JA, Maurer LR, Witt EE, Perez N, Reich A, Bates DW. Telemedicine, COVID-19, and disparities: policy implications. Health Policy Technol. 2020;9(2020):368–71.
16. Albahri, A.S., Jwan K A., Taha, Z.K., Sura, F.I., Hamid, R.A., Zaidan, A.A., Albahri,O.S., Zaidan,B.B., Alamoodi,A.H., and Alsalem, M.A. (2020). IoT-based telemedicine for disease prevention and health promotion: State-of-the-Art. J Netw Comput Appl, 1-59. https://doi.org/10.1016/j.jnca.2020.102873.
17. Jha AK, Sawka E, Tiwari B, Dong H, Chiat D, Ghaemi S, Zhang X, Jha AK. Telemedicine and community health projects in Asia. Dermatol Clin. 2021;39(2021):23–32. https://doi.org/10.1016/j.det.2020.08.003.
18. Zobair KM, Sanzogni L, Sandhu K. Expectations of telemedicine health service adoption in rural Bangladesh. Soc Sci Med. 2019;238(2019):112485. https://doi.org/10.1016/j.socscimed.2019.112485.
19. Avanesova AA, Shamliyan TA. Worldwide implementation of telemedicine programs in association with research performance and health policy. Health Policy Technol. 2019;8(2019):179–91.
20. Suzuki T, Hotta J, Kuwabara T, Yamashina H, Ishikawa T, Tani Y, Ogasawara K. Possibility of introducing telemedicine services in Asian and African countries. Health Policy Technol. 2020;9(2020):13–22. https://doi.org/10.1016/j.hlpt.2020.01.006.

21. Weinstein RS, Krupinski EA. Clinical examination component of telemedicine, telehealth, mHealth, and connected health medical practices. Med Clin N Am. 2018;102(3):533–44. https://doi.org/10.1016/j.mcna.2018.01.002.
22. Botrugno C. Telemedicine in daily practice: addressing legal challenges while waiting for and EU regulatory framework. Health Policy Technol. 2018; https://doi.org/10.1016/j.hlpt.2018.04.003.
23. Lesher AP, Shah SR. Telemedicine in the perioperative experience. Semin Paediatr Surg. 2018;27(2):102–6. https://doi.org/10.1053/j.sempedsurg.2018.02.007.
24. Parimbellia E, Bottalicob B, Losiouka E, Tomasic M, Santosuossob A, Lanzolaa G, Quaglinia S, Bellazzia R. Trusting telemedicine: a discussion on risks, safety, legal implications and liability of involved stakeholders. Int J Med Inform. 2018;112(20180):90–8. https://doi.org/10.1016/j.ijmedinf.2018.01.012.
25. Blue R, Yang AI, Zhou C, Ravin ED, Teng CW, Arguelles GR, Huang V, Wathen C, Miranda SP, Marcotte P, Malhotra NR, Welch WC, Lee JYK. Telemedicine in the era of coronavirus disease 2019 (COVID-19): a neurosurgical perspective. World Neurosurg. 2020;139:549–57.
26. Abuzeineh M, Muzaale AD, Crews DC, Avery RK, Brotman DJ, Brennan DC, Segev DL, Ammary FA. Telemedicine in the care of kidney transplant recipients with coronavirus disease 2019: case reports. Transplant Proc. 2020;52(9):2620–5.
27. Yamin MAY, Alyoubi BA. Adoption of telemedicine applications among Saudi citizens during COVID-19 pandemic: An alternative health delivery. J Infect Public Health. 2020;13(12):1845–55.
28. Samarraie HA, Ghazal S, Alzahrani AB, Moody L. Telemedicine in middle Eastern countries: progress, barriers, and policy recommendations. Int J Med Inform. 2020;141(104232) https://doi.org/10.1016/j.ijmedinf.2020.104232.
29. Mishra V. Telemedicine in chronic care- a case of diabetes management. Health Policy Technol. 2020;9(1):7–22. https://doi.org/10.1016/j.hlpt.2020.01.007.
30. Rotker K, Velez D. Where will telemedicine go from here? Fertil Steril. 2020;114(6):1135–9. https://doi.org/10.1016/j.fertnstert.2020.10.050.
31. Mouchtouris, N., Lavergne, P., Montenegro, T.S., Gonzalez, G., Baldassari, M., Sharan,A., Jabbour, P., Harrop, J., Rosenwasser, R., and Evans, J.J. (2020). Telemedicine in neurosurgery: lessons learned and transformation of care during the COVID-19 Pandemic. World Neurosurg, 140, e387-e394. https://doi.org/10.1016/j.wneu.2020.05.251.
32. Leochico CFD. Adoption of telerehabilitation in a developing country before and during the COVID-19 pandemic. Ann Phys Rehabil Med. 2020;63(6):563–4. https://doi.org/10.1016/j.rehab.2020.06.001.
33. Miller KA, Baird J, Lira J, Eguizabal JH, Fei S, Kysh L, Lotstein D. The use of telemedicine for home-based palliative care for children with serious illness: a scoping review. J Pain Sympt Manage. 2021;62(3):619–36. https://doi.org/10.1016/j.jpainsymman.2020.12.004.

Methodologies for Improving the Quality and Safety of Telehealth Systems

14

Hitesh Kumar Sharma, Tanupriya Choudhury, and Anurag Mor

14.1 Introduction

Telemedicine and e-hospital already proved their existence worldwide in pandemic situations like COVID-19. This technology and various available platforms were required for remote guidance when physical presence for doctors and patients is not possible. Some of the most popular Web/mobile-based telemedicine systems used worldwide are given below.

- Teladoc (US)
- Doctoroo (Australia)
- Livi (UK)
- Practo (India)
- WhiteCoat (Singapore)

In 2018, the market size of telemedicine was USD 34.28 billion. It has been projected in a survey that it will be USD 185.66 billion by 2025, having CAGR of 23.5% in the predicted timeline. As per Telehealth Index [1] by American Well's, 350,000 – 595,000 US physicians will be active on telehealth technology by 2022.

As per the survey of American Well's, following points were identified

- 77% efficient use of time of doctors and patients
- Reduced healthcare cost by 71%

Hitesh Kumar Sharma and Tanupriya Choudhury contributed equally to this work.

H. K. Sharma (✉) · T. Choudhury (✉) · A. Mor
School of Computer Science, University of Petroleum and Energy Studies (UPES), Dehradun, Uttarakhand, India

- 71% effective communication between doctor and patients
- 60% enhancement in doctor and patient relation

Secured storage of patient health e-records and doctor prescription is a big challenge as the popularity and significance of these telemedicine systems are increasing day by day. Many researchers worldwide have proposed one-way, two-way and three-way authentication scheme for secured access of the system but a full secured model for stored records is still a major challenge. Blockchain is an emerging filed in this domain. Some researchers have proposed basic frameworks to make secured these records using blockchain but still lacking in providing proof of concept.

Before COVID-19 pandemic, online education in schools and work from home (WFH) were considered as a myth and society believe that these activities are not possible without face-to-face interaction. In the same way, telemedicine is also considered an impossible process. Most health service providers and patients considered that telemedicine is also a myth in the healthcare sector. However, Digital India Mission started a few years back; this association helped in corona-virus situation and proved that telemedicine is not a myth and it played a phenomenal role in bridging some of the pain of the lockdown. Doctors are consulting patients on mobile app/ phone calls. Govt. of India has also started web portals for telemedicine services (e.g. https://esanjeevaniopd.in/, https://ehospital.gov.in/). The citizens of India are using these facilities and getting the consultancy at their home by good doctors across India. Due to lack of awareness and lack of infrastructure in India, telemedicine systems still require extraordinary efforts from government, doctors, and technical persons for making maximum peoples aware of this system and spread its awareness in their nearby places especially in rural areas. Security of health records saved in the form e-record is again a major challenge in Indian telemedicine systems. Peoples are not actively using these platforms in India, because they are worried about stealing of their health records. A more secured record storage framework with proof of concept will increase people's confidence for using these platforms. Many researchers have also proposed their blockchain-based secured storage framework, but they have proposed a basic framework and not a complete proof of concept.

14.2 Literature Review

The authors [2] have discussed about the emerging telemedical services in India. Here the authors have discussed about the lacking healthcare facilities and how the telemedical services are helping the low-middle income countries like India which are facing the shortage of basic healthcare facilities due to shortage of doctors and infrastructure available. Here, the authors have focused on the objective of telemedical services and its role in providing the adequate healthcare services to both the rural and urban people. Here, the authors are talking about the advent of telemedical services and provides a model whole working is based on the top of a mobile applications and include various functionalities like teleconsultations, video conferences, diagnostics details and used via a public-private partnership model [3, 4]. In 2012, Wu et al. proposed a new model in which they have reduced some exponential operators to minimize computing time and they have also claimed that with reducing computing time their model is more effectively secure for any kind of network attack. After Wu et al.'s work, Debiao et al. in same year 2012 reviewed Wu et al.' s model and found vulnerabilities like an insider attack and an impersonation attack. To overcome these two major attacks in Wu et al.' s scheme they proposed their own model. Wei et al. in [5] analysed both models, Wu et al. [5] and Debiao et al. [6], and they identified an offline password guessing attack is possible in both the authentication schemes. Wei et al. in [5] proposed a new model to remove mainly these security issues. In 2013, Khan and Kumari identified that Zhu [7] as well as Wei et al.'s [5] authentication models were weak to the stolen/lost smart card, offline password guessing and denial-of-service attacks. At the same time, Lee and Liu [8] found session key agreement attack in Zhu [7] scheme. To remove these flaws in previous authentication schemes, they introduced a new scheme to defeat the security attacks like facing session key disclosure, password guessing, and parallel session.

In 2013, Awasthi and Srivastava introduced a three-factor authentication system for TMIS using biometric system and random numbers. Analysing their schemes, Tan in 2014 caught an issue of user anonymity and a reflection attack in their work. Arshad and Nikooghadam in 2014 identified replay attacks and denial-of-service in Tan's scheme. In 2015, Giri et al. [9] reviewed Lee and Liu's [8] user authentication scheme for TMIS and found an offline password guessing attack vulnerability. In the same year, Amin and Biswas 2015 identified some flaws in authentication schemes of Giri et al.'s [9]; these flaws or weaknesses are offline password guessing, lack of user anonymity, and insider attacks, and they proposed a new RSA-based scheme.

In continuous effort, to enhance the security in the previous schemes, Bin Muhaya in 2014 introduced an enhanced authentication and key agreement scheme for TMISs. However, it was proved that Bin Muhaya's scheme also has a weakness for offline password guessing attacks and it is not able to perfect forward secrecy. To remove the security weaknesses of authentication scheme of Bin Muhaya, Arshad et al. in 2015 proposed a new two-factor key agreement scheme and user anonymity preserving authentication for TMISs.

14.3   Tele-Based Healthcare Vs Conventional Method

Conventional clinical treatment and medical care allude to the regular act of giving medical care administrations to the public where a patient either visits or conveyed to a close-by clinic or a centre and gets analysed by an expert specialist [10]. One of the escape clauses of the conventional medical services framework is the way that individuals cannot generally contact a specialist might be because of their tight timetables or some other explanation. Telemedical services are pretty much like the customary method of diagnosing and therapy, however, contrasting with a couple of focuses. It has helped individuals who do not have the chances and headways of clinical consideration who come from a regressive foundation. This framework gives another space and opens up a layer of the structure that ably depicts the administration of well-being-related data across the computational stages and its trade from the advisor to the victim beneficially [11]. It likewise guarantees a decent nature of finding and guess and helps in giving an encounter like a "live" interview to the patients making it easy in its conveyance. Tele-Based healthcare services put together the patient and the doctor on a common platform, and in this way can be expressed as a benefit over the conventional usual methodology of a medical care system:

- Better insight and improved nature of the discussion.
- Less determination/visualization mistakes.
- Modest medical care.
- Medical services at Home (no visits required!)
- Moderate medical care routine.
- Improved assessment of the infections.
- Early revelation of pandemic episodes in nations.

In Fig. 14.1, we have shown the relationship between bioinformatics and information technology. IoT and sensor-based devices with AI-enabled algorithms make telemedicine a successful platform for healthcare.

Fig. 14.1 The relation between bioinformatics, telemedicine, telegenetics, and telegenomics

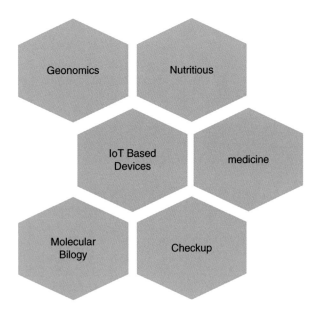

14.4   Blockchain in Telemedicine

Telemedicine is not the solution for all health-related problems, but it can be used for addressing many health issues without any physical movement of patients and doctors. It will help in the reduction of an unnecessary crowd in private and govt. hospitals [12]. Using these kinds of telemedicine platforms a patient who resides in a rural area can get his/her health consultancy from various available prestigious hospitals and world class doctors across the globe. This approach increases the efficiency and availability of expert doctor and medical staff whenever required [13]. But there are many factors that are responsible for less usage of telemedicine systems especially in India.

The following factors are responsible for holding back telemedicine to reach its expected levels:

- Less secure e-records storage mechanism
- Lack of data privacy and poor authentication scheme
- Lack of efficient AI-based expert system

There are many more factors that are responsible for poor reachability of these telemedicine systems in rural society. The most important challenge in all of the above is the lack of awareness and digital illiteracy. Due to these challenges, we are still not able to utilize our existing telemedicine systems. In Fig. 14.2, the author [14] presented a complete flowchart to adopt the blockchain technology at different layers of the telemedicine system. Blockchain can be implemented at any layer as per the complexity of the system. In addition, cost to set up large-scale IoT networks, manage centralized clouds and network all the equipment is substantial. In addition, IoT devices must be impervious to physical and information assaults. Although many of the existing approaches provide security for IoT systems, they are complicated and not suitable for IoT devices that have low resource power. Blockchain builds a peer-to-peer network, lowering central cloud, data centre and networking devices installation and maintenance cost, distributing computation and storage needs over all networked devices [15]. This communication approach addresses the problem of failure. Blockchain addresses data protection issues for IoT networks with the use of cryptographic techniques.

14.5   Methodology

There methodology consists of five-step process enabling blockchain for authentication and storing of data in telemedical healthcare server [16]. The cloud provides interface for enabling the registration of new users and new doctors. Users after registering themselves are allowed to upload their data in terms of health records. Note that the user data is generated by sensors and other medical devices. The registered doctor will then access the cloud and access the user health records, and after examining the records, the registered doctor will upload his prescription report data

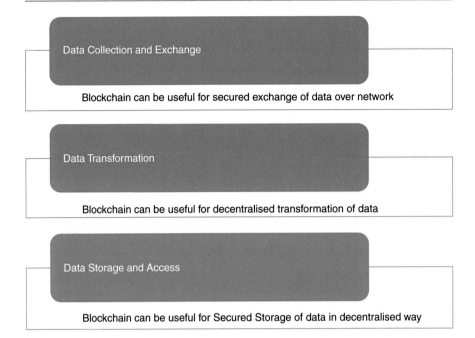

Fig. 14.2 Evaluating the use of blockchain technology in a healthcare system (Ref. [5])

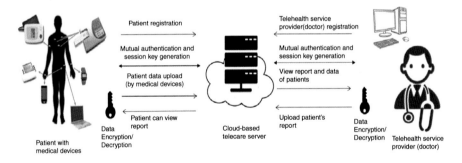

Fig. 14.3 Telemedicine authentication process flow

to the cloud needed for the treatment of the user. The user may easily see his treatment report by re-login and access the cloud. The complete framework for TMIS authentication system is shown in Fig. 14.3.

The scheme is lightweight security protocol for the TMIS [17, 18]. It consists of five phases: (i) user registration phase with medical registration cloud, (ii) doctor registration phase, (iii) user login phase, (iv) doctor login phase, and (v) user treatment report accessing phase. The different phases of the protocol are shown in Fig. 14.1. The storage of the data communication between the patient and the doctor is stored in the cloud-based telecare server [19, 20]. The blockchain technology helps the stored data for providing security between the user and the telehealth service provider.

14.5.1 Phase 1: User Registration Phase with Medical Registration Cloud

- Step 1: In this phase, a user ui (1<i<=m) registers with the Medical Registration Cloud so that the user is able to access various medical services and the diagnosis and treatment from doctors of various specialties. The user chooses his Identification IDi, generates a Random number RDi and then sends [IDi, RD] through a secure channel.
- Step 2: On receiving the user registration request, MRC will use SHA-512 hashing technique to compute S1 =h(IDi||RD||OTP||NID), where OTP is one-time password generated by MRC with validity for this particular session, NID is unique network ID.
- MRC also computes two more values A and B where A=IDi||OTP⊕, B=RD||NID. MRC stores the tuple [S1, A, B] in a table and issues it to the user via a secure channel, thereby completing ⊕ the registration process of the user.
- Step 3: After receiving the above tuple, the user computes OTP′ = ⊕A ||IDi S1′ = h(IDi||RD||OTP). A session key SKuc is then generated between the user and the cloud using S1′ SKuc = h(IDi|| S1′).

14.5.2 Phase 2: Doctor Registration Phase with Medical Registration Cloud

- Step 1: In this phase, similar to the user, each doctor also needs to get registered with MRC before he can start treating the users. A doctor di (1<i<=n) registers with the Medical Registration Cloud; for that he chooses his identification IDdi, his departmental/specialty ID DIDdi and also generates a random number RD. Doctor then sends [IDdi, RD, DIDdi] to MRC through a secure channel.
- Step 2: On receiving the doctor registration request, MRC uses SHA-512 hashing technique to compute S2 = h(IDdi||RDd||NIDd|| DIDdi) and B = DID⊕di NIDd. Thereafter, MRC stores the tuple [S2, B] in a table and issues it to the doctor via a secure channel, thereby completing the registration process of the doctor.
- Step 3: After receiving the above tuple, the doctor computes NIDd′ = B DIDd and S2′ = h(IDdi||RDd||NIDd′|| DID⊕di). A session key SKdc is then generated between the doctor and the cloud using S2′, SKdc = h(IDi|| S2′).

14.5.3 Phase 3: User Login Phase

After the user registration process is completed, user is allowed to login to MRC from anywhere and at all times in order to upload his medical health records and also to access his treatment plan uploaded by his treating doctor. It may be noted that user is only allowed to login when both user and MRC mutually authenticate each other.

- Step 1: User's ui physiological parameters/data via sensors is collected and is stored along with users ID and the random number. This tuple is referred to as (mi) = [datai, IDi, RD].
- Step 2: To ensure confidentiality and privacy of his medical data, user first encrypts his data, then achieves mutual authentication and session key agreement with MRC, then uploads his data to MRC. All the steps to accomplish above are given below:
  - 2a. In order to encrypt his data mi, user ui generates a keyi which is = h(IDi‖NID'), where NID' = B RD
  - 2b. user ui encrypts his data using the key generated in step 2a and generates a message C1 = Ekey1(mi)
  - 2c. user ui generates a message digest by hashing mi using SHA-512 to create MDi, which is the hash code of the message containing the data—MDi = h (mi)
  - 2d. To authenticate itself to MRC, the user creates a digital signature, for which it calculates and sends two quantities, viz. Mi and S3, that are function of user's private key, hash code of message containing the data, and an additional parameter NID that is generated randomly or pseudorandomly and is unique for each signing. Where Mi = SKuc (IDi‖C1‖NID'‖ Sigui) and Sigui = Spri (MDi), where Spri is the private key of the user ui, and S3 = h (SKuc ‖Mi).
- Step 3: MRC after receiving [Mi, S3] will verify the digital signatures sent by the user. For this, MRC first computes its own session key Skuc'=h(IDi‖S1) and then finds S3'=h(Skuc' ‖ Mi). If S3'=S3, then the user's authenticity is verified and the user is allowed to login, else the request is discarded. After the successful log in of the user, all the related parameters, viz. IDi, Sigui, NID, and C1, are stored on the cloud for further processing .

14.5.4 Phase 4: Doctor Login Phase

Doctor needs to login to MRC so that he can access the health records of the user and advise appropriate treatment plan to the user. In this phase, the doctor is first authenticated by MRC using the value of session key.

- Step 1: The doctor tries to login to the MRC via its identity and NID and sends a message [IDdi, NIDd, SKdc] to MRC.
- Step 2: Based on the received login message of the doctor [IDdi, NIDd, SKdc], MRC computes the value of the session key SKdc' = h(IDdi ‖ NIDd ‖ DIDd) and matches with the received session key SKdc. If it matches, MRC believes in the authenticity of the doctor and allows him to login; otherwise, the session is rejected.
- Step 3: MRC now sends the health data of the user to the doctor as CM (already stored on it by the user) to the doctor after encrypting it via the session key SKdc. CM = ESKdc (C1).
- Step 4: After receiving CM, the doctor decrypts CM through the session key and extracts the original health record of user mi. DSKdc = mi.

- Step 5: The doctor examines the health record of the user and accordingly prepares a treatment plan md. The doctor then encrypts both the user health data and the corresponding treatment plan with the keyud to create C2 = EKeyud = (mi, md), where Keyud = h(IDui "IDd).
- Step 6: To authenticate itself, the doctor then creates a digital signature, for which he calculates and sends two quantities to MRC, viz. C3 and S, that are function of session key between doctor and MRC, hash value of (mi, md) encrypted using a private key and doctor's signature. C3 and S are given as C3 = ESKdc(C2, sigd) and S = h(SKdc || C2 || Sigd).
- Step 7: On receiving [C3, S], MRC decrypts the message to extract C2 and sigd. MRC computes S′ = h(SKdc || C2 || sigd). If S′ = S, then MRC stores the C2 and sigd, else stops the session.

14.5.5 Phase 5: User Treatment Plan Checking Phase

- Step 1: In order to get his treatment plan, the user sends [IDi, SKuc] that is his ID along with the session key to MRC.
- Step 2: MRC computes SKuc′ = h(ID || NID || Rd.|| OTP). It checks if SKuc′ = SKuc; if it matches, MRC computes C4 and C5 and sends these values to the user, where C4 = C2 ⊕ IDi and C5 = NID ⊕ IDd.
- Step 3: Based on the received values of C4 and C5, user computes IDd′ = NID C ⊕ 5 and C2′ = C4 ⊕ ID i. The user then decrypts C2 (DKeyud (C2) = (mi, md)) to extract both his health record and the corresponding doctor's treatment plan. The key used for decryption is found by the hash function: h(IDi || IDd).

In all the above the data is stored in the server that need to secure, and it is possible with the help of blockchain technology.

14.6   Conclusion

Telemedicine is not the solution for all health-related problems, but it can be used for addressing many health issues without any physical movement of patients and doctors. It will help in the reduction of an unnecessary crowd in private and govt. hospitals. Using these kinds of telemedicine platform, a patient who resides in a rural area can get his/her health consultancy from various available prestigious hospitals and world class doctors across the globe. This approach increases the efficiency and availability of expert doctor and medical staff whenever required.

Quality of Services (QoS) and safety is highly desired in Tele-Based Healthcare Systems. These systems are directly dealing with the health of general public, so a strong and efficient authentication mechanism is also needed in these systems. Blockchain-based authentication is a proposal that we have proposed in this chapter. Blockchain-based authentication scheme can be implemented in telemedicine and it can secure this system as it secured cryptocurrency.

References

1. https://static.americanwell.com/app/uploads/2019/07/American-Well-Telehealth-Index-2019-Consumer-SurveyeBook2. pdf.(Last accessed on 31st May 2022, 5:45pm IST).
2. Kustwar RK, Ray S. eHealth and telemedicine in India: an overview on the health care need of the people. Journal of Multidisciplinary Research in Healthcare. 2020;6(2):25–36. https://doi.org/10.15415/jmrh.2020.62004.
3. Saha A, Amin R, Kunal S, Vollala S, Dwivedi SK. Review on "Blockchain technology based medical healthcare system with privacy issues". Security Privacy. 2019;2(5):e83. https://doi.org/10.1002/spy2.83.
4. Taneja S, Ahmed E, Patni JC. I-Doctor: an IoT based self patient's health monitoring system. In: 2019 International conference on innovative sustainable computational technologies, CISCT 2019; 2019.
5. Wei HT, Chen MH, Huang PC, Bai YM. The association between online gaming, social phobia, and depression: an internet survey. BMC Psychiarty. 2012;12:92. https://doi.org/10.1186/1471-244X-12-92.
6. Debiao & Jianhua, Chen & Jin, Hu. An ID-based client authentication with key agreement protocol for mobile client–server environment on ECC with provable security. Information Fusion - INFFUS. 2012;13. https://doi.org/10.1016/j.inffus.2011.01.001.
7. Zhu C. Student satisfaction, performance, and knowledge construction in online collaborative learning. Educational Technology & Society. 2012;15:127–36.
8. Kind T, Liu KH, Lee DY, DeFelice B, Meissen JK, & Fiehn O. LipidBlast in silico tandem mass spectrometry database for lipid identification. Nature methods. 2013;10(8):755–58.
9. Giri D, Maitra T, Amin R, Srivastava PD. An efficient and robust RSA-based remote user authentication for telecare medical information systems. Journal of Medical Systems. 2015;39(1):1–9.
10. Sharma A, et al. Health monitoring & management using IoT devices in a Cloud Based Framework. In: 2018 International conference on advances in computing and communication engineering (ICACCE); 2018. p. 219–24.
11. Kamdar N, Jalilian L. Telemedicine: a digital interface for perioperative anesthetic care. Anesth Analg. 2020;130(2):272–5. https://doi.org/10.1213/ANE.0000000000004513.
12. Shamshad S, Mahmood K, Kumari S, Chen CM. A secure blockchain-based e-health records storage and sharing scheme. J Inform Security Appl. 2020;55:102590.
13. Hussien HM, Yasin SM, Udzir SNI, Zaidan AA, Zaidan BB. A systematic review for enabling of develop a blockchain technology in healthcare application: taxonomy, substantially analysis, motivations, challenges, recommendations and future direction. J Medical Syst. 2019;43(10) https://doi.org/10.1007/s10916-019-1445-8.
14. Sharma HK, Patni JC. Pandemic diagnosis and analysis using clinical decision support systems. J Crit Rev. 2020;
15. Gupta S, Sharma HK. User anonymity based secure authentication protocol for telemedical server systems. Int J Inform Comput Secur. 2021;
16. Shailender SHK. Digital cancer diagnosis with counts of adenoma and luminal cells in plemorphic adenoma immunastained healthcare system. IJRAR. 2018;5(12)
17. Patni JC, Ahlawat P, Biswas SS. Sensors based smart healthcare framework using internet of things (IoT). Int J Sci Technol Res. 2020;9(2):1228–34.
18. Purri S, Kashyap N, et al. Specialization of IoT applications in health care industries. In: Proceedings of the IEEE International conference on big data analytics and computational intelligence (ICBDAC). IEEE; 2017. p. 252–6.
19. A. Joshi, et al. Data mining in healthcare and predicting obesity. In: Proceedings of the third international conference on computational intelligence and informatics, pp. 877–888, Hyderabad, India, 2020.
20. Krishnan DSR, et al. An IoT based patient health monitoring system. In: 2018 international conference on advances in computing and communication engineering (ICACCE), p. 1–7.

Application of Bioinformatics in Telemedicine System

15

Hitesh Kumar Sharma, Tanupriya Choudhury, and Anurag Mor

15.1   Introduction

Recent technological advancements are offering users new and easier ways to access healthcare services. With the advent of high-speed networks, low-cost storage, inexpensive telecommunication systems, patient monitoring systems, and cloud computing, telecare medical information system (TMIS) is becoming a reality [1]. Due to the advantage of telehealthcare medical system, we are reaching directly to the patient home over internet or mobile networks and data is stored as electronic medical records (EMR).The major challenge here is ensuring secure access of communication data by patients and doctors; for this we need a secure and efficient way of user access control and the data stored in the cloud so that attacker cannot impersonate the user data and medical server. The confidentiality, integrity and availability need to be ensured. Also, the authentication process should be user friendly so that patients can use it easily. Medical data includes medical images, prescription by doctors, and sensors data which might be tampered by intruders. Our aim is to overcome the limitation of present market scenario and provide the efficient way of communication between user and doctor with the help of blockchain technology in cloud-based medical system. Telemedicine systems can be viewed as an instrument that is being used as an incredible wellspring of diminishing the far distance between distantly dwelled rustic individuals and the medical care administrations. It has heap applications and has reached out in a wide range of clinical consideration applications like conferences, analysis, nursing, prescriptions what's more, treatment, psychiatry and brain research, recovery, what's more, some specific

---

Hitesh Kumar Sharma and Tanupriya Choudhury contributed equally to this work.

H. K. Sharma (✉) · T. Choudhury (✉) · A. Mor
School of Computer Science, University of Petroleum and Energy Studies (UPES),
Dehradun, Uttarakhand, India

administrations. To the best of the World Health Organization's knowledge, telemedicine entails employing information technology (IT) for an evident diagnosis, treatment, and prevention of infection to deliver clinical medical services administered by clinical specialists when distance is a debilitating factor. Additionally, it likewise assists with assessing and work upon the misconstrued or least contemplated messes and sicknesses.

Bioinformatics is one of the main technical domains which can play an important role in security and authentication in TMIS systems.

15.2 Tele-Based Healthcare vs Conventional Method

Telemedicine is not the solution for all health-related problems, but it can be used for addressing many health issues without any physical movement of patients and doctors. It will help in the reduction of an unnecessary crowd in private and govt. hospitals. Using these kinds of telemedicine platforms, a patient who resides in a rural area can get his/her health consultancy from various available prestigious hospitals and world class doctors across the globe. In Fig. 15.1, we have shown a single module of automated heartbeat recording of a patient using bioinformatics sensor. The recorded heartbeat is stored in online database for real-time monitoring by doctors using web/app dashboard of smart care healthcare system [2].

This approach increases the efficiency and availability of expert doctor and medical staff whenever required. But there are many factors that are responsible for less usage of telemedicine systems especially in India [3]. The following factors are responsible for holding back telemedicine to reach its expected levels: (1) Less secure e-records storage mechanism, (2) lack of data privacy and poor authentication scheme and (3) lack of efficient AI-based expert system. There are many more factors that are responsible for poor reachability of these telemedicine systems in rural society. The most important challenge in all of the above is the lack of awareness and digital illiteracy. Due to these challenges, we are still not able to utilize our existing telemedicine systems.

In Fig. 15.2, we have shown a proposed small bioinformatics-based smart healthcare system for maintaining social distance, which will help to reduce spreading of communicable disease. As we have seen in COVID-19, this kind of module integration in smart healthcare system and telemedicine system will be useful.

According to the needs of the general public, Tele-wellness administrations are structured as follows: Keeping Stocks and Stimulating: In this type of telecasted medical treatment, clinical data such as clinical images, patient's profiles, and so on are gathered and then sent to a professional for an expert assessment. It requires a legitimate very much organized arrangement of the clinical record of an individual and a sound/video correspondence of the patient which proves to be useful to the expert for recommending and determination of the treatment. It is otherwise called far off observing or self-appraisal. It helps clinical meetings to survey an individual indirectly based on utilizing numerous innovative devices and gadgets [4]. This assistance assists with giving an effective, recognizable, and cheap method of

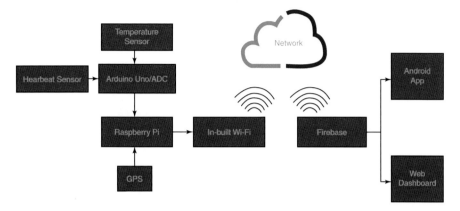

Fig. 15.1 Basic module of a smart healthcare

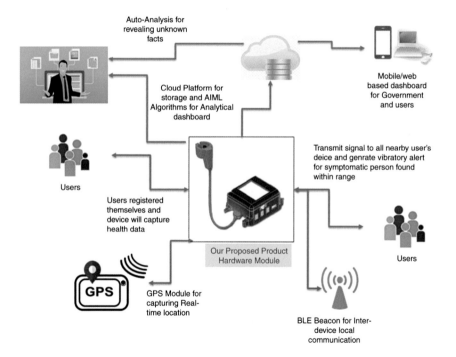

Fig. 15.2 A small bioinformatics-based system for healthcare (proposed)

treatment. It depends on the patient's direct electronic contact with the specialist via videoconferencing or phone call. There's more to telecasted clinical care than just conclusions, guesses, therapy, and advice. There are also follow-up meetings with patients. This allows patients with no difficulties to speak freely with the adviser about issues and their circumstances with no time limit, in contrast to the traditional medical care setup.

15.3   Relation Between Bioinformatics, Telegenomics, Telemedicine, and Telegenetics

Before COVID-19 pandemic, online education in schools and work from home (WFH) were considered as a myth and society believe that these activities are not possible without face-to-face interaction. In the same way, telemedicine is also considered an impossible process. Most health service providers and patients considered that telemedicine is also a myth in the healthcare sector [5]. However, Digital India Mission started a few years back; this association helped in corona-virus situation and proved that telemedicine is not a myth and it played a phenomenal role in bridging some of the pain of the lockdown. Doctors are consulting patients on mobile app/ phone calls. Govt. of India has also started web portals for telemedicine services (e.g. https://esanjeevaniopd.in/, https://ehospital.gov.in/). The citizens of India are using these facilities and getting the consultancy at their home by good doctors across India. Due to lack of awareness and lack of infrastructure in India, telemedicine systems still require extraordinary efforts from government, doctors, and technical persons for making maximum people aware of this system and spread its awareness in their nearby places especially in rural areas. Security of health records saved in the form of e-record is again a major challenge in Indian telemedicine systems. Peoples are not actively using these platforms in India, because they are worried about stealing of their health records. A more secured record storage framework with proof of concept will increase people's confidence for using these platforms. Many Indian researchers have also proposed their blockchain-based secured storage framework but they have proposed a basic framework and not a complete proof of concept [6]. Through the use of remote conferencing, it will bring together analysts, physicians, and patients to accelerate the impact of inherited characteristics. Individual genetic information may also be more readily available to both medical care communities and patients as a result of DNA sequencing's lowering cost [7]. Telecasted medical care still has a lot of research to be done, not just for patients and their advisers, but also in general for the whole mechanical and examination industry.

15.4   Tele-Based System Categories

Telemedicine is a platform that has technical and socio-economic relevance in the healthcare sector. Telemedicine systems have already proved their relevance across the globe but India is behindhand to use this extraordinary and revolutionary platform because of digital illiteracy in rural areas. Peoples living in rural areas are not aware of these life-saving technical platforms. All developed countries in the world are using these platforms to serve high-quality healthcare facilities in minimum timespan and generating revenues to get economic benefits. It is possible for these developed countries just because of digital awareness and proper IT infrastructure available. As I have mentioned earlier, in 2018, the market size of telemedicine was USD 34.28 billion. It has been projected in a survey that it will be USD 185.66 billion by 2025, having CAGR of 23.5% in the predicted timeline. As per Telehealth Index (2019) by American Well's, 350,000–595,000 US physicians will be active on telehealth technology by 2022. Telemedicine and e-hospital already proved their existence worldwide in pandemic situations like COVID-19. This technology and various available platforms were required for remote guidance when physical presence for doctors and patients is not possible.

Some of the most popular Web/mobile-based telemedicine systems are given below.

- Teladoc (US)
- Doctoroo (Australia)
- Livi (UK)
- Practo (India)
- WhiteCoat (Singapore)

In 2018, the market size of telemedicine was USD 34.28 billion. It has been projected in a survey that it will be USD 185.66 billion by 2025, having CAGR of 23.5% in the predicted timeline. As per Telehealth Index (2019) by American Well's, 350,000–595,000 US physicians will be the active on telehealth technology by 2022.

As per the survey of American Well's, following points were identified:

- 77% efficient use of time of doctors and patients
- Reduced healthcare cost by 71%
- 71% effective communication between doctor and patients
- 60% enhancement in doctor and patient relation

The current circumstance of tele-based medical care administrations has demonstrated to be greatly tending to the medical problems of people in general, this with a dream of giving individualization to each resident. Tele-based well-being administrations are limited to gentle sicknesses as well as it is commendable for the therapy of persistent issues also. If you believe Or and Marsh, personalization means that the patient is the only focus of a terms of risk unit. This means that cell phone applications and electronic pre-surgery programs should be combined to cater to the patient's daily schedule and way of life, including eating habits and public activities. Improving the present medical services organizations should incorporate telehealthcare frameworks that involve patients and their family, physicians, and other surgical personnel. Since telehealthcare is meant to be a "familiar consideration", patients and their families should also be prepared before utilizing it. The following are four characteristics that telecasted medical services frameworks should have to be competitive:

- It should be tailored based on patient experiences and their genetic information, if available.
- Those same frameworks should be sufficiently foresighted so that the risks of diseases may be mitigated in advance.
- Telemedicine frameworks should provide patients with preventative estimations they may use to prepare for illness in advance.
- If it is participatory, it should provide the option of connecting a patient with his or her adviser.

15.4.1 Telediagnosis

An affirmation of a possible illness at an off-site location that relies on telehealth techniques for communicating data is called a "telediagnosis" [1]. To diagnose remotely using tele-diagnostics requires access remotely to test findings and restorative histories of a far situated patient who has no physical interaction with the professional performing the evaluation. This technique should be possible by using distinctive correspondence systems, including telephonic conversations and texting. Over the most recent couple of years, numerous propositions have been created for telediagnosis, two of them are clarified as (a) using 3G/4G networks, the mobile telemedicine system (MTS) collects information from multiple devices and transmits it to social security and the medical care provider. MTS may be accessed from anywhere in the world via a high-speed network (3G/4G) and online services to evaluate chronic illnesses. (b) AI, including profound neural organizations, has been ending up being helpful in different infection analysis. A case in point is the discovery of Parkinson's disease, a neurodegenerative condition that affects the brain's engine architecture. An innovative mobile phone-based telediagnosis technique based on brain organization was proposed by Zhang. The possibility of Parkinson's illness classification depends on text perusing and discourse acknowledgment, following these means:

15.4.2 Teleconsultation

If there is not enough data to make an inquiry, then the specialists, specialists, and patients can communicate by telephone [1]. This is a type of tele-diagnostics known as teleconsultation or tele-diagnostics. Disregarding the customary strategies, teleconsultations offer the potential gain of taking outpatient proximity at specific periods of the assessment strategy. Serving medical care offices in provincial zones is a difficult assignment. Teleconsultation offers simplicity to individuals of country territories through media transmission by utilizing electronic administrations. A few electronic frameworks, called virtual polyclinic, were produced for teleconsultation that gives media teleconsultation as well as online medical services records. Patients can utilize these online medical care records to trade information among subject matter experts and professionals.

15.4.3 Telenursing

Telenursing works with attendants to look at and learn about their patients by utilizing electronic frameworks and data of customers, where specialists fill in as experts. As a result of telenursing, patients are more satisfied, and nursing administrations have more capacity [1]. Due to the fact that HbA1c levels are improved, the stress of diet treatment is reduced. Patients convey their well-being-related issues to the specialist, and after discussion, the medical caretaker gives the answers for the patients. The patient offers input to the specialist in the wake of finishing his treatment. Telenursing is given to the patients to telephone nursing and phone care. Phone nursing helps in giving guidance and data, arrangements, side effects to the board, and infection the executives to the patient as per the data of illness given by the patient. Phone care gives strong consideration, instruction, evaluation, and infection to the executives to the patient. A telenursing framework system using web applications was developed for regulating medical care using Internet administrations. This electronic application was created as a structure for nursing care using forefront information advancement. The features of Kawaguchi's telenursing system fuse having the capacity to pick information advancement (on-demand webcam conversations, email, and calls) for intervention according to well-being necessities and care of attendant essentials. It has the office to record under-standing self-checking information as an element of the prosperity record and graphing of oneself noticing information in the prosperity record with the objective that patients can see their specific data with no time limit. Telenursing comprises a medical care place worker and common organization which is associated with an attendant, a doctor, and a patient.

15.4.4 Telerehabilitation

Telerehabilitation is the use of ICT to deliver recovery services to persons who live in remote areas, giving the patient a sense of self-assurance and acceptance. As a result, they are becoming more than just a latent element of their thinking. It allows access to those who live in remote areas or who have transportability difficulties related to a physical impairment, as well as financial considerations. Reduces travel costs and time spent by the patient as well as the social security provider. In tandem with the expansion of telerehabilitation, the movement of care is gaining momentum. Additionally, its different modules enable an ECG, an oximeter, temperature and vital signs as well as a stationary bicycle and language teaching programming in addition to sound and video parts. In this stage, a variety of recovery populations, including muscle health, aspirator health, and brain health, may be effectively treated. It enables clinicians to distantly associate with and pass on understanding thought outside of the helpful setting, thusly shedding the issue of detachment among clinician and patient. Through inquiry, the specialist determines what the patient's problem is, and then provides appropriate addressing components. The recovery process begins with a focus on personal happiness and predetermined intervention settings. Treatment has been given through the expert assets further that appraisal is begun.

15.5 Telemedicine System Authentication

Network security attacks are mainly classified into two main categories. Passive attack and active attack. In passive attack, the attacker only captures data packets sent from sender to the receiver and understands the information passed through these data packets, but the attacker does not modify the data packet flows into the network. But in active attack the attacker captures and modifies also to these data packets and send the modified data packet to receiver on behalf of actual sender. As shown in the following figure, the middle attacker is capturing sender's data. In active attack, the attacker sends his modified packet on behalf of sender. The receiver thinks that the data packet is the actual data packet which was initially sent by the actual sender. There methodology consists of five-step process enabling blockchain for authentication and storing of data in telemedical healthcare server. The cloud provides interface for enabling the registration of new users and new doctors. Users after registering themselves are allowed to upload their data in terms of health records. Note that the user data is generated by sensors and other medical devices. The registered doctor will then access the cloud and access the user health records, and after examining the records, the registered doctor will upload his prescription report data to the cloud needed for the treatment of the user. The user may easily see his treatment report by re-login and access the cloud. The scheme is lightweight security protocol for the TMIS. It consists of five phases: (i) user registration phase with medical registration cloud, (ii) doctor registration phase, (iii) user login phase, (iv) doctor login phase, and (v) user treatment report accessing phase. The storage of the data communication between the patient and the doctor is stored in the cloud-based telecare server. The blockchain technology helps the stored data for providing security between the user and the telehealth service provider.

15.6   Telehealth: Database, Techniques, Approach

In clinical frameworks and their instruments, the application of bioinformatics and calculating originals has opened up a new way of thinking. Methods like this can mimic the natural phenomenon, allowing for the collection of data that will ultimately aid in the development of medical care systems. Endoscopic photographs taken at a distance have been acknowledged as an example acknowledgement framework for defining the synthesis, consistency, and designation of the endoscopic pictures once again in remote container endoscopy. Toxins for cardiovascular medical treatments are also determined using this method. It is self-evident, with the development of computational force the information has likewise developed immensely preposterous years. For that, one needs to admire the idea of Big Data and Fog Data for the equivalent. Information withdrawal, information mining, and information evaluation are the need of great importance which should be taken up by the clinical clique. In the past, a low-power, encased machine was used for information mining and information analysis, which relied on unprocessed data from multiple wearable sensors used for tele-based health services [4].

15.7   Challenges

In India, before COVID-19 pandemic, online education in schools and work from home (WFH) was considered as a myth and society believe that these activities are not possible without face-to-face interaction. In the same way, telemedicine is also considered an impossible process. Most health service providers and patients considered that telemedicine is also a myth in the healthcare sector. However, Digital India Mission started a few years back; this association helped in corona-virus situation and proved that telemedicine is not a myth and it played a phenomenal role in bridging some of the pain of the lockdown. Doctors are consulting patients on mobile app/ phone calls. Govt. of India has also started web portals for telemedicine services (e.g. https://esanjeevaniopd.in/, https://ehospital.gov.in/). The citizens of India are using these facilities and getting the consultancy at their home by good doctors across India. Due to lack of awareness and lack of infrastructure in India, telemedicine systems still require extraordinary efforts from government, doctors, and technical persons for making maximum peoples aware of this system and spread its awareness in their nearby places especially in rural areas. Telemedicine is not the solution for all health-related problems, but it can be used for addressing many health issues without any physical movement of patients and doctors. It will help in the reduction of an unnecessary crowd in private and govt. hospitals. Using these kinds of telemedicine platforms a patient who resides in a rural area can get his/her health consultancy from various available prestigious hospitals and world class doctors across the globe. This approach increases the efficiency and availability of expert doctor and medical staff whenever required. But there are many factors that are responsible for less usage of telemedicine systems specially in India.

The following factors are responsible for holding back telemedicine to reach its expected levels:

- Lack of awareness
- Digital illiteracy
- Internet availability
- Lack of data privacy and security mechanism
- Lack of efficient AI-based expert system

There are many more factors that are responsible for poor reachability of these telemedicine systems in rural society. The most important challenge in all of the above is the lack of awareness and digital illiteracy. Due to these challenges, we are still not able to utilize our existing telemedicine systems.

15.8 Conclusions

Telemedicine is a platform that has technical and socio-economic relevance in the healthcare sector. Telemedicine systems have already proved their relevance across the globe but India is behindhand to use this extraordinary and revolutionary platform because of digital illiteracy in rural areas. Peoples living in rural areas are not aware of these life-saving technical platforms. All developed countries in the world are using these platforms to serve high-quality healthcare facilities in minimum timespan and generating revenues to get economic benefits. It is possible for these developed countries just because of digital awareness and proper IT infrastructure available. As I have mentioned earlier, in 2018, the market size of telemedicine was

USD 34.28 billion. It has been projected in a survey that it will be USD 185.66 billion by 2025, having CAGR of 23.5% in the predicted timeline. As per Telehealth Index (2019) by American Well's, 350,000–595,000 US physicians will be active on telehealth technology by 2022. It is no secret that genetics and telemedicine are two rapidly emerging fields that promise to deliver new configurations of medical treatment with no limit to distance or time restrictions. In a few medical services sectors, telemedicine is now being used in précised medication by including it into genomic and genetic research fields. Analysts, doctors and patients will be able to collaborate via remote conference to better understand how inherited characteristics and genomes affect the diagnosis and treatment of diseases.

References

1. Qazi S, Tanveer K, ElBahnasy K, Raza K. Chapter 10: From telediagnosis to teletreatment: the role of computational biology and bioinformatics in tele-based healthcare. In: Jude HD, Balas VE, editors. Telemedicine technologies: Academic Press; 2019. p. 153–69.
2. Sharma HK, Patni JC. Pandemic diagnosis and analysis using clinical decision support systems. J Crit Rev. 2020;
3. Gupta S, Sharma HK. User anonymity based secure authentication protocol for telemedical server systems. Int J Inform Comput Secur. 2021;
4. Shailender SHK. Digital cancer diagnosis with counts of adenoma and luminal cells in plemorphic adenoma immunastained healthcare system. IJRAR. 2018;5(12)
5. Patni JC, Ahlawat P, Biswas SS. Sensors based smart healthcare framework using internet of things (IoT). Int J Scientific Technol Res. 2020;9(2):1228–34.
6. Taneja S, Ahmed E, Patni JC. I-Doctor: An IoT based self patient's health monitoring system. In: 2019 International conference on innovative sustainable computational technologies, CISCT 2019, 2019.
7. Sharma HK, Patni JC, Ahlawat P, Biswas SS. Sensors based smart healthcare framework using internet of things (IoT). Int J Sci Technol Res. 2020;9(2):1228–34.

Role of Telemedicine in Children Health

16

Avita Katal, Niharika Singh, Susheela Dahiya,
and Hitesh Kumar Sharma

16.1 Introduction

Telemedicine is the use of electronic information and communication systems to offer and sustain patient services where the patients are isolated by a large distance. The use of the telephone for appointments between physicians and patients, as well as the use of radio to link emergency services to medical centres, are on the commonplace side of the spectrum. On the other end of the telemedicine continuum are mainly experimental developments such as telesurgery, in which surgeons gain visual and tactile input to direct robotic instruments in performing surgery at a remote location. Telemedicine was not widely used a century ago due to inefficient, expensive, and inconvenient technologies. Telemedicine has established a solid foundation as a stable, helpful, and viable application as a result of advancements in telecommunications and information technology. Telemedicine has a broad range of applications that include a wide range of networking technologies. This broad dissemination allows telemedicine technologies to be used by people from all walks of life, regardless of their access to the Internet. Technologists, engineers, physicians, and entrepreneurs are constantly collaborating to create innovative and more efficient telemedicine technologies. Telemedicine is a well-understood term these days. A variety of audio, visual, and data communication systems and implementations occur at these two ends of the spectrum. These, such as immersive videoconferencing, which allows doctors to hear, view, ask, and advice remote patients in real time for medical and clinical purposes, are comparatively costly. Others, built on store and forward technology, allow digital images and other material to be stored and sent reasonably and cheaply to consultants who can collect and decode them whenever it is convenient, giving

A. Katal (✉) · N. Singh · S. Dahiya · H. K. Sharma
School of Computer Science, University of Petroleum and Energy Studies (UPES),
Dehradun, Uttarakhand, India

© The Author(s), under exclusive license to Springer Nature
Switzerland AG 2022
T. Choudhury et al. (eds.), *Telemedicine: The Computer Transformation of
Healthcare*, TELe-Health, https://doi.org/10.1007/978-3-030-99457-0_16

those on both ends of the communications connection greater scheduling flexibility. These various innovations have a number of existing and future applications in professional education, science, public health, and management, in addition to medical care. Costs for expensive information and communication investments could be spread out more evenly for such multiple applications.

16.1.1 Telemedicine for the Health of the Children

The definition of the requirements of the young and, as a result, the formulation of plans for their health promotion are critical elements in both developed and developing country policies. Government and non-governmental organizations in least developed countries support these activities as well. If the interests of the weakest are not taken into consideration, the same concept of welfare cannot be considered general. Children are, in some respects, the most helpless members of our society, but they still have the highest importance. They are the citizens of tomorrow, and all future initiatives must begin with this premise, regardless of the other goals sought. Telemedicine cannot necessarily be characterized as the distribution of treatment from one location with higher health requirements to another with fewer resources, or as the passive transfer of information from one source to a less fortunate recipient. This is a part of what telemedicine is expected to achieve, but it is unlikely to be the most significant. Telemedicine, on the other hand, can be a two-way sharing of information and expertise. It provides access to healthcare regardless of where you are from, mitigating the pressure on the child, improving their chances of avoiding sickness, and attempting to better their standard of living. In other words, it will inspire the child to require fast and greater assistance in immediate or life-threatening occurrences; to obtain urgent counselling even if the child lives in the centre of nowhere; to spend little moment in the treatment workplace or in the clinic; and to having spent more top-notch time doing the things that children are supposed to do, thereby lowering the number of children who wished to be or accept assistance. When a significant proportion of diseases necessitate direct medical intervention, the telehealth structure and gadget chosen for delivering medical services for child's welfare should be viewed as "a process of increasing children's care standards". As we can see, the child's empowerment in the control of his or her own well-being (and therefore of his or her quality of life) is mostly a process of coping interventions that assist the child in understanding his or her state of health and how to relate and convey his or her own pain to caregivers or other individuals. Communication often entails receiving constant input from the partner in order to provide a closed loop in which problems and solutions can be revealed on a regular basis. As a result, two major methods must be considered:

(i) The use of a telemedicine system to transmit reports about a child's well-being to healthcare providers.

(ii) The utilization of information and communication technology (ICT) to collect health data, encourage healthier habits, avoid risky activities, and detect diseases in their early stages.

The constructive position of the child may or cannot be used in these two techniques. In the most recent case, there can be open communication among the clinic and the child's next of family members: a parent can seek medical consultation using a mobile app that can better determine their child's health status, submitting reports to the surgical department or a local hospital. The same ICT resources that can improve the health of a child can also be a cause of problems that may have a negative effect on his or her health. An unprecedented number of depressive symptoms and suicide attempts in children and teenagers have been attributed to machine- or Internet-mediated abuse; therefore, children should have access to the telemedicine. First and foremost, it will assist children in taking an active part in the regulation of their own welfare, which is intended to enhance their quality of life during their childhood and as potential adults. Second, telemedicine services can assist children in establishing proper contact networks with health professionals, allowing them to transmit and receive information in a manner that is understandable to them.

16.2   Literature Review

The authors in [1] showed successful use of a telehealth device in the homes of children with complicated medical problems by a caregiver. Caregivers were at ease with and happy with the equipment. Clinicians found the gadget beneficial for collecting data to guide patients' treatment plans. They lay the groundwork for further research on the benefits of telehealth in the homes of other groups with specific healthcare requirements.

The authors in [2] have explored the use of telemedicine for the paediatric sleep. They also demonstrated the use of telemedicine in different domains related to children, difficulties, as well as rethinking paediatric sleep in the context of telemedicine.

The authors in [3] have demonstrated the use of telemedicine for the children that are dependent on ventilator. Their goal was to evaluate the impact of telemedicine in promoting the early and permanent discharge of such patients to home care.

The authors in [4] describe a new creative and comprehensive paediatric emergency telemedicine service developed at a big metropolitan university medical facility. According to initial research, patients who use teleconference have shorter appointment times, greater drug management, and decreased chances of PED diagnosis and eventual hospitalizations.

16.3   Financial Impact of Telemedicine

Even though the expense of a programme is considerable, telehealth has the potential to result in substantial cost savings and economic benefit. Stakeholders are interested in the entire financial effect of this innovation. This is a difficult procedure since various aspects must be considered while evaluating a programme. Economic assessments of telemedicine are hampered by methodological concerns such as the inability to analyse all costs, the difficulties estimating the economic advantage, and the viewpoint from which economic advantages are examined. While the use of creativity has been demonstrated in brief trials with specific client groups to be cost efficient, present healthcare system constraints like financing and credentialing expenditures may limit these benefits. However, by choosing the correct point of view and outcome indicators, and time off work, it may be able to demonstrate effectiveness.

16.3.1 Expenses

The cost of a telecommunication programme varies considerably based on the type of therapy and the technology employed. Hardware at both the source and remote locations, and also annual loss and a rough estimate of future expenditures, must all be factored into the cost calculation. Technology, software support, administrative expenditures, training, licence fees, programme upgrades, and the amount of time available for both originating and remote site providers to perform services are all key issues. Costs that are more difficult to quantify must also be addressed. When calculating expenses, it should be kept in mind that even equivalent programme may have varying estimates. On the basis of both the evaluation techniques and the technology utilized, a comparison of two ICU studies revealed a nearly fourfold range in predicted programme costs [5, 6].

16.3.2 Return on Investment

Before implementing a telemedicine programme, all costs must be examined. Benefits will differ depending on who is conducting the evaluation: a physician, a patient, a hospital, a payer, a policy analyst, or a healthcare utilization researcher. The university may gain from direct billing, contract payments, and extramural funding, while patients may value travel, time off from work, and convenience more. Providers may find that they don't require as much specialized office space as they once did. The money savings from fewer emergency room visits and hospitalization might be considerable. Currently, only a few financially viable telemedicine businesses offer electronic visits to a wide range of clients. The provision of subspecialist services is the greatest example of commercially viable telemedicine operations. Radiology services like NightHawk and intensive care services like Visicu are the most well-known of these [7]. Both of these firms went public and were later acquired by larger for-profit healthcare corporations. Specialists on Call is an example of a corporation that offers neurology, psychiatry, and acute care services. More recently, telehealth has begun to penetrate the broader paediatric market, with businesses like NuPhysicia offering video visits through Walmart's immediate care facilities, and Walgreens just announcing a similar initiative with MDLive [8]. The introduction of for-profit enterprises like MDLive, Doctors on Demand, and Teledoc is another fascinating trend. These for-profit telehealth companies provide low-acuity visits using videoconferencing technology, either over the phone or in combination with audiovisual computer encounters. Such meetings are frequently held outside the family's primary care doctor's office, and reports from these visits may or may not be received by the main care physician, resulting in fragmented treatment.

16.3.3 Sustainability

The lack of evidence of telemedicine's long-term viability has hampered its wider adoption. Business modelling is crucial and must be utilized in the advancement of a training plan. Grant-funded pilot projects may fail if the criteria for justifying future financial support are not linked with the initial initiative and stakeholder goals, showing the significance of cost and benefit alignment with all partners and consumers. Payment is a critical aspect in ensuring the long-term viability of services. Although some projects have failed due to a lack of funding, public opinions may be shifting.

16.4 Infrastructure for Paediatric Telemedicine

The technological requirements of a telehealth programme will vary depending on whether the business plans to conduct asynchronous or synchronous telemedicine. Synchronous includes people at two or more locations interacting in real time. Asynchronous telemedicine entails capturing medical data at one location and then passing the data to another site or locations for subsequent examination by a medical practitioner.

Remote monitoring is a crucial aspect of telehealth since it allows specialists to keep eye on patients in real time while also allowing people to self-monitor chronic conditions including asthma, diabetes, and heart disease. Figure 16.1 shows the infrastructure of telemedicine.

16.4.1 Equipment

It may be necessary to use dedicated turnkey videoconferencing devices in addition to software-based videoconferencing solutions for PCs, tablets or cell phones.

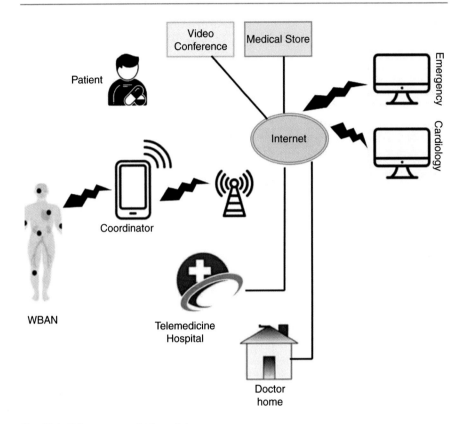

Fig. 16.1 Infrastructure of telemedicine

While allowing experts to freely speak, the technology should be able to give adequate audio-video clarity for the patient's evaluation. Depending on the demands of the telehealth programme, hardwired or portable peripheral medical devices should be able to connect through some technology.

Interoperability with current telemedicine services and technology is a significant factor when picking technology for the telehealth programme. The system should enable the H.264 video reduction code, the G.711 audio reduction standards, H.261 compression algorithms standard compliance, or any other superior benchmark for achieving great audio and video. The solutions must adhere to current organizational, legal, and legal needs.

16.4.2 Connection

The connection created between the locations engaged in the call determines the quality of a telemedicine conversation. As a result, the business should allocate sufficient bandwidth to fulfil the telehealth programme's objectives. The organization must be able to include point-to-point connection both inside and outside the health-care facility. The majority of telemedicine encounters currently take place via an Internet connection at a fast speed. When a location lacks the necessary architecture for optimized Internet, telemedicine interactions may employ an integrated services digital network link.

16.4.3 Security and Privacy

Other regulatory regulations include the 1996 Health Insurance Portability and Accountability Act (HIPAA) [9]. The aim of HIPAA is to safeguard people's medical information while also directing various institutions to employ contemporary technology to optimize the efficacy and usefulness of client therapy. The Security Rule is adaptable, allowing covered entities to create policies, processes, and technologies that are appropriate for their scale, architecture, and risk of exposing protected health information to their customers. Between the devices involved in the communication, the majority of telemedicine systems employ point-to-point encryption. A frequent way for strengthening the privacy of a telemedicine Internet connection is to use virtual private tunnels. Although the confidentiality and the authentication of the Internet determine the security of the telemedicine contact, each covered organization shall establish adequate measures to ensure the security of patient information, such as data security, accessibility, and security tracking.

16.5   Application Areas

16.5.1 Children with Medical Complexity (CMC)

It uses a lot of resources in the healthcare system. Despite making up just 5% of the population in the USA, they account for more than 60% of all children's healthcare spending [10]. Multiple medical comorbidities, dependency on medical technology, major functional impairments, financial strain on caregivers, and disconnected medical treatment are all typical among people with Alzheimer's disease. Costs and logistics of transportation may cause delays in obtaining treatment and assessment in emergency rooms (EDs). Furthermore, CMC are prone to rapid changes in physiologic condition, which commonly need the use of hospital-based healthcare.

When compared to phone discussions between patients and providers, telehealth technology enables for more comprehensive distant experiences. Telehealth engagements may include the use of ancillary equipment such as a stethoscope, otoscope, or camera to transmit data that is equivalent to or better than in-person assessments. A growing number of studies in adult and paediatric populations have demonstrated feasibility, decreased treatment costs, and high physician satisfaction when using telehealth. The published studies focused solely on the usage of videoconferencing and found that it improves family happiness while lowering travel costs. Few studies have looked into the role of a remote inspection device, and none have described how a CMC home caregiver may utilize one.

16.5.2 Telemedicine for Asthma Management

Telehealth offers a one-of-a-kind chance to overcome the challenges of providing asthma care in a traditional environment. Patients and doctors have utilized RPM (remote patient monitoring) and mobile health to educate them, track ailments and adherence to medication, verify intravenous access, or even completely replace doctor's visits. School-based telemedicine, in particular, has been found to improve physical activity, lung function, and asthma awareness while lowering asthma symptoms, missed school days, ED visits, and hospitalization. An ongoing telemedicine facility is very useful as in-person appointments for asthmatic follow-up care in a recent research. Remote spirometry testing for asthmatic children has also been shown to be helpful via telemedicine [11]. Paediatric-trained specialists and specialized treatment are available through both clinical visits and telemedicine-assisted spirometry testing. The intervention would be significant to parents, clinicians, and school officials if an effective school-based telemedicine (SBTM) asthma programme reduced healthcare usage. Because this possible advantage might result in fewer lost school days and maybe higher academic performance. SBTM might be utilized to create asthma treatment models for both chronic and acute asthma. Both approaches provide beneficial possibilities for students, care takers, and educators. School nursing coverage and resources are typically insufficient to aid in the managing of acute asthma attacks. An SBTM facility that offers severe asthma visits will allow nursing personnel and/or employees to get real-time guidance from of the child's doctor, avoiding unnecessary trips to the ER or other acute health professionals. Acute guidance given during an exacerbation, on the other hand, might significantly shorten the time it takes for EMTs to arrive and/or transfer to the ED. Telemedicine can help with chronic asthma treatment by increasing access to both general and specialized asthma treatment. Children in high-risk neighbourhoods, in particular, may lack accessible access to experts, transportation, and other barriers to treatment. Some of these significant impediments might be addressed by an SBTM asthma programme. An SBTM approach might provide further access to education for nursing staff by actively engaging in instructional materials such as webinar, videoconferencing, and other continuities, in addition to chronic asthma treatment. These chances are critical since disparities in school nurse training between urban and rural areas are highlighted, with village staff having less opportunity to participate in asthma education programme. In a school context, both synchronous and asynchronous telemedicine can be employed. Creating a continuous, active video link between such a patient at an originating site, including a university or hospital, and a doctor at a remote location is referred to as synchronous telemedicine [12]. The most common applications of synchronous telemedicine are in the school context and for various urgent paediatric healthcare models. Asynchronous telemedicine makes use of recorded video, which is frequently accompanied with a thorough medical history form and, where necessary, imaging. Halterman et al. [13] employed asynchronous telemedicine for asthma in the school context and found it to be more suited for chronic illness management. Tele presenters, or trained experts, are widely employed in both synchronous and asynchronous telemedicine consultations to help with the visit. During the visit, the telepresenter assists the patient by assuring that the lighting and telehealth gear are in working condition, as well as aiding the patient examination with peripherals such as a stethoscope, examination camera, and other telemedicine gear.

16.5.3 Telemedicine for the Paediatric Trauma Patient

Telemedicine currently includes a variety of delivery methods for different types of clinical treatment. Pre-hospital (field examination and transfer), in-hospital (emergency department, inpatient/ICU), and residence follow-up and retraining are all part of trauma therapy. Telehealth can be a beneficial tool for early assessment, evaluation, and treatment in the prehospital situation. One research, for example, looked into the practicality of a portable ultrasound that can transmit live pictures in healthy participants and comes with a transmission equipment backpack. The gadget was able to send live photos over a local cellular network or through satellites in remote areas. Telemedicine help during transportation can improve patient care in a similar way. In simulated trauma patients, according to Charash et al. [14], the victims' vital signs improved drastically when they arrived by the ambulance outfitted with real-time camera and oxygen saturation monitoring that was wirelessly related to a doctor's workstations at a county hospital. A juvenile catastrophe centre's accessibility to the paediatric skills of both the paediatric critical care doctor and the paediatric surgeons is a demonstrated benefit. By using professionals' presence online to assist in the treatment of wounded kids in relatively distant and urgent accessibility facilities is predicted to improve results as well. A telemedicine programme, on the other side, can boost hospital revenue and transfers. Over a seven-year period, Dharmar et al. [15] investigated the financial implications of a telemedicine programme in a major hospital for children. In the post-telemedicine era, the percentage of patients moved from regional institutions increased from 143 to 285, leading in a $1.6 million rise in the sector's average annual wage.

16.5.4 Telemedicine for Paediatric Cardiology

Telemedicine is increasingly being utilized to enhance the efficiency of paediatric cardiology care in hospitals where paediatric cardiologists are not available. Initial results indicate that tele cardiology is accurate, improves patient care, is cost-effective, improves echocardiography quality, and saves needless neonatal transfers in areas where paediatric cardiologists are not available. In bigger urban regions, paediatric tele-echocardiography is also being employed in community hospitals. Tele-echocardiography offers the ability to deliver real-time diagnostics to newborn institutions that don't have their own paediatric cardiologists on staff [16]. Many newborns in rural regions, small towns, and community hospitals may not have rapid access to paediatric sonographers or paediatric cardiologists for echocardiography interpretation. This can lead to subpar echocardiogram quality, a delay in medical intervention, unnecessary patient transportation, and higher medical costs. Telemedicine is increasingly being utilized to enhance the efficiency of paediatric cardiology care in hospitals where paediatric cardiologists are not available. Telecardiology, according to early studies, is accurate, improves patient care, is cost-effective, improves echocardiography quality, and reduces needless transfers of neonates to regions where paediatric cardiologists are not available.

16.5.5 Use of Telemedicine in Paediatric Sleep

Diminished travel time and expenses, less school unlucky deficiencies, less missed work time for guardians, and uniting numerous guardians advantageously, like guardians, sitters, instructors, and grandparents, who may all give care to a kid and give alternate points of view, are generally possible advantages of consolidating telemedicine into paediatric rest rehearses.

Because full assessments were difficult to complete, funding was irregular, and many physicians were focused with their in-office practices before the COVID-19 outbreak, few paediatric sleep medicine practitioners employed telemedicine consultations. Since (COVID-19) pandemic, telemedicine in paediatrics has been a popular topic in an effort to lower the risk of sickness for children. Prior to the COVID-19 outbreak, few practitioners employed telemedicine for routine visits since comprehensive assessments were difficult to do. Many doctors were focused with their in-office practices due to a lack of consistent pay.

In one research, moms of healthy term babies were sent regular emails or text messages with brief safe sleep movies for 60 days [17]. When contrasted with control treatments, the scientists found that this mobile health treatment increased self-reported compliance to four newborn safe sleep habits.

In juvenile obstructive sleep apnoea (OSA) [18], telemedicine through phone calls and follow-up visits has also been examined. The nurse-led telephone visit was evaluated by 55 of these parents, and 100% of them were "completely happy", feeling that the phone conversation follow-up offered ease, tailored care, and assurance. Only 11 of the 55 children were later seen at the clinic [18].

Telemedicine via the phone has also been utilized to treat insomnia. After five phone conversations and 6 months of follow-up, a randomized controlled study in which 61 children with insomnia and attention deficit hyperactivity problem, a telephone-coached intervention for sleeplessness resulted in a reduction in sleep issues and an enhancement in psychological adjustment [19]. Following that, the insomnia treatments were tried on adolescents with neurological issues, with parents indicating that the phone calls were both effective and practical.

16.6   Case Studies

Table 16.1 shows the case studies in the domain of paediatric telemedicine.

16.7   Research Challenges in Paediatric Telemedicine

Telemedicine has been a major success, as seen by the rapid growth of its application in paediatrics over the previous decade. However, it is not without its drawbacks. These include technological barriers, provider issues, patient problems, financial issues, credentialing and licencing barriers and legal issues. Figure 16.2 shows the research challenges in paediatric telemedicine.

16.7.1 Technological Barriers

For telehealth to be effective, foundation should be set up at both the counselling site and the destinations mentioning conference. Many towns, however, lack a broadband connection with adequate capacity to perform successful telehealth exchanges. This is particularly true in rural and underdeveloped communities, where telemedicine can help bridge important gaps in specialist or critical care availability. For example, in a paediatric cardiovascular home telehealth initiative, researchers discovered that availability to high-quality landlines and mobile phones

Table 16.1 Case studies in the domain of paediatric telemedicine

Name of the company	Category	Solution	Target people
Acorn Pediatrics	Telehealth	During the pandemic, virtual visits imply reduced exposure to patients and workers. Telemedicine also allows parents who work outside the house to schedule appointments during the evenings, as well as patients whose parents may not be in the same physical area	Children
ZZ Pediatrics	Telehealth	Able to view inside a child's ears and send an antibiotic prescription if an infection is present When a kid has breathing problems, one can use the pulse ox to check oxygen levels and persuade parents to try steam instead of coming to the ER	Children
Forest Hills Pediatric Associates	Telehealth	Virtually all of the providers began seeing patients. The practice began doing remote visits on a regular basis as well as on demand	Children
Active KidMD	Remote monitoring	Offering virtual visits, and both the medical staff and the families have been pleased with the ability to communicate via telehealth	Children
Dekalb Pediatric Center	Telehealth	Patients can be cared for afar, and virtual behavioural health visits can be held	Children

Fig. 16.2 Research challenge in paediatric telemedicine

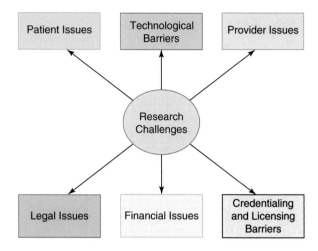

for data transmission was so inconsistent that certain eligible participants were unable to be registered due to a lack of stable telephone services. In addition, some services, such as telehealth for radiology or echocardiography, need a high degree of system quality to ensure that images can be appropriately analysed by consultation specialists. These services may be hard to perform due to a lack of high-quality equipment.

16.7.2 Provider Issues

One of the most significant roadblocks to telehealth adoption has been clinicians' reluctance to employ the technology in patient care. Many clinicians find that telehealth is difficult to integrate into their daily workflow, that it takes time away from their already hectic schedules, and that it typically provides little benefit beyond a typical phone conversation. Many community hospital physicians are wary of depending on consultants they don't know, and they don't want to feel supervised or reprimanded as a result of needing to seek advice from others. Interestingly, consultant physicians have indicated concerns about being accused of stepping on the toes of community physicians in polls. Furthermore, the application of telehealth for different providers thinks that transferring sicker children is safer. Students would like to go to university hospitals as quickly as possible and wouldn't want to waste too much time at hub locations or risk having their transfer denied. Another reason for physician opposition is a lack of knowledge with telehealth and the equipment. When traffic is low, it is tough to keep providers competent with the equipment. Fear of seeming inadequate in front of other institutions' physicians, as well as patients and their families, makes practitioners who utilize telehealth technology seldom even more afraid to utilize it. Even among those clinicians who see the general advantage of telehealth, many do not regard it as required or effective for their specific practice, and hence are hesitant to adopt it, even at institutions that promote it.

16.7.3 Patient Issues

Patient and parent opposition to telemedicine seem to be far less of a barrier than provider reluctance. There are significant obstacles for patients that must be overcome. Concerns include dangers to privacy and security, the capacity to communicate effectively with doctors using technology, and the loss of face-to-face contact with physicians. Patients and guardians who use telehealth for home observing should approach the essential hardware, have the actual smoothness to utilize it fittingly, and have adequate well-being education and numeracy abilities.

16.7.4 Financial Issues

Financial hurdles to telehealth might come from a variety of places. To begin with, organizations or practices interested in telehealth must first invest in the appropriate technologies. In addition, costs for equipment upkeep, personnel training, and technical support are ongoing. Providers and hospitals in underprivileged and rural areas may find these expenses particularly difficult to bear. The most major monetary hindrance is the absence of clear and reliable repayment for telehealth, just as an absence of profit from speculation. There is as of now no normalized repayment technique for telehealth experiences, and both government and private back up plans stand up to obstructions. Even though a payer may reimburse, due to the time-consuming nature of the procedure, some providers and organizations fail to do so. As a result, many telehealth initiatives rely on grant money, which is usually limited in time and may not be enough to ensure long-term viability. Furthermore, proof of return on investment is noticeably lacking.

16.7.5 Credentialing and Licencing Barriers

The certification procedure for providers is one of the most significant impediments to telemedicine mentioned in the literature. The credentialing procedure for a certain hospital frequently entails a significant quantity of documentation and might take months. Completing documentation for each possible spoke hospital where a clinician would conduct telehealth consultation might be time-consuming for a clinician at a hub hospital. There is also a lot of variety in the licencing requirements for physicians who work in telehealth. Licensure is done at the state level, and the site of service is usually the site where a patient meets with a clinical clinician face to face. Whether a consultant needs complete licensure in all jurisdictions where they work, merely their home state's licence, or a specific telehealth licence is very varied.

16.7.6 Legal Issues

Telehealth brings up a number of legal problems that many providers and organizations are concerned about. One point to consider is medico legal responsibility. Clear liability protection must be in place at both locations, for example, to protect experts counselling on patients remotely as well as individuals who follow their advice. Telehealth is a hybrid of face-to-face and telephone meetings, and in principle, treatment should be better than telephone contacts due to the consulting physician's greater capacity to envision the patient. Telephone malpractice lawsuits, on the other hand, have been found to be extraordinarily expensive in terms of settlements, and to cause severe morbidity and even mortality—in fact, the most common damage was death, which occurred in 44% of the claims examined [20]. Understandably, providers and organizations may be concerned about the medico-legal liability concerns, particularly if they are concerned about the Return on Investment. What would happen if the technology failed is likewise uncertain.

16.8   The Future

In paediatrics, telemedicine offers a wide range of uses. As innovation advances and costs fall, telemedicine will improve research, instruction, admittance to mind, crisis reaction, and the conveyance of general and forte paediatrics in an assortment of settings. It will expand correspondence among families and clinical specialists really focusing on their youngsters' overall paediatrics in local area-based practice. Payment, cross-state licence, and liability are the most major roadblocks. More study is needed to evaluate the appropriate applications of telemedicine, the consequences for patient safety and quality improvement, as well as the cost-effectiveness of alternative payment schemes like Accountable Care Organizations (ACOs). Telemedicine's biggest strength is its capacity to reach medically underprivileged groups despite distance and time constraints. This strength should allow telemedicine to be used in a variety of paediatric situations.

16.9   Conclusion

Telemedicine is described as the transmission of health evidence from one place to other using digital technologies in attempt to enhance a patient 's medical overall health. Telemedicine's attractiveness stems from its capacity to transcend geographical and time obstacles to make healthcare more cost-effective and accessible. This novel technique provides advantages for both parents and children in a paediatric context. Time away from work is reduced, transportation costs are reduced, and long-term health management can be carried out with minimal disruption. This chapter has not only covered the introduction to telemedicine but also the use of telemedicine for the children's health. The chapter also covered the detailed information about the financial impact of telemedicine and its infrastructure and application areas. The chapter also covered the case studies and concluded with the barriers of paediatric telemedicine and the future of telemedicine in the domain of children's health.

References

1. Notario PM, Gentile E, Amidon M, Angst D, Lefaiver C, Webster K. Home-based telemedicine for children with medical complexity. Telemed J e-Health. 2019;25(11):1123–32. https://doi.org/10.1089/tmj.2018.0186.
2. Paruthi S. Telemedicine in pediatric sleep. Sleep Med Clin. 2020;15(3S):e1–7. https://doi.org/10.1016/j.jsmc.2020.07.003.
3. Muñoz-Bonet JI, López-Prats JL, Flor-Macián EM, Cantavella T, Bonet L, Domínguez A, Brines J. Usefulness of telemedicine for home ventilator-dependent children. J Telemed Telecare. 2020;26(4):207–15. https://doi.org/10.1177/1357633X18811751.
4. Kim JW, Friedman J, Clark S, Hafeez B, Listman D, Lame M, Eid DA, Sharma R, Platt S. Implementation of a pediatric emergency telemedicine program. Pediatr Emerg Care. 2020;36(2):e104–7. https://doi.org/10.1097/pec.0000000000002044.
5. Kumar G, Falk DM, Bonello RS, Kahn JM, Perencevich E, Cram P. The costs of critical care telemedicine programs: a systematic review and analysis. Chest. 2013;143(1):19–29. https://doi.org/10.1378/chest.11-3031.
6. Franzini L, Sail KR, Thomas EJ, Wueste L. Costs and cost-effectiveness of a telemedicine intensive care unit program in 6 intensive care units in a large health care system. J Crit Care. 2011;26(3):329.e1–329.e3296. https://doi.org/10.1016/j.jcrc.2010.12.004.
7. Mullaney T. The sensible side of telemedicine. Bloomberg Businessweek June 25, 2006. Available at: www.businessweek.com/stories/2006-06-25/online-extra-the-sensibleside-oftelemedicine. Accessed June 01, 2021.
8. Reardon M. Are the stars aligning for telemedicine's success? July 19, 2009. Available at: http://news.cnet.com/8301-1001_3-10290067-92.html. Accessed June 01, 2014.
9. US Department of Health and Human Services. Summary of the HIPAA privacy rule 2003. Available at: www.hhs.gov/ocr/privacy/hipaa/understanding/summary/index.html. Accessed June 01, 2021.
10. Simon TD, Berry J, Feudtner C, Stone BL, Sheng X, Bratton SL, Dean JM, Srivastava R. Children with complex chronic conditions in inpatient hospital settings in the United States. Pediatrics. 2010;126(4):647–55. https://doi.org/10.1542/peds.2009-3266.
11. Perry TT, Marshall A, Berlinski A, Rettiganti M, Brown RH, Randle SM, Luo C, Bian J. Smartphone-based vs paper-based asthma action plans for adolescents. Ann Allergy Asthma Immunol. 2017;118(3):298–303. https://doi.org/10.1016/j.anai.2016.11.028.
12. Ronis SD, McConnochie KM, Wang H, Wood NE. Urban telemedicine enables equity in access to acute illness care. Telemed J e-Health. 2017;23(2):105–12. https://doi.org/10.1089/tmj.2016.0098.
13. Halterman JS, Fagnano M, Tajon RS, Tremblay P, Wang H, Butz A, Perry TT, McConnochie KM. Effect of the School-Based Telemedicine Enhanced Asthma Management (SB-TEAM) program on asthma morbidity: a randomized clinical trial. JAMA Pediatr. 2018;172(3):e174938. https://doi.org/10.1001/jamapediatrics.2017.4938.
14. Charash WE, Caputo MP, Clark H, Callas PW, Rogers FB, Crookes BA, Alborg MS, Ricci MA. Telemedicine to a moving ambulance improves outcome after trauma in simulated patients. J Trauma. 2011;71(1):49–55. https://doi.org/10.1097/TA.0b013e31821e4690.
15. Dharmar M, Sadorra CK, Leigh P, Yang NH, Nesbitt TS, Marcin JP. The financial impact of a pediatric telemedicine program: a children's hospital's perspective. Telemed J e-Health. 2013;19(7):502–8. https://doi.org/10.1089/tmj.2012.0266.

16. Sable CA, Cummings SD, Pearson GD, Schratz LM, Cross RC, Quivers ES, Rudra H, Martin GR. Impact of telemedicine on the practice of pediatric cardiology in community hospitals. Pediatrics. 2002;109(1):E3. https://doi.org/10.1542/peds.109.1.e3.
17. Moon RY, Corwin MJ, Kerr S, Heeren T, Colson E, Kellams A, Geller NL, Drake E, Tanabe K, Hauck FR. Mediators of improved adherence to infant safe sleep using a mobile health intervention. Pediatrics. 2019;143(5):e20182799. https://doi.org/10.1542/peds.2018-2799.
18. Walijee H, Sood S, Markey A, Krishnan M, Lee A, De S. Is nurse-led telephone follow-up for post-operative obstructive sleep apnoea patients effective? A prospective observational study at a paediatric tertiary centre. Int J Pediatric Otorhinolaryngol. 2020;129:109766. https://doi.org/10.1016/j.ijporl.2019.109766.
19. Corkum P, Lingley-Pottie P, Davidson F, McGrath P, Chambers CT, Mullane J, Laredo S, Woodford K, Weiss SK. Better nights/better days-distance intervention for insomnia in school-aged children with/without ADHD: a randomized controlled trial. J Pediatric Psychol. 2016;41(6):701–13. https://doi.org/10.1093/jpepsy/jsw031.
20. Katz HP, Kaltsounis D, Halloran L, Mondor M. Patient safety and telephone medicine: some lessons from closed claim case review. J Gen Internal Med. 2008;23(5):517–22. https://doi.org/10.1007/s11606-007-0491-y.

Telemedicine: The Immediate and Long-Term Functionality Contributing to Treatment and Patient Guidance

17

Sudhanshu Mishra, Disha Sharma,
Shobhit Prakash Srivastava, Khushboo Raj,
Rishabha Malviya, and Neeraj Kumar Fuloria

17.1 Introduction

"Tele" is a Greek term that describes "distance," and "mederi" is a Latin phrase that refers "to heal." Telemedicine has been dubbed "healing by wire" by Time magazine. While it was originally regarded as "futuristic" and "experimental," telemedicine is now a practice and here to stay. Telemedicine may be used for several purposes, including hospital care, training, science, management, and human health. Formalized paraphrase Families in remote and isolated areas around the world fail to get appropriate, high-quality specialized healthcare services [1]. Inhabitants within those areas also have little access to specialized hospitals, because medical specialists are most inclined to be clustered in dense urban areas.

S. Mishra
Department of Pharmaceutical Science & Technology, Madan Mohan Malaviya University of Technology, Gorakhpur, Uttar Pradesh, India

D. Sharma (✉)
Gahlot Institute of Pharmacy, Navi Mumbai, Maharashtra, India

S. P. Srivastava
Dr. M C Saxena College of Pharmacy, Lucknow, Uttar Pradesh, India

K. Raj
Department of Pharmacy, ARKA Jain University, Tata Nagar, Jamshedpur, Jharkhand, India

R. Malviya
School of Medical and Allied Sciences, Galgotias University,
Greater Noida, Uttar Pradesh, India

N. K. Fuloria
Faculty of Pharmacy, AIMST University, Semeling, Kedah, Malaysia

267

T. Choudhury et al. (eds.), *Telemedicine: The Computer Transformation of Healthcare*, TELe-Health, https://doi.org/10.1007/978-3-030-99457-0_17

The World Health Organization (WHO) defines Telemedicine as, "The delivery of healthcare services, where distance is a critical factor, by all healthcare professionals using information and communication technologies for the exchange of valid information for the diagnosis, treatment and prevention of disease and injuries, research and evaluation and for the continuing education of healthcare providers, all in the interests of advancing the health of individuals and their communities" [2].

Telehealth refers to the use of a virtual environment built on technologies to provide different facets of health education, monitoring, surveillance, and medical treatment. Telemedicine is the largest component of telehealth and is the fastest-growing field of healthcare. Broadly speaking, telemedicine is the practice of treatment by a remote electronic device. There have been discrepancies in the distribution of telemedicine [3]. In nature, the great majority of hospital-based service provision is doctor-to-doctor, with expert specialists delivering specialized treatment to sometimes rural, foreign, or non-specialist doctors. In comparison, patient-to-doctor medical treatment is a rising market, and patients can access physicians by direct-to-consumer providers. Withstanding this, telemedicine is still to be broadly adopted owing to stringent legislative requirements and a scarcity of supportive payment systems. Faced with the latest pandemic, hospitals have also been driven to expand their use of telehealth facilities to the detriment of conventional face-to-face patient interactions. Scholars have studied the benefits and drawbacks of telemedicine in comparison to conventional patient visits for many years. Throughout a pandemic, telemedicine can vastly enhance patient access to high-quality, low-cost therapies while maintaining physical separation for both patients' and physicians' safety [4].

Telemedicine is now much more available than it has ever been, thanks to advances in smartphone and tablet technology. According to a Pew Research Centre survey from 2019, 69.90 Americans should use the web. Furthermore, 81% of Americans now own a smartphone, almost 75% own desktop or notebook computers, and about 50% own tablet computers or e-readers. This expansion of mobile communications coverage has been crucial to the development of telemedicine [5]. As a result, any use of the Internet in healthcare is also now commonplace. Any use of patient health records helps all patients and physicians to store and view medical documents. Patients can display results using these services [6].

The latest research has well established the effectiveness of telemedicine as a way of delivering high-quality healthcare. Powell et al. interviewed patients after telemedicine encounters with their primary care providers in the form of primary care and discovered that almost all participants examined considered telemedicine interactions to be acceptable with certain acute care needs, and a majority indicated that they will always continue to use telemedicine rather than in-person encounters throughout the possibility [7]. According to a report that assessed the viability of using a smartphone for wound infection follow-up after an appendectomy, the responsiveness and accuracy for monitoring wound infection complications were 100% and 91.67%, respectively. Moreover, research that used texting as a method of follow-up following colorectal procedure discovered that no postoperative risk went undetected in the trial, and also proposed that symptomatology follow-up survey questions using texting might theoretically substitute the conventional postoperative follow-up examination [8]. Finally, telemedicine technologies such as Tele-stroke services, which offer stroke resources to hospitals requiring specialists in stroke care, have proven highly popular and continue to develop in the United States.

Telemedicine has developed slowly in the latest days, with just 8% of Americans using it in 2019. Major obstacles to broader acceptance involved minimal insurance, patients' and physicians' lack of engagement with telemedicine technology, and, more importantly, little persuasive arguments for replacing in-person treatment even outside rural medicine [9]. Amid all the challenges many health services have also been developing in telemedicine capability, hoping that it will become even more common in the potential. Even then, this technological innovation, like all innovative technologies, faces major obstacles while realizing its maximum capabilities. Understanding the sector as it develops is a huge challenge. When considering the advancement of technology such as e-mail and mobile phones, it is clear that adequate knowledge and awareness of the technologies in the context of the possibilities that they provide is missing as in the developed world [10]. Transnational companies, for instance, have a 71% failure rate in applying Western information communication technologies (ICTs) to emerging countries. Furthermore, calling is mainly constructed for urgent purposes rather than for informal chat. As a result, subscribers spend even less per service than they already do in developing countries, making it difficult to serve those territories and yet remain profitable [11].

17.2   Types of Telemedicine

All telemedicine applications have one commonality: a client (e.g., a patient or a healthcare worker) gets a perception from someone who knows more when the parties are separated in space, time, or both; expertise in the relevant field is required. Telemedicine can be classified based on two factors [3, 12]:

- The interaction between the client and the expert
- The type of information being transmitted.

Components of telemedicine are shown in Fig. 17.1, while various types of telemedicine are summarized in Fig. 17.2.

17.3   Positive and Negative Aspects of Telemedicine

Positive Aspects: Telemedicine has the potential to improve access to information for both health professionals and patients, as well as the general public. For example, electronic search engines such as PUBMED, MEDLAR, and others have demonstrated their potential in allowing any health professional to stay up to date on any

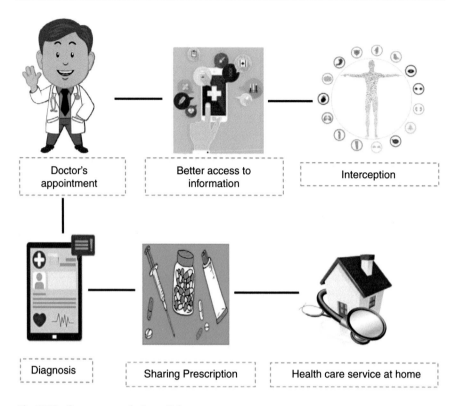

Fig. 17.1 Components of telemedicine

Fig. 17.2 Various types of telemedicine

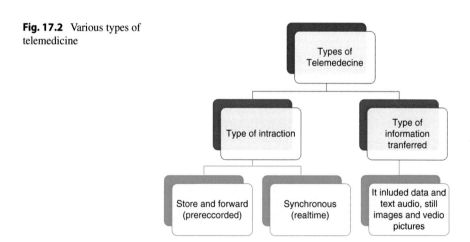

case-related information within a fraction. Similarly, patient data is kept and can be made by allowing for quick and immediate data transfer between general practitioners and hospitals [11].

Telemedicine also helps to improve access to services and elevate the care of delivering. Also, patients will be benefited from increased convenience and time savings. Improved access to care between and within regions, which had earlier been denied due to socioeconomic restrictions, particularly in developing countries, and the willingness for specific services to be centralized in urban centers can be possible and also it is less cost-effective [13].

Negative Aspects: It may lead to the failure in the relationship of health professionals and between the health professionals and patients due to various reasons such as sometimes the whole consultation is not possible to be performed especially in those cases where palpitation is an important part of examination [14]. Video consultancy may not be sufficient in these types of cases. Also, there is a chance of threat that highly skilled staff at the remote location will consider that their autonomy is endangered by the use of telemedicine, or even worse, that they will become nothing more than technicians, going to act merely as the hands of the specialist, who will start receiving all the praise and recognition for conducting a consultation [15].

17.3.1 The Positive Aspect of Telemedicine

In addition to priority, telemedicine has supported the public health emergency by enabling for the rapid mobilization of great numbers of healthcare personnel and the supply of facilities in places where local hospitals and healthcare centers are unable to fulfill the demands. During this virus outbreak, telemedicine was being used to provide healthcare information to both noninfected people and sick individuals [16]. Telemedicine's use for chronic disease therapy is gaining popularity, with studies demonstrating that it can effectively treat diseases including diabetes and congestive heart failure [17].

The expanded use has sparked debate over incorporating telemedicine into healthcare professional credentialing, support for telemedicine and redesigning clinical care models, among other aspects [18].

Several possible advantages of telemedicine can indeed be imagined, which include [19, 20]:

- Better access to information.
- Availability of frequently unavailable coverage.
- Management that enables to facilities and care delivery.
- Enhanced clinical practice.
- Quality management of treatment strategies.
- Lower cost of healthcare.
- To offer information to patients for them to consider the essence of their illness, its prognosis, the causes for such inquiries, and the impact of any therapy.

- To disseminate information to the people, including the underprivileged: for particular, as a component of health awareness or health promotion to individuals, classrooms, and medical facilities.
- Telemedicine may also provide virtual lectures on well-being and illness. These types of presentations have the ability to solve problems owing to illiteracy.
- Enhanced availability to primary care telemedicine may strengthen direct connections to primary care.
- It can also increase access to healthcare services at home.
- Tracking and recovery at residence.
- Home supervision and management of patients suffering from multiple diseases will increase medical safety and efficiency. The five aspects below show how telemedicine can help with those advancements.
- Increased exposure to skilled nursing telemedicine has the potential to increase access to hospitals. It can also increase access inside and between hospitals.

17.3.2 Provision of Previously Unavailable Treatment

The Norwegian government launched a nationwide telemedicine network in the 1980s. The primary purpose was to provide residents of remote, rural areas with an alternative to travelling due to local shortages of specialist treatment. Overall, this strategic effort was vindicated and has since been repeated in other parts of the country [21].

17.3.3 Provision of Previously Unavailable Treatment

Patients and the public, in general, will benefit from this information. In several countries, computers in classrooms, households, offices, and local libraries provide access to electronic data information over the Internet. This is an example. Has provided an opportunity to include a "superhighway" of wellness and illness knowledge that could be used for a variety of purposes [22].

17.3.4 The Negative Aspect of Telemedicine

Limitations to telemedicine that have been identified include a lack of knowledge about the efficacy and safety of telemedicine in light of current circumstances, patient preferences for seeing their provider rather than someone with whom they may not have an established relationship, a lack of understanding about how to access telemedicine visits, and a lack of knowledge about hematology (including alternative respiratory muscle activity, breath effort, and expression), the occurrence of a patient cough (whether dry or sustainable), oropharynx analysis through the camera, and patient-directed lymph nodes to evaluate for significant lymphadenopathy [23].

While telemedicine has many potential benefits, it also has some drawbacks. The following are the key pitfalls of telemedicine that can be anticipated [24, 25]:

- A deterioration in the interaction between the health patient and the provider.
- A decline in the availability of healthcare professionals.
- Problems surrounding the accuracy of medical details and operational and procedural complexities.
- Physical and emotional causes.
- Depersonalization.
- Separate consultation process.
- Failure to complete the whole consultation.
- The diminished trust of patients and health practitioners.
- Different expertise and expertise needed by health professionals are some of the factors that can trigger a deterioration in the relationship between the health provider and patient as opposed to regular face-to-face consultations [26].

Relationship breakdown between a health provider and a patient: It should not be believed that using teleconsultations would lead to deterioration in the patient-doctor relationship. Concerns over the accuracy of health records as previously said, the Internet contains a plethora of medical knowledge. This can be categorized into three broad categories [27, 28]:

- Textbook-style material provided by medical institutions and some other research institutions.
- Analyses of peer-reviewed papers and even whole documents in medical journals health brochures and articles owned by individuals.
- Charity associations or particularly unique groups.
- Difficulties of management and bureaucracy: The fact that telemedicine has the ability to improve healthcare quality does not guarantee that it will be enforced [29].

In 1994, the Western Governors' Association Telemedicine Action Report identified six.
"telemedicine hurdles" that could stymie the adoption of this form of healthcare delivery [30, 31].

- Issues with technology planning and management.
- Issues with telecommunications restrictions.
- Issues with compensation for telemedicine services due to unavailable or incompatible policies.
- Issues with licensure and certification due to competing interests in providing quality of healthcare, restricting professional duties, and adopting policy frameworks.

17.4   Physician Perspective of Telemedicine

Healthcare delivery is regulated by a three-tier structure and health is the primary responsibility of the society. Quality and access to healthcare within urban and rural areas are distinct. In India, poverty, prosperity, and civil war are primarily influenced by the northeastern states [32]. Restricted infrastructure in the area and weak connectivity with the rest of the world were the key constraints of development and growth in these states [33]. A telemedicine platform that can be incorporated with the current healthcare delivery system can bridge the gap of healthcare in rural and urban areas.

There have been several studies conducted on telemedicine like in Apollo TeleHealth Services offered 116 clinicians who perform telemedicine. A total of 51 experts participated in the survey. Seventy-one patients enrolled in the study [34]. The patients were connected through different means like either via e-mail, telephone call, or videoconferencing with a specialist. Patient symptoms ranged from headache to consultation and/or care in Orthopedics, Neurology, Cardiology, Psychology, Urology, Dermatology, General Medicine, Obstetrics and Gynecology, Rheumatology, and Oncology [35]. The length of treatment provided by telemedicine varies from one visit to as long as 1 year based on the quality of the care given to the patient. All the doctors had telemedicine experience; 55% of the patients had 10-20 consultations a day and 22% had more than 20 consultations per day. Sixty-five per cent of participants invested 1-2 h per day of their time on telemedicine consultation. Both the doctors were pleased with the TSC procedure. Ninety-four percent of respondents responded that they had desirable outcomes on the diagnosis of a patient's disease [5]. Recall percent of patients in this sample was 71%. Approximately 94% of services are open to telemedicine promotion.

The questions set out in this analysis were appropriate in pursuing the topic of telemedicine from the point of view of the patient and the doctor. The self-reporting methodology was used for data collection and is deemed sufficient for the measurement of physicians' decision to implement telemedicine technology. This method of gathering data via a questionnaire was and is successful [36]. This would boost telemedicine treatment and make it simpler, more affordable, and easier to use. Telemedicine may help both the physician and the patient, but little is understood about the financial benefit of both the doctor and the patient. The analysis was carried out with all these points in view.

Doctors who use this service can treat the patients without a face-to-face consultation with a specialist and deliver comparable results. Using store-and-forward technologies rather than videoconferencing, this site offers year-round expert diagnostics and management advice. The cases shall be replied to within 24 h of their request. There are advantages in terms of improved availability, decreased time, expense, and professional isolation. However, the penetration remains low, possibly due to lack of understanding, the expanded workload for referral professionals, and lack of financial rewards [37].

As the part of the telecommunication, there is ample evidence of a high degree of patient satisfaction, although several studies have methodological weaknesses.

Overall, there is no evidence of efficacy and cost-effectiveness. Good data exists for diagnosis, home treatment, and specialized consultation with a general physician with patients present. All offer evidence that video consulting has an important role to play, but does not avoid the need for a face-to-face consultation [3]. Video consulting contradicts conventional professional positions, especially those of nurses, and may enhance the skills and job satisfaction of health workers.

More importantly, the conventional division between primary and secondary treatment is undermined by telehealth. This may be a source of opposition, but it may ultimately be one of its strengths. Appropriately tailored video consultation has a great potential to enhance the delivery of primary healthcare in Australia, especially in rural and remote areas [7, 38].

17.5   Patient Perspective of Telemedicine

Telemedicine is a general concept that includes a variety of innovations, from digital X-rays to over-the-phone appointments, videoconferencing, and remote surgery results. In other words, it is the use of cellular technologies to offer medical care or facilities [39]. It provides access to medical services through video calls, e-mails, access to medical records and remote diagnostics, like rural care in the near future. Advances in the field are intended to encourage the vast majority of the world to be beyond the scope of medical treatment. This will dramatically alter the direction of growth of many countries [40]. This will radically affect the pattern of development of many communities. Telemedicine offers independence by making it possible for patients and people to receive medical services. Rather than wasting several hours or days commuting to a health clinic, medical advice and consultation may be accessed more locally, freeing up time and making it possible to get care [41].

To date, economic analyses of cost-saving approaches such as telemedicine have almost entirely taken the provider's perspective. From a public policy point of view, however, the calculation of patient (consumer) welfare improvements from healthcare advances could be at least as significant, provided that public funds strongly subsidize health insurance through Medicare and Medicaid reimbursements and provide funding for facilities and services. Innovation that offers small cost savings to the provider could lead to substantial losses in the well-being of the customer. Patient welfare must be taken into account in determining the social welfare benefits of such innovation [42].

From the patient perspective, various examples have shown positive result in telemed scenario. A few studies have been released on the use of instantaneous video and emerging media to help in periprocedural treatment in liver disease. A case report highlighted a good example of gastroenterologist-led teleproctoring using simple video technologies to allow a surgeon to conduct sclerotherapy for hemostasis in the setting of a variceal bleed. Some other case report identified the transfer of smartphone images from surgical trainees to an attending physician to make a real-time decision about a potentially problematic liver acquisition, which took place 545 km away from the university hospital [43]. A retrospective clinical study identified the viability and effective usage of high-resolution digital macroscopic imaging and virtual delivery between liver transplant centers in the United Kingdom to expand the use of such split liver transplantation, a situation in which comprehensive knowledge of vessel anatomy is required for innovative medical preparation. Similarly, the unregulated case series from Greece documented the viability and efficiency of macroscopic image delivery to help in the assessment of liver transplant grafts. In different cases telemedicine has been proven to be efficient in the treatment of cardiovascular disease; however, an in-depth review of its efficacy in some areas, such as patient satisfaction and cost-effectiveness, is important [44].

Telemedicine is commonly used in most countries addressed as a method to improve access to healthcare by eliminating proximity to fair justice. However, technical limitations and lack of digital literacy have persisted as a major problem in the successful introduction of this virtual technique. While telemedicine is exciting in terms of its potential to improve access and quality, the ease and adoption of this modality of treatment are important for its dissemination.

17.5.1 Drawback from Patients

Physical and mental factors: Sometimes there are chances that patient has low vision or hearing power so that he/she may face difficulties in following the instructions that are presented in a video consultation or sometimes it might happen that patient is illiterate and not able to understand the written language or sign.

Derealization: The images of both the healthcare worker and the patient are projected onto a monitor during a teleconsultation, and all interactions between the two parties are indirect. Because our perceptions of what we see on a monitor are heavily influenced by our television viewing experience, a teleconsultation may not be perceived as genuine by either party. Research suggests that elderly patients do not always believe that a physician appearing on what appears to be a television set can see and pay attention to them adequately [45].

Reduce Patients confidence: There are possibilities that the patient is not very much habitual of handling technologies or videoconferencing, etc. especially in the rural part of the country. There are chances that they might be not able to open the video link and hesitate to consult their healthcare professionals.

17.6 Current Scenario of Telemedicine

Telemedicine has helped to strengthen uptake and has demonstrated considerable progress in improving access to health services, encouraging patient disease control and enabling screening in-between visits to healthcare. While the future is promising, more research is required to find optimal ways to implement telemedicine especially remote monitoring within routine clinical care. We call on specialist societies to put out a strong political statement that legislative changes are needed to address regulatory and reimbursement challenges. Telehealth has the ability to expand the boundaries of the practices of providers by removing the proximity barrier. Along with the adoption of a new mode of treatment, there is a transition, and the literature mentions different responses to this change. One research reported extreme opposition to change, while others showed an acceptance of the change. Older patients typically do not welcome transition, but new surveys have established generational adoption of technologies and mHealth in general [46, 47].

Predominantly, chronic illness treatment has focused on a sequence of return trips to hospitals scheduled at arbitrary hours. Telemedicine also provides for faster, more regular virtual appointments, and the potential to integrate various providers into the care of the patient. Frequent weight checks in patients with congestive heart failure or daily blood glucose checking in patients with diabetes can prevent hospital and emergency service visits, relieve the burden on the healthcare system, and minimize the total cost of chronic disease management. Telemedicine is making steady strides and the demand for this service is growing in the face of the emerging pandemic [45]. As such, federal and state laws need to rapidly respond to the increased need for telemedicine and preserve their capacity to deliver the six primary facets of the human right to health. This is a unique moment for America, and telemedicine legislation has to be adapted more effectively than ever during the COVID-19 pandemic.

Telemedicine has a wide range of uses in in-hospital care, education, science, management, and public health. Globally, people living in rural and remote areas are unable to receive timely, high-quality speciality medical services. Residents in these regions also have under-standard access to specialized healthcare, largely because specialist doctors are more likely to be based in areas of the dense urban population [27]. Telemedicine has the ability to cross this gap and facilitate healthcare in these remote areas.

Given the tremendous promise, traditional telemedicine research methods can be overwhelming given the rapid and growing usage of emerging technology for patients and health systems. As such, the classical approach of randomized controlled trials to assess the feasibility of intervention or change of patient delivery is therefore not practicable. We accept that there is a need to reevaluate the definition of what constitutes a high-quality study of telemedicine. For example, practical and applied science-based experiments that assess feasibility, scalability, and expense, in comparison to traditional clinical outcomes, may be better suited and more widely embraced.

17.7   Limitations of Telemedicine

Telemedicine medicines are not advantageous for everybody since they will not suit 870 and every patient circumstance, so we must use natural medicine over the telemedicine structure.

Limitations for patients as well as the healthcare provider [47]:

17.7.1 Limitations for Patients

Defending medical data: Criminals and hackers can also gain access to this patient's medical information, — particularly if the patients acknowledge telemedicine and a public network via an encrypted channel.

Care delays: When a patient needed emergency treatment, the telemedicine may be delayed in the treatment particularly since a doctor cannot provide lifesaving care on laboratory test digitally.

17.7.2 Mission for Healthcare Worker/Providers

Licensing issue: State law varies from state to state for adding a license to the health workers and also the clinical may not be able to practice telemedicine across the state lines concerning the health worker belonging to other state and the patients at the other state.

Concerns about technology: For the study of patients' physical problems, using the correct applications for telemedicine therapy is insufficient; doctors must utilize a very advanced form of application for telemedicine medication for this study.

Being unable to evaluate patients using a digital platform: The healthcare provider simply looks at the test reports of the patients that are available on the website, but he or she cannot physically examine the patients or even see the complaints accurately. Sometimes the patients and healthcare provider do not cooperate with each other through the platform provided by the telemedication.

17.8 Future Prospective

Telemedicine allows citizens in both rural and urban areas to access healthcare at their leisure. This leads to a method of caring for two patients who do not have access to a reliable transportation system. Patients with serious illnesses can visit a virtual office that is more convenient for them and avoid travelling.

Telemedicine encourages cost-cutting in health-care services by:

- Improving staff distribution and healthcare resources within the healthcare facility.
- Increasing the number of primary care providers.
- Increasing the patient engagement and outcomes.
- Avoiding unnecessary offices, rooms, and patient admissions.

In the current scenario, there is an unexplored market for telemedicine for virtual chronic disease management; it is under-utilized as compared to other services such as telebehavioral health and speciality telemedicine. People with the chronic diseases must see their doctors on a regular basis, and by targeting this patient demographic with telemedicine, the number of emergency room visits can be reduced.

The second growing field is the "hospital at home" or "hospital on wheels" model; this model is useful for patients who meet the criteria for hospitalization but is stable at home due to some emotional factors.

The use of an e-hospital system should be encouraged in order to deliver the greatest healthcare system possible to a patient who is resting at home and can contact and discuss their difficulties. It would be helpful for the person having corporate jobs or staying alone or may help in conditions like the COVID-19 lockdown phase.

17.9   Conclusion

Various pandemics, like as COVID-19, have struck mankind over the last few decades. The improvement and usage of telemedicine administrations are vital, as these administrations permit us to proceed to supply high-quality healthcare whereas keeping up the hone of physical removal to avoid the spread of these infections. The benefits of telemedicine incorporate comfort, expanded get to care from a separate, particularly for patients living in rustic zones, and diminished healthcare costs. Presently is time for us to execute these administrations and make the utilization of telemedicine standard. Telemedicine in these farther regions permits for convenient treatment of crisis cases. Hence, it contributes towards inaccessible crisis basic care in arrange to spare lives in pivotal cases. Also, the rising propels have presently empowered telemedicine to exchange expansive sums of clinical informatics information counting pictures, and test reports to the particular specialized well-being experts in a few genuine cases. It is now known that telemedicine will before long be fair another way to see well-being proficient.

Acknowledgments Authors are highly thankful to Dr. M C Saxena College of Pharmacy, Lucknow, India, ARKA Jain University, Department of Pharmacy, Jamshedpur, India, School of Medical and Allied Sciences, Galgotias University, Greater Noida, India, and Faculty of Pharmacy, AIMST University, Semeling, Kedah, Malaysia, for providing library facilities for literature survey. Conflict of InterestAuthors have no conflict of interest.

Funding Authors have received no funding from any Govt or non-Govt organization.

References

1. Ganapathy K. Telemedicine in India—the Apollo experience. online information source www.thambraj.com 2002.
2. Bashshur R, Armstrong PA, Youssef ZI. Telemedicine; explorations in the use of telecommunications in health care. CC Thomas; 1975.
3. Dasgupta A, Deb S. Telemedicine: A new horizon in public health in India. Indian J Commun Med. 2008;33(1):3.
4. Mechanic OJ, Persaud Y, Kimball AB. Telehealth systems. In: StatPearls. Treasure Island, FL: StatPearls Publishing; 2020. [Updated 2020 Sep 18].

5. Kichloo A, Albosta M, Dettloff K, Wani F, El-Amir Z, Singh J, Aljadah M, Chakinala RC, Kanugula AK, Solanki S, Chugh S. Telemedicine, the current COVID-19 pandemic and the future: a narrative review and perspectives moving forward in the USA. Family Med Commun Health. 2020;8(3)

6. Malapile S, Keengwe J. Information communication technology planning in developing countries. Educ Inf Technol. 2014;19(4):691–701.

7. Hjelm NM. Benefits and drawbacks of telemedicine. J Telemed Telecare. 2005;11(2):60–70.

8. Coulter A, Entwistle V, Gilbert D. Sharing decisions with patients: is the information good enough? BMJ. 1999;318(7179):318–22.

9. Norum J, Pedersen S, Størmer J, Rumpsfeld M, Stormo A, Jamissen N, Sunde H, Ingebrigtsen T, Larsen ML. Prioritisation of telemedicine services for large scale implementation in Norway. J Telemed Telecare. 2007;13(4):185–92.

10. Kristensen GB, Nerhus K, Thue G, Sandberg S. Standardized evaluation of instruments for self-monitoring of blood glucose by patients and a technologist. Clin Chem. 2004;50(6):1068–71.

11. Acharya RV, Rai JJ. Evaluation of patient and doctor perception toward the use of telemedicine in Apollo Tele Health Services, India. J Family Med Primary Care. 2016;5(4):798.

12. Khongji P. J North East India Stud. 2017;7(1):47–58.

13. Croteau AM, Vieru D. Telemedicine adoption by different groups of physicians. In: Proceedings of the 35th Annual Hawaii International Conference on System Sciences 2002 Jan 10. IEEE. p. 1985–93.

14. Muir J. Telehealth: the specialist perspective. Aust Fam Physician. 2014;43(12):828.

15. Raven M, Butler C, Bywood P. Video-based telehealth in Australian primary health care: current use and future potential. Aust J Prim Health. 2013;19(4):283–6.

16. Baigent MF, Lloyd CJ, Kavanagh SJ, Ben-Tovim DI, Yellowlees PM, Kalucy RS, Bond MJ. Telepsychiatry:'tele'yes, but what about the 'psychiatry'? J Telemed Telecare. 1997;3(Suppl. 1):3–5.

17. Wootton R, Yellowlees P, McLaren P, editors. Telepsychiatry and e-mental health. London: Royal Society of Medicine Press; 2003 Jan 1.

18. Dillon E, Loermans J. Telehealth in Western Australia: the challenge of evaluation. J Telemed Telecare. 2003;9(Suppl. 2):15–9.

19. Kmucha ST. Physician liability issues and telemedicine: Part 3 of 3.

20. Van Velsen L, Wildevuur S, Flierman I, Van Schooten B, Tabak M, Hermens H. Trust in telemedicine portals for rehabilitation care: an exploratory focus group study with patients and healthcare professionals. BMC Med Inform Decis Mak. 2015;16(1):1–2.

21. Perednia DA, Allen A. Telemedicine technology and clinical applications. JAMA. 1995;273(6):483–8.

22. Cameron AE, Bashshur RL, Halbritter K, Johnson EM, Cameron JW. Simulation methodology for estimating financial effects of telemedicine in West Virginia. Telemed J. 1998;4(2):125–44.

23. McCue MJ, Mazmanian PE, Hampton CL, Marks TK, Fisher EJ, Parpart F, Malloy WN, Fisk KJ. Cost-minimization analysis: a follow-up study of a telemedicine program. Telemed J. 1998;4(4):323–7.

24. Zincone LH Jr, Doty E, Balch DC. Financial analysis of telemedicine in a prison system. Telemed J. 1997;3(4):247–55.

25. Capalbo SM, Heggem CN. Valuing rural health care: Issues of access and quality. Am J Agric Econ. 1999;81(3):674–9.

26. Ahmed A, Slosberg E, Prasad P, Keeffe EB, Imperial JC. The successful use of telemedicine in acute variceal hemorrhage. J Clin Gastroenterol. 1999;29(2):212–3.

27. Croome KP, Shum J, Al-Basheer MA, Kamei H, Bloch M, Quan D, Hernandez-Alejandro R. The benefit of smart phone usage in liver organ procurement. J Telemed Telecare. 2011;17(3):158–60.

28. Mammas CS, Geropoulos S, Saatsakis G, Konstantinidou A, Lemonidou C, Patsouris E. Telepathology as a method to optimize quality in organ transplantation: a feasibility and reliability study of the virtual benching of liver graft. Stud Health Technol Inform. 2013;190:276–8.

29. Kruse CS, Soma M, Pulluri D, Nemali NT, Brooks M. The effectiveness of telemedicine in the management of chronic heart disease—a systematic review. JRSM open. 2017;8(3):2054270416681747.
30. Scott Kruse C, Karem P, Shifflett K, Vegi L, Ravi K, Brooks M. Evaluating barriers to adopting telemedicine worldwide: a systematic review. J Telemed Telecare. 2018;24(1):4–12.
31. Serper M, Volk ML. Current and future applications of telemedicine to optimize the delivery of care in chronic liver disease. Clin Gastroenterol Hepatol. 2018;16(2):157–61.
32. Tsai CH, Kuo YM, Uei SL. Influences of satisfaction with telecare and family trust in older Taiwanese people. Int J Environ Res Public Health. 2014 Feb;11(2):1359–68.
33. Bishop TF, Press MJ, Mendelsohn JL, Casalino LP. Electronic communication improves access, but barriers to its widespread adoption remain. Health Aff. 2013;32(8):1361–7.
34. Breen P, Murphy K, Browne G, Molloy F, Reid V, Doherty C, Delanty N, Connolly S, Fitzsimons M. Formative evaluation of a telemedicine model for delivering clinical neurophysiology services part I: utility, technical performance and service provider perspective. BMC Med Inform Decis Mak. 2010;10(1):1–2.
35. Kruse CS, Mileski M, Moreno J. Mobile health solutions for the aging population: a systematic narrative analysis. J Telemed Telecare. 2017;23(4):439–51.
36. Thirthalli J, Manjunatha N, Math SB. Unmask the mind! Importance of video consultations in psychiatry during COVID-19 pandemic. Schizophr Res. 2020;
37. Ganapathy KN. Apollo Hospitals, Chennai, Telemedicine in India-the Apollo experience. Neurosurgery on the Web. 2001.
38. Proctor E, Silmere H, Raghavan R, Hovmand P, Aarons G, Bunger A, Griffey R, Hensley M. Outcomes for implementation research: conceptual distinctions, measurement challenges, and research agenda. Adm Policy Ment Health Ment Health Serv Res. 2011;38(2):65–76.
39. Bashshur RL. On the definition and evaluation of telemedicine. Telemed J. 1995;1(1):19–30.
40. Craig J, Petterson V. Introduction to the practice of telemedicine. J Telemed Telecare. 2005;11(1):3–9.
41. Grigsby J, Sanders JH. Telemedicine: where it is and where it's going. Ann Intern Med. 1998;129(2):123–7.
42. Ekeland AG, Bowes A, Flottorp S. Effectiveness of telemedicine: a systematic review of reviews. Int J Med Inform. 2010;79(11):736–71.
43. Hailey D, Roine R, Ohinmaa A. Systematic review of evidence for the benefits of telemedicine. J Telemed Telecare. 2002;8(Suppl. 1):1–7.
44. Thrall JH, Boland G. Telemedicine in practice. In: Seminars in nuclear medicine 1998;28(2):145–157. WB Saunders.
45. Gustke SS, Balch DC, West VL, Rogers LO. Patient satisfaction with telemedicine. Telemed J. 2000;6(1):5–13.
46. Sanders JH, Bashshur RL. Challenges to the implementation of telemedicine. Telemed J. 1995;1(2):115–23.
47. Nittari G, Khuman R, Baldoni S, Pallotta G, Battineni G, Sirignano A, Amenta F, Ricci G. Telemedicine practice: review of the current ethical and legal challenges. Telemed e-Health. 2020;26(12):1427–37.
48. Whitten P, Kingsley C, Grigsby J. Results of a meta-analysis of cost–benefit research: is this a question worth asking? J Telemed Telecare. 2000;6(Suppl. 1):4–6.

Web Application Based on Deep Learning for Detecting COVID-19 Using Chest X-Ray Images

18

Ali Mansour Al-Madani, Ashok T. Gaikwad,
Zeyad A. T. Ahmed, Vivek Mahale, Saleh Nagi Alsubari,
and Mohammed Tawfik

18.1   Introduction

The Covid-19 virus is one of the epidemics that spread worldwide in December 2019, and according to reports, it first appeared in Wuhan, China [1]. This Covid-19 virus has infected many people in different countries of the world and affected the economy of most countries due to preventive measures against the risk of contracting the symptoms of this disease. Covid-19 is the most prevalent cause of these symptoms: fever, dry cough, and tiredness [2]. Aches, headaches, nasal congestion, throat or discomfort, and diarrhea are all possible side effects of a prescription. However, the symptoms are only somewhat noticeable [3].

The coronavirus disseminated infection everywhere throughout the world. It isolated many people and disabled numerous enterprises, which have affected the nature of human life. Coronavirus is named based on the marks of crown-like appearance when seen under the microscope.

A coronavirus is an enormous group of hazardous infections that may cause extreme and contagious sicknesses; MERS and severe acute respiratory syndrome are examples of new viral infections reported in late 2012 (SARS) [2]. COVID-19 examination is difficult due to the lack of a ubiquitous diagnostic system. Most doctors use X-rays to diagnose most diseases, such as pneumonia, pulmonary infections, pulmonary swellings, and bulges lymph nodes.

From this standpoint. Because of the limitations and difficulties they face in examining the COVID-19, we used artificial intelligence to detect cases of the

A. M. Al-Madani (✉) · Z. A. T. Ahmed · S. N. Alsubari · M. Tawfik
Department of Computer Science, Dr, Babasaheb Ambedkar Marathwada University, Aurangabad, Maharashtra, India

A. T. Gaikwad · V. Mahale
Institute of Management Studies and Information Technology, Aurangabad, Maharashtra, India

© The Author(s), under exclusive license to Springer Nature   283
Switzerland AG 2022
T. Choudhury et al. (eds.), *Telemedicine: The Computer Transformation of Healthcare*, TELe-Health, https://doi.org/10.1007/978-3-030-99457-0_18

novel virus (Covid-19) using CNN-based X-ray pictures. Identifying the infection and risk of COVID-19 virus by utilizing techniques is the best way to prevent spreading early. CNN is most commonly used for medical image recognition and classification, which helps diagnose diseases with high accuracy. This system will substitute for the mechanism used in the world's countries through slide testing kits that need 24 h for the results to appear and diagnose the case. If the disease is spotted quickly, the impact on overall results and the number of setbacks caused by COVID-19 disease will be lower. This study developed a web application based on deep learning to test chest X-ray scans and detect whether the person has COVID-19, pneumonia, or is normal. This application provided an easy and cheap technique to diagnose chest diseases. The advantage of this web application can be used anywhere, which helps people in remote areas with high accuracy results.

The rest sections are: The second section presents the prior studies related to COVID-19 identification, including cases from chest X-ray images. The methodology and the dataset utilized in this research are discussed in Sect. 18.3. The outcome and discussion are presented in Sect. 18.4. Finally, in Sect. 18.5 the conclusion is discussed.

18.2 Literature Review

Since COVID-19 inception, several researchers have developed artificial intelligence systems and several methods for predicting the behavior of this virus and the detection of infection. Most medical studies have indicated that most coronavirus patients have an infection in the lung (COVID-19). A literature study reveals many artificial intelligence efforts to examine COVID-19. Here are some of the previous studies related to predicting lung diseases.

Narin et al. [4] applied the pre-training models for COVID-19 detection. They used 100 images; 50 cases were affected by COVID-19, and 50 were not affected. Inception-V3 and Inception-ResNetV2 were used for classification. The classification result using Inception-V3 was 97% accuracy, Inception-ResNetV2 was 87% accuracy, and the best performance was done using ResNet50 98% accuracy on validation data.

Abbas et al. [5] used DeTraC deep learning model for X-ray images classification. The output of the model has two classes: positive and negative. Dataset was gathered from around the world's various hospitals. The accuracy of the model was 95.12%.

In Hall et al. [6], deep learning to COVID-19 detection based on X-ray chest pictures has been employed. A set of data was used with 135 patients with COVID-19 and 320 cases of pneumonia. 102 COVID-19 patients and 102 cases of pneumonia were trained for 10 times cross-validation. The Resnet50 model has been utilized. 95% of the accuracy has been obtained from this model.

Wang et al. [7] used COVID-19 pre-training models predicting X-ray pictures-based. They used the CXR dataset: normal 8851, 9576 for pneumonia, and 140

COVID-19. The ResNet-101 and ResNet-152 pre-training deep learning have been used to achieve 96.1% accuracy on validation data.

Yoo et al. [8] developed CNN with Decision-Tree Classifier for COVID-19 detection using chest X-ray images. They used CXR images collected from normal cases and abnormal cases. The result of the first decision tree is 98%, the second decision tree is 80%, and 95% for the third decision tree.

Ozturk et al. [9] proposed and developed a binary classification model for COVID-19 patients and normal people. They tried to implement three classes: COVID-19, No-Findings, and Pneumonia. The accuracy result of the binary classification was 98.08%, but the accuracy for multi-class cases was 87.02%.

Kumar et al. [10] proposed an ML-based classification model with ResNet152 for COVID-19 and Pneumonia patients' classification based on chest X-ray pictures. The classification result obtained 97.3% precision with Random Forest, and the XGBoost classification reached 97.7%. Ioannis et al. [11] proposed and developed a DL model for binary classification (COVID-19 and No-Findings). The model achieved 98.75% accuracy, and for three classes, it achieved 93.48% accuracy; they used 224 confirmed COVID-19, 504 normal, and 700 pneumonia radiology images.

Nayak et al. [12] applied pre-training models for detecting COVID-19 using X-ray images. Eight pre-trained COVID-19 patients and normal cases have been implemented: AlexNet, GoogleNet, MobileNet-V2, VGG-16, ResNet-34, Inception-V3, SqueezeNet, and ResNet-50. ResNet-34 achieved the best 98.33% precision performance.

Zhang et al. [13] classified COVID-19 and Pneumonia using the ResNet model. The dataset collected of 100 CXRs images, the model achieved the best accuracy of 72%.

Karakanis et al. [14] proposed deep learning models with X-ray pictures. The first model used binary classification: positive and negative cases, and the second model has 3 classes COVID-19, normal and pneumonia. For binary classification, the precision and performance achieved were 98.7%, sensitivity 100%, and specificity 98.3%. Multi-class precision and performance achieved 8.3% precision, sensitivity 99.3%, and specificity 98.1%.

Toraman et al. [15] proposed a method for detecting COVID-19. The first model is based on a binary classification of positive and negative cases. The second model has implemented three classes: COVID-19, No-Findings, and Pneumonia. The accuracy for binary classification was 97.24%, but the accuracy for multi-class cases was 84.22%.

Heidari et al. [16] developed a deep learning model with chest X-ray images for the predicted COVID-19. The model includes three classes—COVID-19, infected with pneumonia, and normal. The public dataset, which contains 8474 2D X-ray photographs, 415 COVID-19 photographs, 5179 other lung disorders, and normal 2880, was used. The precision of the CNN-based CAD system is 94.5%.

Jain et al. [17] implement a deep learning model for detecting covid-19 based on X-ray images. They used an available online dataset which consists of 1215 images. They increased the number of samples to 1832 images using data augmentation techniques. The result of classification accuracy is 97.77%.

By looking at previous studies, we find that our system is the best, as it got 98.75% ≈ 99% accuracy for multi-class, and a web application was also designed by using flask to make it easier for the user to use.

18.3 Methodology

18.3.1 Dataset

In this study, X-ray chest images were collected from various public sources for people suffering from COVID-19 disease and pneumonia and healthy cases. The COVID-19 patients There were 219 X-ray images, 1345 images of patients with pneumonia, and 1341 images of healthy cases. The X-ray images of pneumonia patients were collected from the Kaggle [18]. The COVID-19 X-ray images of patients were collected from the GitHub repository [19]. The X-Ray images of the Normal case were collected from Kaggle [20].

18.3.2 Preprocessing

The pre-processing was done by dividing the dataset into three parts: 85% for training, 5% for testing, and 10% for validation. Table 18.1 describes how many images are in each class and how many images are in training, validation, and testing (Figs. 18.1–18.3).

Table 18.1 Dataset breakdown [18–20]

Classes name	Dataset	Training	Validation	Testing
COVID-19	219	186	21	12
Normal	1341	1139	134	68
Pneumonia	1345	1143	134	68

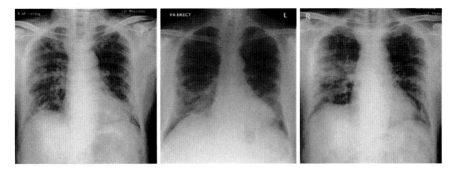

Fig. 18.1 X-ray Covid-19 images [18–20]

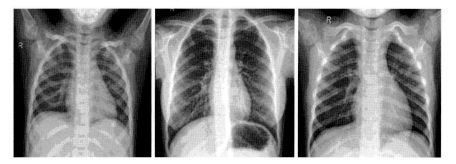

Fig. 18.2 X-ray normal images [18–20]

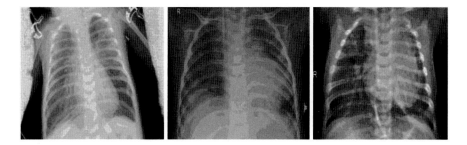

Fig. 18.3 X-ray pneumonia images [18–20]

18.3.3 ConvNet Models

Convolutional neural network (ConvNet) is similar to a multi-layer perceptron network. CNN is most commonly used for image classification, recognition, and video analysis [21, 22]. The CNN model provided a number of the hidden layers used for feature extraction from images or videos [23]. The flattening or fully connected layer converts the data from the hidden layers into a one-dimensional array. The classification layer is used to determine the output based on the possibilities of the class [24]. The basic components of the main CNN model are the convolutional layer, activating function, pooling layer, and flattening layer.

18.3.4 Convolutional Layer

The convolutional layer is an important part of the CNN model, which is used to learn the neural network by extracting features from the input image. There is a set of filters in the convolutional layer, also known as a kernel.

18.3.4.1   Pooling layer
The pooling layer is used since the convolutional layer's number of parameters must be reduced while preserving the features extracted from the input image. In

addition, it was used to avoid overfitting the CNN model. The idea of the pooling layer can be interpreted as the process of reducing the matrix size to reduce the weight of the neural network and speed up the training process. There are two types of pooling layers.

The max-pooling is most widely used because it extracts the features of the greatest values in the filter and minimizes the size of the feature map.

18.3.4.2 Fully Connected Layer

This layer is the last in the convolutional network, which consists of a multi-layer perceptron where neurons are fully bound to all nodes of the previous layer.

The reason for its existence, in the end, is because the final classification process is done in it (Fig. 18.4).

Training and Validation of the Model

The training of models has been done using python language with deep learning libraries; Keras and TensorFlow on Lenovo laptop named LEGION have GEFORCE GTX 1650, 4GB GPU.

Three pre-trained models were used in this work: Inception-V3, InceptionResNetV2, and MobileNet. The input image size to the models is (224*224*3). The pre-training should custom the top layers according to the needs of our problem. The find-tuning has been done by adding two dense layers on the top of the model architecture—the first layer of 1024 neurons. The Kernel regularizes L2(0.015) has been used to reduce the weights, and the bias is set as False. The layer 1024 neurons followed by (0.4) dropout layer with batch-normalization. The prediction layer used the SoftMax function. The output of this model will be in three classes: Covid-19, Normal, and Pneumonia. An early-stopping strategy has been used to monitor the validation loss with ten patients, stop training, and save the best performance accuracy. The models have trained on 100 epochs, with batch size 80. The RMSprop optimizer has been used to reduce the error.

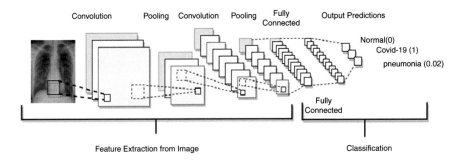

Fig. 18.4 Convolutional Neural Network (Detecting COVID-19)

18.4   Results and Discussion

18.4.1 Training and Testing

COVID-19 is one of the most dangerous diseases nowadays, the cost of the test is high, and it is not available everywhere. This study developed a cheap and easy application to examine the chest X-ray image, which helps doctors diagnose Covid-19 easily and quickly. This application can examine three types of lung radiographs, and then it shows the result of either normal, pneumonia, or corona virus infected. Most studies used either Normal or COVID-19 [25, 26]. Using two classes, the misclassification may happen because of lung disease similarities such as pneumonia and COVID-19. So, there is a need to develop an application to diagnose the different types of lung diseases and detect COVID-19, which helps doctors give the patient the right treatment. In this study, three types of model architecture were experimented with to reach a high classification accuracy that enabled us to access the coronavirus and pneumonia detection, which will be used to develop the web application. This proposed model is capable of being used in the cloud as future work and secure using blockchain technology to keep the privacy of the patients that provide a decentralized database [27–29].

This model can also be developed to classify different lung diseases that may appear due to the spread of new types of respiratory viruses. This application can classify new viruses in one of the two affected categories, making doctors further investigate [30]. But if samples of the new disease are available, we can update and develop the application to classify more than four or more diseases that may affect the lung.

The InceptionResNetV2 model achieved 97.92% accuracy, the InceptionV3 model achieved 97% accuracy, and the MobileNet achieved 98.75% accuracy on the Validation Data. The best performance got in the study was 98.75% by using MobileNet. Figure 18.5 shows the plot of the accuracy of training and validation. Figure 18.6 shows the loss of training and validation (Table 18.2).

Fig. 18.5 Training and validation accuracy

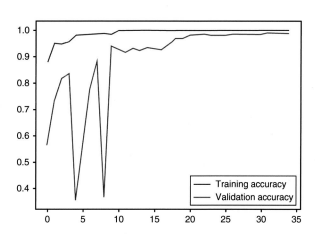

Fig. 18.6 Training and validation loss

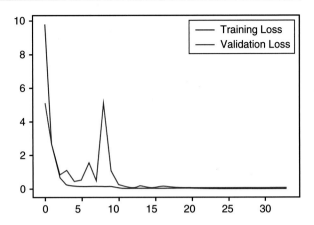

Table 18.2 Result of the models

Model name	Training accuracy	Validation accuracy	Sensitivity	Specificity
InceptionV3	100%	97.23%	99%	99%
InceptionResNetV2	99.12%	97.92%	99%	95%
MobileNet	100%	98.75% ≈ 99%	100%	100%

18.4.2 Confusion Matrix

The confusion matrix table has shown in Fig. 18.7 classification of three classes: COVID-19, Pneumonia and Normal. First True positives (TP): the model has correctly predicted, 21 cases have COVID-19. True Negatives (TN): the model has correctly predicted, 134 cases are Normal. False Positives (FP): the model falsely predicted 0 cases. False Negatives (FN): the model falsely predicted 0 cases. The Pneumonia TN model has correctly predicted 130 cases have Pneumonia, and FN model has falsely predicted 4 cases as normal cases but have Pneumonia. The confusion matrix table of the InceptionV3 and InceptionResNetV2 are shown in Figs. 18.8 and 18.9, respectively. Comparing the confusion matrix of the three pre-training models shows the classification results by describing the number of cases for each class. MobileNet has high-performance overall models that have 0 FP COVID-19 cases. InceptionV3 also has a good result, but the FP of Pneumonia cases is higher than MobileNet. InceptionResNetV2 has 1 case as FP. The web app was developed based on MobileNet because of the high accuracy with 0 FP cases.

The equation that has been used to calculate and evaluate the COVID-19 detection model is as follows:

- "Accuracy = (TP + TN)/(TP + FP + TN + FN)
- Specificity = TN/(TN + FP).
- Recall (Sensitivity) = TP/(TP/FN).
- Precision (PPV) = TP/(TP + FP).
- F1-Score = (2 * PPV * Sensitivity)/(PPV + Sensitivity)" where:
- True Positive (TP) is the number of X-ray image cases the model correctly preceded as positive COVID-19.

Fig. 18.7 Confusion
matrix of MobileNet

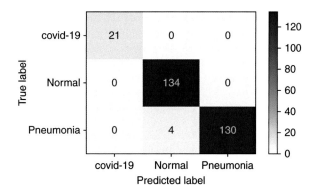

Fig. 18.8 Confusion
matrix of
InceptionResNetV2

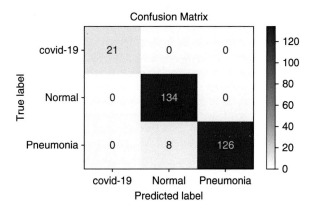

Fig. 18.9 Confusion
matrix of InceptionV3

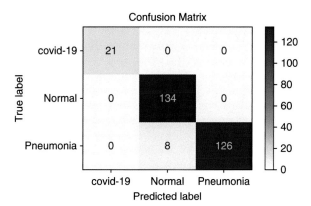

- True Negative (TN) is the number of X-ray image cases the model correctly predicted as Negative-COVID-19; it is classified as normal.
- False Positive (FP) is the number of X-ray image cases that incorrectly detect C as normal but have COVID-19.
- False Negative (FN) is the number of X-ray image cases incorrectly predicated as COVID-19, but they are normal.

18.4.3 Web Applicataion for Detecting COVID-19 Using Chest X-Ray Images

Developed a web application in Python using the needs of the platform called Flask. It has been used as a back-end deep learning model to develop the application by saving the model file in .h5 format. HTML, Js, and CSS have been used for developing the user interface. The user can select the chest X-ray image by using the button (Select X-Ray image) on the web page and uploading it as shown in Fig. 18.10; after that, click on the examine button. The result will appear whether it is normal, COVID-19, or pneumonia, as shown in Fig. 18.11.

The program was created and programmed on python, one of the most popular languages in programming used to train CNN models. The more significant effort focuses on the algorithm's partial focus on colors and changes in one of the X-ray images introduced into the system. The result is based on the algorithm's rules to show that the person has been infected with coronavirus or no. The maximum diagnostic time for a single image is 5 s, unlike the usual diagnosis, which takes at least 24 h for the test results to appear.

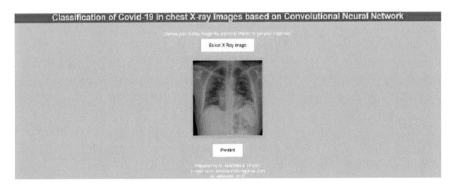

Fig. 18.10 Home page screenshot of WebApp

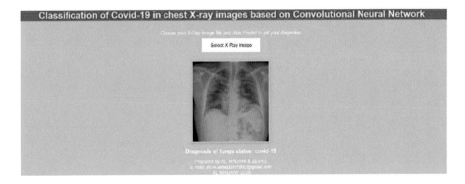

Fig. 18.11 prediction result

As mentioned in Table 18.1, accuracy, specificity, positive predictive value (PPV), sensitivity, and negative prediction value (NPV) are the metrics used to assess the X-ray images' model.

18.5   Conclusion

Coronavirus is one of the most dangerous viruses that have swept the world, which has confused people and governments and caused a complete closure of commercial and governmental activities. Turn the focus around on creating an easy technique test to predict the COVID-19. This test should be available anywhere. Thus, the use of special chest X-rays has become faster and more accurate in detecting lung diseases. This study developed a web app based on a deep learning model. This web app can predict lung diseases such as COVID-19 or pneumonia and normal if they do not suffer from an infection of lung diseases using a chest X-ray. This study compared the results of three pre-training models; InceptionV3 achieved 97.23%, InceptionResNetV2 achieved 98.33, and MobileNet achieved 98.75% ≈ 99% accuracy on validation data. The best performance was done by MobileNet, which achieved 98.75% ≈ 99%. An X-ray chest image is uploaded to a website using this web software. The application tests the image-based trained model, and the result has been shown to the user through the UI. This study will provide an easy-to-use and high-performance application for detecting COVID-19 disease.

References

1. https://www.cidrap.umn.edu/news-perspective/2019/12/news-scan-dec-31-2019
2. World Health Organization (WHO).
3. Hemdan EED, Shouman MA, Karar ME. Covidx-net: a framework of deep learning classifiers to diagnose COVID-19 in x-ray images. arXiv preprint arXiv:2003.11055. 2020
4. Narin A, Kaya C, Pamuk Z. Automatic detection of coronavirus disease (covid-19) using x-ray images and deep convolutional neural networks. Pattern Anal Appl. 2020;24(3):1207–20. arXiv preprint arXiv:2003.10849
5. Abbas A, Abdelsamea MM, Gaber MM. Classification of COVID-19 in chest X-ray images using DeTraC deep convolutional neural network. Appl Intell. 2021;51(2):854–64. arXiv preprint arXiv:2003.13815
6. Hall LO, Paul R, Goldgof DB, Goldgof GM. Finding covid-19 from chest x-rays using deep learning on a small dataset. arXiv preprint arXiv:2004.02060. 2020.
7. Wang N, Liu H, Xu C. Deep learning for the detection of COVID-19 using transfer learning and model integration. In: 2020 IEEE 10th International conference on electronics information and emergency communication (ICEIEC). IEEE; 2020. p. 281–4.
8. Yoo SH, Geng H, Chiu TL, Yu SK, Cho DC, Heo J, et al. Deep learning-based decision-tree classifier for COVID-19 diagnosis from chest X-ray imaging. Front Med. 2020;7:427.
9. Ozturk T, Talo M, Yildirim EA, Baloglu UB, Yildirim O, Rajendra Acharya U. Automated detection of COVID-19 cases using deep neural networks with X-ray images. Comput Biol Med. 2020;121:103792. https://doi.org/10.1016/j.compbiomed.2020.103792.
10. Kumar R, Arora R, Bansal V, Sahayasheela VJ, Buckchash H, Imran J, et al. Accurate prediction of COVID-19 using chest X-Ray images through deep feature learning model with SMOTE and machine learning classifiers. medRxiv. 2020

11. Apostolopoulos ID, Mpesiana TA. Covid-19: automatic detection from x-ray images utilizing transfer learning with convolutional neural networks. Phys Eng Sci Med. 2020;43(2):635–40.
12. Nayak SR, Nayak DR, Sinha U, Arora V, Pachori RB. Application of deep learning techniques for detection of COVID-19 cases using chest X-ray images: a comprehensive study. Biomed Signal Process Control. 2021;64:102365. https://doi.org/10.1016/j.bspc.2020.102365.
13. Zhang J, et al. Viral pneumonia screening on chest X-rays using confidence-aware anomaly detection. IEEE Trans Med Imaging. 2020;40(3):879–90. https://doi.org/10.1109/tmi.2020.3040950.
14. Karakanis S, Leontidis G. Lightweight deep learning models for detecting COVID-19 from chest X-ray images. Comput Biol Med. 2021;130:104181. https://doi.org/10.1016/j.compbiomed.2020.104181.
15. Toraman S, Alakus TB, Turkoglu I. Convolutional capsnet: a novel artificial neural network approach to detect COVID-19 disease from X-ray images using capsule networks. Chaos Solitons Fract. 2020;140:110122. https://doi.org/10.1016/j.chaos.2020.110122.
16. Heidari M, Mirniaharikandehei S, Khuzani AZ, Danala G, Qiu Y, Zheng B. Improving the performance of CNN to predict the likelihood of COVID-19 using chest X-ray images with preprocessing algorithms. Int J Med Inform. 2020;144:104284.
17. Jain G, Mittal D, Thakur D, Mittal MK. A deep learning approach to detect coronavirus with X-Ray images. Biocybern Biomed Eng. 2020;40(4):1391–405.
18. https://www.kaggle.com/paultimothymooney/chest-xray-pneumonia.
19. https://github.com/ieee8023/covid-chestxray-dataset/
20. https://www.kaggle.com/paultimothymooney/chest-xray-pneumonia
21. Al-madani AM, Gaikwad AT, Mahale V, Ahmed ZAT, Shareef AAA. Real-time driver drowsiness detection based on eye movement and yawning using facial landmark. In: 2021 International Conference on Computer Communication and Informatics (ICCCI); 2021. p. 1–4. https://doi.org/10.1109/ICCCI50826.2021.9457005.
22. Howard AG, Zhu M, Chen B, Kalenichenko D, Wang W, Weyand T, et al.. Mobilenets: efficient convolutional neural networks for mobile vision applications. arXiv preprint arXiv:1704.04861. 2017
23. Rahimzadeh, M., & Attar, A. (2020). A new modified deep convolutional neural network for detecting COVID-19 from X-ray images. arXiv preprint arXiv:2004.08052.
24. Minaee S, Kafieh R, Sonka M, Yazdani S, Soufi GJ. Deep-covid: predicting covid-19 from chest X-ray images using deep transfer learning. Med Image Anal. 65:101794. arXiv 2020, arXiv:2004.09363
25. Shi F, et al. Large-scale screening of covid-19 from community acquired pneumonia using infection size-aware classification. Phys Med Biol. 2020;66(6):065031. arXiv preprint arXiv:2003.09860
26. Russell J, Echenique A, Daugherty S, Weinstock M. Chest x-ray findings in 636 ambulatory patients with covid-19 presenting to an urgent care center: a normal chest x-ray is no guarantee. J Urgent Care Med. 2020;14(7):13–8.
27. Tawfik M, Almadani A, Alharbi AA. A review: the risks and weakness security on the IoT. IOSR J Comput Eng (IOSR-JCE). 2017;
28. Al-madani AM, Gaikwad AT. IoT data security via blockchain technology and service- centric networking. In: 2020 International Conference on Inventive Computation Technologies (ICICT), Coimbatore, India; 2020. p. 17–21. https://doi.org/10.1109/ICICT48043.2020.9112521.
29. Al-Madani AM, Gaikwad AT, Mahale V, Ahmed ZAT. Decentralized E-voting system based on Smart Contract by using Blockchain Technology. In: 2020 International conference on smart innovations in design, environment, management, planning and computing (ICSIDEMPC), Aurangabad; 2020. p. 176–80. https://doi.org/10.1109/ICSIDEMPC49020.2020.9299581.
30. Bai HX, Hsieh B, Xiong Z, Halsey K, Choi JW, Tran TML, Pan I, Shi L-B, Wang D-C, Mei J, et al. Performance of radiologists in differentiating covid-19 from viral pneumonia on chest CT. Radiology. 2020;296(2):200823.

Telemedicine in Healthcare System: A Discussion Regarding Several Practices

19

Shaweta Sachdeva, Aleem Ali, and Salman Khalid

19.1 Introduction

Telemedicine means healing the patients at a distance. The institution of medication uses telemedicine as a tool for collecting electronic data and to communicate for supply and gives support for comfort care when patients were residing far away. Telemedicine helps in most common applications like X-rays, CT scans, cardiology, orthopedics, dermatology, and psychiatry to keep the record of patients and gives more benefit to the patients. In some cases, video briefings and records of particular patients are kept for further processes to treat patients in an advanced manner as shown in Fig. 19.1. Group of doctors, instructors, and analysts "meet" over huge separations through VSAT systems.

Telemedicine also stores the electronic records of the patient, get to the libraries and databases on the Internet. Telemedicine emerged initially to serve provincial populaces, any people which are geographically dispersed—where it takes more time to travel for the finest remedial care. Presently, it is being utilized in standard pharmaceuticals organizations, to permit specialists of the world to share costly assets and important conclusions. In 1997, telemedicine progressively became worldwide in its reach; there were so many dynamic programs around the world, especially in Israel, India, Taiwan, Japan, and the USA. The significance of transmission capacity can be seen in any case. With 28.8 kbps dial-up connections, the

S. Sachdeva (✉) · A. Ali
Department of CSE, Glocal University Saharanpur, Saharanpur, Uttar Pradesh, India
e-mail: aleem@theglocaluniversity.in

S. Khalid
IT Department King Saud Medical City, Riyadh, Saudi Arabia
e-mail: sakhalid@ksu.edu.sa

© The Author(s), under exclusive license to Springer Nature Switzerland AG 2022
T. Choudhury et al. (eds.), *Telemedicine: The Computer Transformation of Healthcare*, TELe-Health, https://doi.org/10.1007/978-3-030-99457-0_19

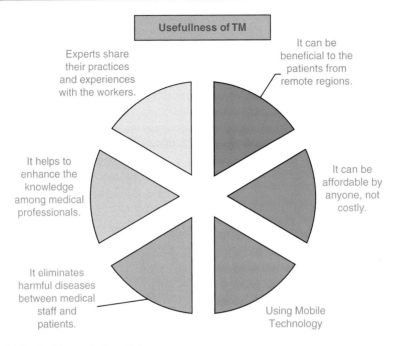

Fig. 19.1 Usefulness of telemedicine

transmission of standard X-ray takes 30 min in all, with a T1 line at 1.5 Mbps it takes 30 s, and with a large speed DS3 circuit, it takes one moment as shown in Fig. 19.2. Therefore, telemedicine is efficient and easy to use.

19.2 Primary Components in Telemedicine

In telemedicine, transmission media is used to diagnosing well-being conditions, treatment, as well as taking care of patients. This is an expert-based healthcare system particularly for inaccessible areas that are understaffed. There are three fundamental components of telemedicine: Tele-Consultation, Tele-Mentoring, and Tele-Monitoring.

(i) **Tele Consultation**: This is one of the foremost broadly known categories of telemedicine. It fundamentally introduces to the online visit where an interview between the specialist and client takes place. It can be done through videoconferencing or by essentially putting away a specific picture and sending it to the healthcare provider for further interpretations.

(ii) **Tele Mentoring**: This may be a situation where one restorative professional gets mentorship from another, who may well be more specialized to discover

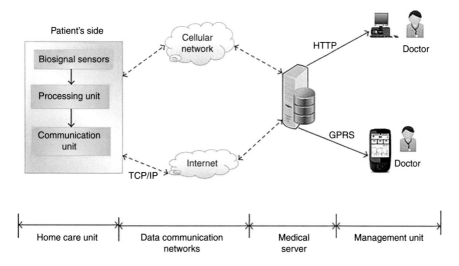

Fig. 19.2 Telemedicine system [1]

ways of making a difference in a patient. A good professional may be a specialist who has a deep understanding of an area and is trying to provide medical
assistance in a specific location. The main thing is to associate with well-being
institution that will have one of their tutors give help online.

(iii) **Tele Monitoring:** This is done for getting information in domestic areas by
using biosensors. It can be done by an electronic scale, a vital-sign screen, a
glucometer, or any other gadget that can successfully screen bio-parameter.
The specialist points out that, the test starts to begin for regulating treatment or
gives medicine to the patients. This frame of telemedicine permits away to be
effortlessly checked from domestic, without having to travel to the well-being
facility.

19.3 Key Elements Needed for Successful Telemedicine Program

If any organization is offering or planning to offer telemedicine programs, the following elements may be considered.

19.3.1 Cooperative Tools

These tools help any well-being of an organization to connect with the patients such
as tablets, Smartphone, laptops, etc.

19.3.2 Protocols and Procedures

It helps well-being organizations, providers, and employees for making further decisions to take action and to ensure all the activities performed under policies/laws. These protocols are also needed for taking major decisions and actions and making guidelines for any organizations to collect day-to-day activities.

19.3.3 Scope of Services (SOS)

Does it conclude what types of services are provided remotely to patients? It provides consultancy, follow-up appointments, and post appointments. It is more important to establish SOS and to think about the Centers for Medicare & Medicaid Services (CMS) and Conditions of Participation. The rules and regulations are different for each facility type, so it makes sure that the telemedicine program is in consent with CMS requirements.

19.3.4 Secure Communication Method

Secured communication is the most important element in the telemedicine system. The use of information technology like videoconferencing helps to provide healthcare remotely. It is very much important that communication with patients be secured while creating, transmitting, or storing information that is received from patients and scanned into EMR(Electronic Medical records) [2].

19.3.5 Agreement Between Organization and Patients

All the risks and benefits of telemedicine services must be cleared or informed to patients and provide them official consent for security purposes. Once the norms are understood by the patients, the documentation is done by the patients on form in a proper manner.

19.3.6 Authentic Documentation

In telemedicine system, documentation is complete and accurate; there is no exemption in case of documentation for the patient case and ensure to provide proper services by any healthcare organization. Authenticity is a must for every patient.

19.4 Review of Literature

In paper [3], Whitten et al. proposed a definition of telemedicine and discussed the applications. Telemedicine application is used and identified as the utilization of advanced communication developments, the internal setting of clinical prosperity, which gives care to patients [4]. It engaged both doctors and patients to get more and more advantages of this application. Such communication development of telemedicine progresses and incorporates with computerized equipment, allowing specialists and other comparable prosperity specialists to supply complex healthcare and take advantage of thousands of patients who live miles missing from the location [5]. The endless telemedicine applications comprise persistent care, preparing, inquire about the treatment, and open well-being to analyze, regulate care, send and get well-being data, analyze X-rays, and teach well-being experts. Telemedicine applications were easily handled with innovative gadgets for healthcare conveyance, medicines prescriptions, medications, and pictures of medical sciences [6].

In paper [4], Aryza et al. proposed that the various administrations uses telemedicine as a framework of telemedicine called E-health, a later breakthrough in telemedicine innovation examined in detail afterward. Moreover, several essential E-health applications approve how telemedicine is important for away from patients and available through any computer (i.e., personal computers and portable workstation of computers, laptops, etc.) connected to the Web [7]. Within the community, it proves how telemedicine was presented to the community and the primary means of it were utilized for healthcare purposes. It shows the truth of this paper that only concentrates on early things of telemedicine applications and additionally it emphasizes on various initial organizations [8, 9]. It remains energetic and commonly utilized interior healthcare applications and other comparative circumstances where benefits from these devices can still be seen.

In paper [10], Imran Sarwar et al. proposed the system for remote patient monitoring using gadgets like smartphones. It is developed for the rural Indian population who undergo hypertension and hypotension. This system is designed to capture pre-cardiac detained situations for people and is prescribed to take precautions from medical/healthcare. These systems used biomedical sensors and microprocessor for performing analysis and get treated.

In paper [11], Seetharam et al. proposed the system for telemedicine for diabetics patients in rural areas. According to the results of ICMR (Indian Council of Medical Research's) researchers evaluated that 62.4 million people are suffering from diabetes. Many efforts have been done for diabetic patients in urban areas, while 70% of the population lived in rural areas. This percentage of evaluation is increased day by day due to lack of awareness in people living in rural areas, limited access to healthcare treatment due to transportation problems, and lack of trained doctors in diabetes. The screening for diabetes is done in rural areas which results in undiagnosed and improper treatment to the patients. The research came up with a diabetes healthcare model to care for patients in a more affordable manner using a mobile van facility having types of equipment to diagnose and in case of emergency they can communicate to experts through trained technicians using satellite communication using VSAT. The research concluded that the cost-effectiveness of healthcare can be achieved through telemedicine projects.

In paper [12], UmaRani et al. proposed a research model named as knocking telemedicine technology for healthcare professionals using different survey methods to evaluate the usage impact of various discrete networks on telemedicine capabilities in India. The ICT infrastructure in India slightly shifted from conventional technical components to high-speed fiber-optic broadband connectivity networks. The study also states it not only marked improvement, but leads to advancement and sustainability in existing telemedicine capabilities as well.

Telemedicine plays a vital role in pandemic for those patients who don't have any option for treatment. With the use of ICT dealt with telemedicine the patients communicate easily with the doctors and get exact treatment for their illness.

19.5   A Modern Means of Telemedicine: E-Health

In the twenty-first century, the world has transformed into a wide-ranging called "cyber-planet." Telemedicine is a standard instrument used with Internet-based curative destinations. WebMD.com, Medlineplus.gov, Medscape.com, and Mentalhelp.net were some of these Internet-based resources. At present, E-health helps patients; people live in any community that is suffering from some mental illness.It can also utilize E-health administrations to get reports on numerous mental problems or medications.

In other words, the number of questions can be replied to by experts with the data given on E-health websites. On the other hand, one of the most common conditions is examined as on-line who utilize E-health in troubled areas, particularly among young generation people. As well as, details of specialists were available who resides near to them and who were specialized in a specific field of mental disorder can be brought to their computer screens to view. These help more patients to get the leading number of curative care from the proper sort of supplier.

In contrast, E-health organizations additionally have the potential to improve the concern of "Tele competence" as shown in Fig. 19.3. Tele competence is the

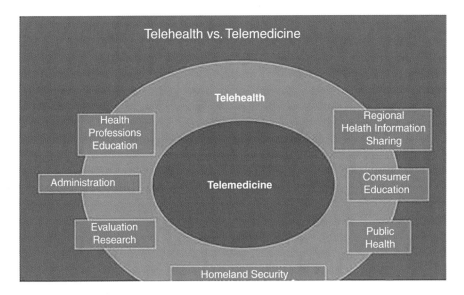

Fig. 19.3 Telehealth vs tele-medicine

premise, has ability to set the guidelines and rules that affect the performance of organizational estimation in telemedicine inside the E-health field. It recognized that E-health fulfills the requirements of all citizens, healthcare buyers, restorative pros and cons, healthcare specialists, and so on. E-health organizations incorporate a group of organizations with additional features such as prosperity instruction, nursing, and pharmaceutical medication or refills through eprescribing.Walgreens.com is one of the E-health company that engages the direct refilling plan of pharmaceutical drugs in their corporate areas. E-mail is another sort of E-health feature which gives a channel by which suppliers and patients can communicate and cost-effective strategy to be discussed around the understanding status of patient and expert suggestions. Hence, e-health organizations are important to those people who affect in enduring to organize healthcare. With more use of the Internet, and online surfing, searching is useful for health-related information. According to both patient's and practitioner's points of view, E-health organizations have basic recommendations for their medical problems and treatment too.

19.6 Applications of Telemedicine

19.6.1 Real-Time Consultation

Live telemedicine is also called real-time telemedicine, i.e., consultation which provides a better way of meeting between doctor-patient anytime on the Internet. Live telemedicine is two-way communications including videoconferencing and video call as seen in Fig. 19.4. It provides a way for experts and patients to communicate

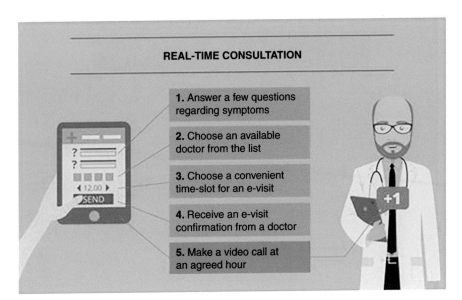

Fig. 19.4 Real-time consultation

with each other in real time. The live telemedicine technique helps experts to evaluate the history of patients; visual examinations, psychiatric evaluations, and medical tests can also be done.

19.6.1.1 Remote Patient Monitoring(Tele-Monitoring)

The second way of telemedicine is called tele-monitoring. It permits healthcare experts to screen patient's medical data from long distances, more regularly than not while to determined to go to their own house shown in Fig. 19.5. With more distant, checking is done especially for consistent conditions like heart sickness, diabetes, and asthma. It gives license to patients to screen themselves for these conditions existed for a long time. Nowadays, essential data can be shared with specialists and other healthcare specialists remotely with telemedicine. Cutting-edge adapt can transmit actual essential data to specialist, allowing them to supply a better level of care and keep an eye out for the foremost reliable signals of convenience.

19.6.1.2 Store-and-Forward Practices

The third application of telemedicine is store-and-forward practices. It helps to understand records of the patient and essential data easily accessible over long partitions as shown in Fig. 19.6. All kinds of essential data (e.g., helpful imaging, the test comes around, bio-signals) can be transmitted over large distances. The advantage of this kind of telemedicine is that it does not require synchronous thought to transmit the data. An expert, caregiver, or specialists can collect the essential data, exchange it, and transmit it for point-by-point audit by another expert in a short time [13]. This kind of non-concurrent organization is utilized by various patient-focused telemedicine stages to understand minor helpful issues. Various fields like pathology, radiology, dermatology, and other specialized cured regions depend day by day on the outline of telemedicine. Various systems exist to help to sort all the

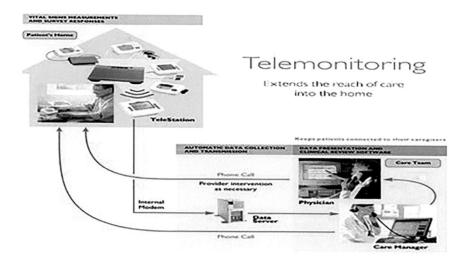

Fig. 19.5 Tele-monitoring

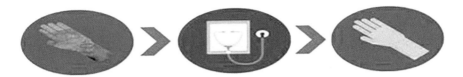

Fig. 19.6 Store-and-forward practices

information into a single record. It shows superior towards the reality that not all electronic prosperity record systems are interoperable. Distant coming records to telemedicine utilized and help to make faith to the favored industry that makes better stages which can take part and communicate easily.

19.6.1.3 Discussion Between Masters and Essential Caregivers

Telemedicine can make stride communications between groups of people to help. A specialist can get data without traveling. Secured videoconferencing makes it helpful for specialists to collaborate on the given cases, with or without the closeness of the calm inside the reporting circle. It can share essential information quickly and completely in advance to assist experts in different fields. In many medicated centers, hospitals, and clinics, video interviews were performed with cameras that permit a separate expert to initiate an up-close view of a patient's condition easily through telemedicine.

19.6.1.4 Medical Imaging

In today's scenario, X-rays, CT checks, and other pictures are scattered from one corrective expert to another through medical imaging shown in Fig. 19.7. Radiology and other indicated symptom justify exceptional thought in telemedicine. Broadband transmission speed allows these pictures to be sent from their point of capture to the specialists and experts who require them for further process of treatment. This also allows healthcare specialists to centralize both the securing and examination of such essential information despite remote challenges. For results, a regional clinic may convey X-rays on-site, transmit them to a cardiologist a hundred miles away, get profitable treatment after examining the patient detail, and revert the reports to hours.

19.6.1.5 Telemedicine Networks

Depending on the financial assets, the telemedicine network helps to collect information about patients according to the requirements of experts as shown in Fig. 19.8. Inside the joining States, various medical centers and clinics utilize given frameworks to share information for concern to experts. These can be controlled over the Internet or on the network to utilize committed information lines [14]. Nowadays, there are hundreds of such frameworks working inside the US, interfacing lots of different healthcare facilities through telemedicine networks.

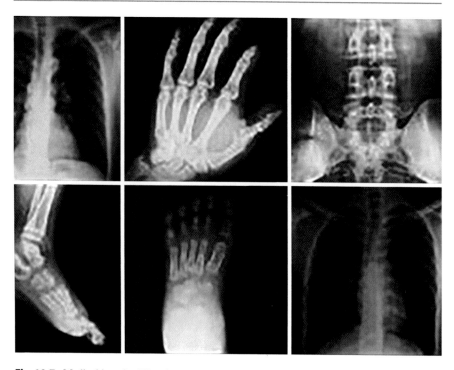

Fig. 19.7 Medical imaging(X-ray)

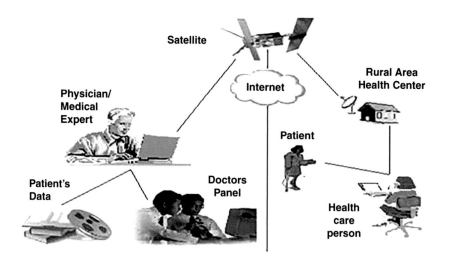

Fig. 19.8 Telemedicine network [15]

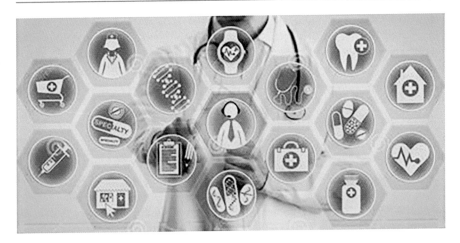

Fig. 19.9 Treat different patients

19.6.1.6 Reaching Out to Patients

Telemedicine is a valuable technique for healthcare experts who have different ways to associate with patients in their own homes. Web-based organizations help in such a way to understanding passages, allow patients to share essential information, and answering the questions of patients by expert/specialists (Fig. 19.9). More energetic bonding can be made through this technique that specialists can collect data from their residential of the body such as pacemakers, fetal heart screens, and pneumonic systems. Resolved passages can be utilized to support health-focused flexible apps or teaching materials, such as articles and recordings. Patients may communicate with specialists in virtual visits, face-to-face, from their own homes through this technique.

19.7 How Do Telehealth and Telemedicine Work?

Telehealth may be a wide umbrella that covers the innovations that give clinical and authoritative back for patients and doctors. Telehealth characterizes as the back given for long remove clinical healthcare, quiet and proficient health-related instruction, and open well-being and well-being organization by the utilization of electronic data and media transmission technologies. Cases of telehealth incorporate nonclinical administrations comprising regulatory meetings, provider training, and proceeding therapeutic instruction in conjunction with clinical administrations. Other agenda of telehealth is to incorporate live-interactive videoconferencing, further observing, and store-and-forward imaging [16].

Telemedicine, on the other hand, suggests the conveyance of clinical care via electronic communications. In the 1970s, term was coined by the World Wellbeing Organization (WHO) as a mode of substantial trade of restorative data relating to the conclusion, treatment, and anticipation of illness and wounds using data and communication innovations to move forward patients' well-being status. Telemedicine cannot be considered a partitioned restorative forte; on the opposite, it is considered a device to be utilized by healthcare suppliers to spread the conventional therapeutic hone past the dividers of the normal medical practices.

Telemedicine has proceeded to broaden as more specialties can utilize this approach and the innovation itself gets to be more inescapable and reasonable. Telemedicine applications and administrations incorporate mail, two-way video, remote apparatuses, phones, and other communication innovation tools [17]. Illustrations of telemedicine incorporate gathering treatment, nursing intelligence, instruction and preparing, televisits to community well-being laborers, and restorative picture transmission. This too incorporates tele-consultations such as teleradiology, tele-dermatology, tele-neurology, and tele-pharmacy. In outline, telehealth could imply of integration of media transmission frameworks into the hone of ensuring and advancing well-being, whereas telemedicine is the consolidation of these systems into corrective pharmaceuticals.

Telehealth may be more extensive extend of inaccessible healthcare administrations that are not essentially related to the clinical field which is called farther nonclinical administrations such as training, medical instruction, and authoritative gathering whereas telemedicine is a portion of the remote services that is related to the clinical field. The telemedicine application may well be completely different categories such as persistent care, proficient instructions, and persistent instructions, investigates, opens well-being, and healthcare organization as shown in Fig. 19.10. Mechanical progression has made several versatile well-being gadgets, which are accessible indeed in resource-limited ranges. Substituted insights can proficiently address the need of specialists and the deluge of complex information created by m-Health and telemedicine as well as advanced imaging modalities.

Services are given in three primary ways with the assistance of fake insights:

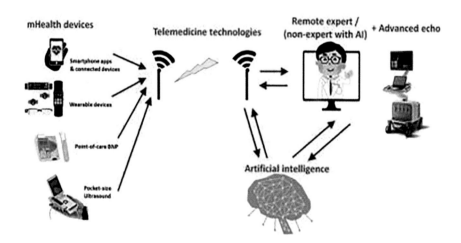

Fig. 19.10 Telehealth works with artificial intelligence

(i) Videoconferences and tele-robotic frameworks with real-time transmissions between well-being suppliers and patients(consultations and methods), and between well-being patients and doctors.

(ii) Inaccessible understanding observing, in which extraordinary electronic gadgets transmit quiet well-being data to well-being care centers.

(iii) Store and forward: Through electronic medias, it transmits information like recordings, computerized pictures stored in tele-radiology, tele-pathology, tele-dermatology applications, etc. between patients and essential care suppliers and therapeutic specialists for getting better medical consultants and treatment.

19.8 Case Study: Apollo Hospital Using ICT Tools and VSAT

19.8.1 Objectives of the Study

- To analyze the mode of operation of telemedicine system used in Apollo Hospital
- To give the best practices and challenges faced at Apollo Hospitals due to telemedicine
- To offer the suggestions for improvement in their basic practices

19.8.2 History of Apollo Hospitals

Apollo Group of Hospital is one of the best hospitals that attract and treat patients from several parts of India, as well as from abroad. The hospital has specialized and trained doctors in different areas of medicine. Apollo has set up 85 telemedicine centers across different locations in India. Apollo hospital has worked with large corporate and government hospitals to make small clinics and information centers for keeping the records electronically and treats the patients remotely.

19.8.3 Mode of Operation of Telemedicine

Apollo Telemedicine Networking Foundation (ATNF) is one of the foundations made for telemedicine having many centers across the country and works in combination with the ISRO(Indian Space Research Organization) to provide specialty medical access to those patients residing in rural communities. With the help of this network, services are provided in different fields like cardiology, dermatology, radiology, nephrology, and general consultation. ATNF is Web-based software used for transmitting various reports, i.e., electrocardiograms, images CT scans reports, MRI reports, ultrasound pictures, and other reports also. The office assistant checks the list of scheduled tele-consultations online and provide to the doctors on a whiteboard, according to the appointments given to the patients. The consultations take place between given timings and then for reviewing tele-consultations, the medical case records are received from the Medical Records Department. When Web-based software is not working properly, then prescriptions are sent via E-mail or fax to the remote areas, where a printout is given to the patients.

A doctor can diagnose every patient using computer-aided transmission of audiovisual data in a distant location. In remote areas, telemedicine provides tertiary healthcare to people through a virtual reduction in distance. Text, sounds, pictures, and videos are used, then merged and interconnected completely in a new way. For example, use of live video-conferencing is used to examine the patients electronically, transmission of patient records and X-rays, and recording of ECG reports over telephone are possible and this is termed as digital convergence concept. Doctors in rural areas get access to experts through telemedicine and guide on complex conditions. When a patient is in the worst condition, the clinical authority creates a patient medical file with examination reports and photos and finally uploads it to the cloud of ATNF. With the help of videoconferencing a patient gets the specialist consultation. Also in a remote center of telemedicine, patients can interact directly with the doctors. This facility allows one or more patients to interact directly living at two different locations by using audio and video support through digital communication.

In this telemedicine project, i.e., ATNF software shown in Fig. 19.11 can be used into three stages. Firstly the data is retrieved and transferred from the consultation center, secondly fixing up a tele-consultations appointment by accepting the records of the patient, and lastly evaluating and viewing post consultation details of patients. Any doctor can use GEMSIT, i.e., General Electric Medical software easily for getting medical records of the patient as it is available for doctors. Through this software, each patient has been given one identification number, i.e., UHID (unique health identification number) through which the patient avail services given by Apollo Hospital. Each patient's records are saved on a centralized server through the cloud based on UHID number and then data consistency is maintained. To

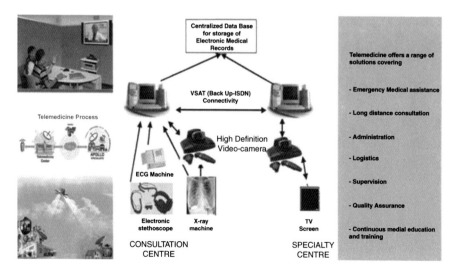

Fig. 19.11 Process of ATNF

maintain privacy, only the tele-consultant is present, also the telemedicine administrators are available for the translation process which helps the patients to understand the complete process.

19.8.4 Challenges in Telemedicine

- As telemedicine increases widely, this challenge is becoming more difficult to handle. For Apollo hospital it is very difficult to relocate the doctors to rural areas and willing to devote their time to treat rural area patients.
- As telemedicine is a new and different process to adapt by patients in different locations, it is limited to the short-term financial viability of the hospital.
- Financial resources are provided by the Indian government for medical care to the rural poor. Even the government can give support privately to hospitals like Apollo to improve their infrastructure in hospitals.
- Telemedicine system started in Apollo hospitals did not generate enough funds; hence there was a shortage of funds for changes to the business model in hospitals.
- It becomes difficult to find a physician with knowledge of different languages to communicate with patients. India is a country with many languages that are more common in rural areas.
- As telemedicine involves two or more parties, it becomes complicated to know who is liable when something goes wrong.
- ISRO is one of the established networks through which the number of hospitals was increased with satellite connections for telemedicine to over large continent, still large rural areas are not connected to various cities, because satellite connections are too costly, and some areas do not have a strong broadband network.

19.9 Conclusion

Amid this worldwide widespread, telehealth is rising as a successful and economical arrangement for safety measure, avoidance, and treatment to stem the spread of COVID-19. As the number of cases of novel coronavirus SARS-CoV-2 is expanded day by day within the Joined together States, the family physicians are expended with attempting to allow the best care for their patients whereas securing themselves and their staff. That is why telehealth has ended up such a valuable apparatus for giving care for these patients. Telehealth/telemedicine create the path between individuals, doctors, and well-being frameworks, empowering everybody, particularly symptomatic patients, to remain at domestic and communicate with doctors through virtual channels, making a difference to diminish the spread of the infection to mass populaces and the restorative staff on the frontlines. By sending telehealth arrangements and programs, individuals who are enduring other therapeutic sicknesses amid this time can get care from domestic, without entering restorative offices, minimizing their chance of contracting the infection.

References

1. Abo-Zahhad M, et al. A wireless emergency telemedicine system for patients monitoring and diagnosis. Int J Telemed Appl. 2014;2014(380787):11.
2. Breen GM, et al. An interpersonal examination of telemedicine: applying relevant communication theories. E-Health Int J. 2007;3(1):18–23.
3. Whitten, et al. Health professionals to provide complex healthcare. HHS Public Access Peer-Rev J. 2010:59–71.
4. Aryza S, et al. A novelty design of minimization of electrical losses in a vector controlled induction machine drive. IOP Conf Ser Mater Sci Eng. 2018;300(1)
5. Matusitz, et al. An evolutionary examination of telemedicine: a health and computer-mediated communication perspective. Soc Work Public Health. 2010;25(1):59–71.
6. Kaur G, et al. A review on telemedicine services in India. Int J Adv Manage Technol Eng Sci. 2018;8(1):214–8.
7. Malasinghe LP, et al. Remote patient monitoring: a comprehensive study. J Ambient Intell Human Comput. 2019;10:57–76.
8. Mohan V, et al. Telemedicine in diabetes care: in rural India, a new prevention project seeks to fill in the screening gap. IEEE Pulse. 2014;5(3):22–5.
9. Ramadhani S, et al. Post-genesis digital forensics investigation. Int J Sci Res Sci Technol. 2017;3(6):164–6.
10. Bajwa IS, et al. Virtual telemedicine using natural language processing. Int J Inform Technol Web Eng. 2010;5(1):43–55.
11. Seetharam K, et al. Application of mobile health, telemedicine and artificial intelligence to echocardiography. Echo Res Pract. 2019;6(2):41–52.
12. UmaRani P, et al. A case study on telemedicine practices implemented with respect to Apollo hospitals. Int J Appl Environ Sci (IJAES). 2015;10(1):23–8.
13. Ali A, Singh N, Verma P. M/M/1/n+Flush/n model to enhance the QoS for Cluster Heads in MANETs. In: Published in International Journal of Advanced Computer Science and Applications (IJACSA), U.K. ESCI, Scopus; 2018.
14. Ali A, Singh N. QoS analysis in MANETs using queueing theoretic approaches: a review. Int J Latest Trend Eng Technol (IJLTET). 2016;7(1):120–4. UGC listed
15. Parveen N, Ali A, Ali A. IOT based automatic vehicle accident alert system. In: 2020 IEEE 5th International Conference on Computing Communication and Automation (ICCCA), 30–31 Oct. 2020. Greater Noida: IEEE; 2020. p. 330–3. https://doi.org/10.1109/ICCCA49541.2020.9250904. (Scopus Indexed).
16. Sachdeva S, Ali A. A hybrid approach using digital Forensics for attack detection in a cloud network environment. Int J Future Gener Commun Netw. 2021;14(1):1536–46.
17. Kaur R, Ali A. A Novel blockchain model for securing IoT based data transmission. Int J Grid Distrib Comput. 2021;14(1):1045–55.

Telemedicine: Present, Future and Applications

20

Harshad S. Kapare, Karishma M. Rathi, and Sonali D. Labhade

20.1 Introduction

In today's era tremendous advancements are happening in healthcare systems. Telemedicine is one of the approaches that are excellent applications of advanced technology. The World Health Organization (WHO) defines telemedicine as, "Delivery of healthcare services, where patients and providers are separated by distance. Information exchange for the purpose of diagnosis and treatment of diseases, research, evaluation and for the continuing education the is carried by ICT in telehealth practice which can contribute in achievement of health coverage in remote areas, vulnerable groups and ageing populations with quality, cost-effective, health services A study performing detailed assessment of various definitions of telemedicine showed that there are four main perspectives those categories all the available definitions of the term. The four bases that withhold all the core definitions of this term are Medical, Technological, Spatial and Benefits [1–3].

Telemedicine approach/programmes are classified into two categories:

1. Synchronous Programmes—It includes a live interactive session between the patient and healthcare provider, e.g. a virtual appointment via technological media with a camera.
2. Asynchronous Programmes—Exchange of information between the patient and healthcare provider in the form of images, videos, written and audio content, etc. via telecommunication and internet [1].

H. S. Kapare (✉) · K. M. Rathi · S. D. Labhade
Dr. D. Y. Patil Institute of Pharmaceutical Sciences and Research, Pimpri,
Pune, Maharashtra, India

20.2 Origin and History of Telemedicine

The term Telemedicine was devised in the year 1970. It is commonly misconceived that the development of the idea of telemedicine also took place in the 1970s despite the fact that the concept came into existence even long before the invention of telephone and radio [1]. The origin of the core idea of the concept of telemedicine dates centuries back when, ancient African villages blew smoke signals to make the neighbouring villages are of the prevailing disease, i.e. the purpose of exchanging important information was fulfilled. Similarly, some European settlements used bonfires to make adjoining villages aware of the bubonic plague in the Middle Ages [4]. In the last five centuries, the field of telemedicine witnessed technological development resulting in the capacity of exchanging any amount of information.

The invention of Guttenberg's printing press in 1452 opened a way to distribute important information [5]. The parameter distance creates a necessity for telemedicine and its options.

The advancement in the field of transportation with the invention of locomotive in 1819 and the invention of stethoscope in 1825 are some noteworthy events in telemedicine which helped counter one of the most important barriers, i.e. distance.

The next important event in the advancement of telemedicine is the invention of telegraph in the year 1844, which led to the invention of electrocardiography by Wilhelm Einthoven. Einthoven also invented the telecardiogram. The invention of the telephone in 1875 led to leaps in the field of telemedicine. The earliest records of the usage of telephone in the exchange of medical information dates back to the early 1900s—the Netherlands used telephone to transmit heart rhythms [1]. Similarly, telephone was used to transmit to radio consultation centres all over Europe. Wilhelm Einthoven himself transmitted electrocardiogram tracings via a telephone network in 1906 [2]. Furthermore, several significant inventions that complimented the execution of telemedicine were seen in the field of transportation, like the invention of automobile and airplane [5]. Following down the timeline, the invention of satellites created even more convenience in the telemedicine field. The beginning of utilization of television for transmission of information was seen in the 1950s in the Nebraska Project (Omaha). The project involved 2 close-circuit TVs set up in 2 hospitals for conduction of interviews involving patient monitoring and consultations with the patients from psychiatric ward [2]. The records show wide utilization of satellites in the field for various purposes—The National Library of Medicine invested in the research of the reliability of telemedicine via satellite communication [4].

The establishment of a microwave video link between MGH and Logan airport in Boston for radiology, dermatology and cardiology related consultations for airport employees and passengers [6]. NASA (National Aeronautics and Space Administration) has made important contributions to the arena of telemedicine with a chain of projects conducted in the decade of 1960. The projects were conducted for the benefit of astronauts. They were successful in providing medical assistance by using telemetric data transmitted from the spacesuits. This enabled them to monitor various vitals like heart rate, blood pressure, and ECG [6]. Furthermore, NASA also designed telemedicine instrumentation packs containing various equipment like endoscope, macro-imaging lens, electrocardiograph, ophthalmoscope, blood pressure sensor, electronic stethoscope, pulse oximeter, etc. for the purpose of monitoring physiological actions of the spaceship boarders [6].

NASA also brought the Space Technology Applied to Rural Papago Advanced Health Care (STARPAHC) project on the Papago Indian Reservation in Arizona, USA, into action in 1972. The project involved a two-way microwave transmission to the Public Health Service Hospital and a van equipped with medical instruments and 2 paramedics.

It also established the 'Spacebridge' project after the earthquake disaster in Armenia which allowed telemedicine consultation between medical centres in the USA and Armenia [4].

In the late 1960s and 1980s, the introduction of the internet and the World Wide Web helped the practice of telemedicine. MIT Media Laboratory successfully developed prototypes of the low-cost portable telemedicine kit targeting patients in developing countries as part of the Little Intelligent Communities (LINCOS) project. The purpose of the LINCOS project was to deploy not only the telemedicine systems, but also high-speed internet, telecommunications and distant education to rural areas of developing countries where people suffer from a shortage of doctors or medical specialists, in 2000 [6].

However, now in the technologically advanced times and the reduced cost of computing there is a surge in fibre optic cable, virtual reality, immersive environments, haptic feedback and nano-technology, and these are proving to be the new promising advances of the present.

20.3 Advancements and Applications of Telemedicine

In earlier times, telemedicine was thought to be a secondary method which could only be used in emergencies and was considered inferior as the practitioner could not interact with the patient by being physically present [7]. Nevertheless, as time went by and advanced technologies were developed, the general opinion regarding telemedicine changed, and is still changing [7].

The beginning of advancements in telemedicines can be traced back to 1906 when a telecardiogram was created. It transmitted electrocardiograms through telephone lines [2]. In the 1950s, closed circuit TV was installed in two hospitals which were 150 kms away. Through this, the doctors interacted with psychiatric patients and interviews were held [2]. In 1968, a microwave video link was created which helped in consultations of cardiology, radiology and dermatology [6]. In the 1960s to 1970s, NASA conducted various telemedicine experiments as the well-being of astronauts in space was essential for the success of space missions. Telemetric transmission of data was used to monitor heart rate, blood pressure, and ECG from their space suits. However due to limited development in technology at that time and high cost of digital data transmission, the advancements were slowed down, which rapidly picked up pace in the 1990s as a result of fast developing information and telecommunication technologies [2].

Today, the development of wireless local area networks, wireless personal area networks and 4G network has made it easier to access highly advanced telemedicine data transmission and medical databases [6]. The further increase in computer power and development of optic fibre cable and strong satellite communication has now increased safety, speed, and efficacy of telemedicine [5]. In India, the Department of Information Technology, Indian Space Research Organization, Ministry of Communications and Information Technology along with state governments and many other medical and technical institutes of the country have taken an initiative to launch various telemedicine joints throughout the country [8]. India's Ministry of External Affairs is also helping other countries to enable telemedicine healthcare under South Asian Association for Regional Cooperation (SAARC). Director General of Health Services has taken an initiative to develop electronic information resources throughout the country for medical field known as National Medical Library's Electronic Resources in Medicine Consortium [8].

There are four main categories in telemedicine application range:

- Telemedicine among medical facilities with practitioners.
- Telemedicine among one medical facility and one household.
- Telemedicine among medical facilities without doctors.
- Telemedicine among co-medicals and households [7].

Some of the general applications of telemedicine are shown in Fig. 20.1. Due to telemedicine, transmission of data is possible from within ambulances to hospitals

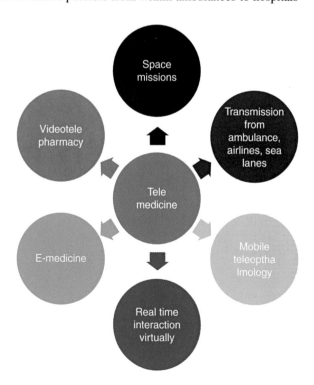

Fig. 20.1 General applications of telemedicine

which saves time and makes it easier to provide first aid, which in turn can save many lives. In the future we might see the same system in airlines and sea lanes [7]. Various institutes and eye hospitals in India, with ISRO's support under national blindness control programme, have established a mobile tele-ophthalmology service to help with early diagnosis and treatment of eye diseases. Many have established mobile tele-hospitals, mobile clinics as well as virtual channels that provide medical assistance instantly with an option of real-time interaction with doctors.

Overview of applications of telemedicine is shown in Fig. 20.1. The government has also launched an e-medicine system to reach all remote areas [8]. Telemedicine allows people from all types of geographic areas to reach healthcare whenever needed [8]. This allows healthcare delivery and makes up for the lack of infrastructure in areas owing to geographical infirmities [2]. Most of the time patients from these areas face long delays as they have to travel vast distances which can sometimes prove fatal. Another issue faced by them can be the unavailability of the same doctor who treated them last time. This can lead to differences in treatment method and understanding as well as difficulty in maintaining proper follow-up. This is where telemedicine plays an important role [8]. Telemedicine enables distribution of healthcare staff and resources throughout the system. It also increases availability of doctors due to reduced unnecessary hospital admission and emergency room visits [1]. Tele-dermatology is also a convenient and upcoming application of mobile telemedicine [1]. Home monitor teaching is also an imminent method for e-learning. Continuing education is important in the medical field to keep up with the rapid advancements in research and development. E-learning allows everyone to gain knowledge without restrictions of time and place, as has been true for all the students who are attending online classes in today's situation [2]. Telemedicine improves the quality of life in the long run as it provides instant and reliable healthcare which can turn out to be a lifesaver in situations where time is of essence and also reduce damage which could have been caused due to delay [9]. It was observed that in telemedicine, computer systems had a positive effect on the patient–healthcare provider relationship as patients were able to be more honest and were comfortable with the professional without feeling intimidated with physical presence. Depending on computer systems and electronic equipment for correctness of results and vital signs was also found to be reassuring for the patients [10]. With telemedicine technology, sky labs and space shuttles are well connected in real time and doctors are able to monitor astronaut's health, well-being, and extend support in various remote and extreme environments [5]. Developments like wearable ECG sensors and motion analysis systems make telemedicine easier [6]. Video telepharmacy is also an application of telemedicine through which pharmacists can dispense medicines as well as counsel patients without being physically present. This is helpful in cost reduction and is more efficient and patient specific [11, 12].

In this anxious situation of COVID-19 where the main problem is limited access to healthcare services, telemedicine can prove to be a breakthrough. These problems of uneven distribution of healthcare, lack of vigilance, and rise in costs are not going to end even after the pandemic. We need to make more use of telemedicine beyond the role as an emergency connectivity tool [13].Telemedicine is also very cost-effective and will help the country's economy in the situation we are facing today [14].

For the promotion and enhancement of the applications and utilization of telemedicine certain approaches like introducing incentive facilities to physicians, cost of telemedicine can be given health insurance coverage, etc. Flat rate charging systems can also be introduced to reduce the communication cost. The promotion for advancement in R&D technology, research promotion, lowering the cost of medical facilities and equipment could be an essential task for tele home care approaches. In some cases the malpractice issues are possible so that the laws from the concerned authorities can be introduced and implemented to control and resolve such issues. The patient's medical records are now shifting from paper based to computerized platforms with the guidelines and initiative by the health ministry which would facilitate telemedicine more significantly. The improvement in the internet facility in terms of security features also needs to be addressed with applications like Medical ID card system, Digital signature, certification authority, virtual private network, etc. to secure privacy as well as efficient applications of telemedicine [7].

Some of the future scopes of telemedicine are shown in Fig. 20.2.

The Indian government has already started taking initiative in national level projects on telemedicine and its planning and implementation is also modernized by the healthcare system by utilization of mobile and telecentres throughout the country specifically in areas where poor healthcare access is identified. ISRO initially started

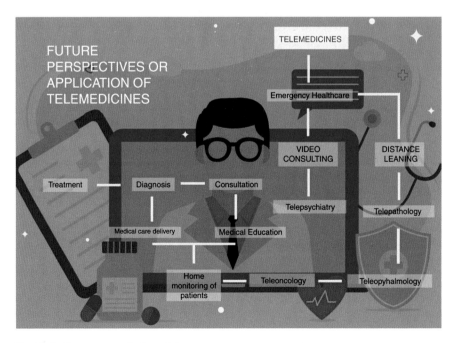

Fig. 20.2 Future scope of telemedicine

a telemedicine programme in 2001 and connected remote areas throughout India. Currently there are around 384 hospitals with 60 specialty hospitals connected under this programme in wide areas like general medicine, cardiology, ophthalmology, etc. ISRO has also provided communication software and hardware systems, equipment with satellite bandwidth, etc. The funds were allotted to hospitals for facility and manpower support. The various MoU's are signed with NGO's for effective implementation of the same. Recently around 139 telemedicine nodes are operational on INSAT-3A satellite and some on INSAT-3C and INSAT-4A. Efforts are continued by ISRO for maintenance. The testing and troubleshooting is now operated by monitoring mode established in DECU Ahmedabad [15].

The Ministry of health and family welfare has also taken up the initiatives for implementation of ONCONET project inspired from the success of Kerala ONCONET project model. Several regional and peripheral network centres planned to facilitate the National Cancer Control Program. Some initiatives also came up with the National Rural Health Mission.

This model gave several advantages in oncology practice with reducing the number of emergency visits at hospitals, unnecessary admissions, early diagnosis, routine follow-up, etc. Not only doctors but all healthcare professionals are involved in the service of ONCONET programme [16]. The department of information technology has also launched various projects in telemedicine in the development of a Web-Based Telemedicine System for Chronic Diseases, E Health Visualization and E-Health Associated Field, Advanced ICT for Health Care, etc. with various government organizations. It has also collaborated at international level with the European Union (EU) in various fields including e-governance and e-health. A MoU was also signed with Afghanistan to set up a telemedicine facility [17].

Globally in US occurrence of chronic diseases is at a faster rate which reflects 75% of the total healthcare expenditure and 70% of all deaths [18]. Recent data reveals telemedicine has captured the market in chronic disease management. It reduces certain obstacles like frequent visiting, number of admissions and emergency room load. The concept of hospital at home model is also becoming popular for patients who meet the specific criteria and can be stably treated at home for diseases like pneumonia, chronic obstructive pulmonary disease, etc. This model is found cost-effective, less treatment duration, etc. [19–21]. Success of telemedicine is also found in the conditions like radiology, intensive care, stroke and psychiatry, etc. in terms of mortality rate compared to conventional models [22, 23].

Several issues are also reported with this shift from conventional orientation to virtual platform with several factors like age, sex, etc. The younger generation is more open to this telemedicine platform and development than older generations since they are not familiar and comfortable with these technology platforms.

Telemedicine procedure is not a self-contained area; in this the open discussion as well critical evaluation and testing are essential procedures and it will be worthless if there is no proper involvement and acceptance by both patients and physicians [24, 25].

Video telemedicine is one of the technological advancements reported to have a more efficient and beneficial way of diagnosis and treatment [26]. Service provision with cost reduction is also one benefit out of this. Other benefits of this technology are also reported like increased productivity and market share with novel development in practice of medicine that further create a competitive healthcare environment. Instead physical visit video telemedicine provides advantages in terms of patient counts nurse practitioners can assist physicians [27]. Telemedicine service now became business demand [28]. The concept of virtual health has existed for a longer period but there are not yet systematic approaches and communication methodology. This concept of telemedicine could help establish the interconnection and systematic approach in virtual healthcare. This can also help in maintaining the proper healthcare records electronically specific for patients and medical history details, etc. FluNet database is an example for the same which is a global monitoring database for influenza. Telepharmacy is also an emerging concept which is having equivalent benefits as telemedicine. Use of smart card technology is a platform which can interconnect the telemedicine and telepharmacy that also collaborate physicians and pharmacists to achieve the motive of the virtual platform. In telepharmacy, video telemedicine is found to be a beneficial remote area for patient counselling [29].

20.4   Future of Telemedicine

Telemedicine allows people from all types of geographic areas to reach healthcare whenever needed. This allows healthcare delivery and makes up for the lack of infrastructure in areas owing to geographical infirmities [1, 2]. Most of the time patients from these areas face long delays as they have to travel vast distances which can sometimes prove fatal. Another issue faced by them can be the unavailability of the same doctor who treated them last time. This can lead to differences in treatment method and understanding as well as difficulty in maintaining proper follow-up. In future these types of problems can be solved by telemedicine [8]. In this anxious situation of COVID-19 where the main problem is limited access to healthcare services, telemedicine can prove to be a breakthrough. As the pandemic extends for the unforeseeable future, the role of telemedicine will remain a vital component for continued healthcare delivery [30].

Video telepharmacy is an application of telemedicine through which pharmacists can dispense medicines as well as counsel patients without being physically present. This is helpful in cost reduction and is more efficient and patient specific. In today's condition of social distancing and sanitization, this can prove to be very helpful [11]. These problems of uneven distribution of healthcare, lack of vigilance, and rise in costs are not going to end even after the pandemic. We need to make more use of telemedicine beyond the role as an emergency connectivity tool in the future as telemedicine holds great potential to solve all our future problems [13]. Telemedicine will enable distribution of healthcare staff and resources throughout the system. It will also increase availability of doctors due to reduced unnecessary hospital admission and emergency room visits. Home monitor teaching can also be an imminent method for e-learning. Continuing education is important in the medical field to keep up with the rapid advancements in research and development. E-learning allows everyone to gain knowledge without restrictions of time and place, as has been true for all the students who are attending online classes in today's situation. Various institutes and eye hospitals in India have established a mobile tele-ophthalmology service to help with early diagnosis and treatment of eye diseases. Many have established mobile tele-hospitals, mobile clinics as well as virtual channels that provide medical assistance instantly with an option of real-time interaction with doctors. Tele-dermatology is also a convenient and upcoming application of mobile telemedicine [1, 2]. We need to popularize and normalize the use of telemedicine more and more in the future and spread awareness about it so that people come to trust this method and understand the benefits of telemedicine. The government has also launched an e-medicine system all over the country. We need to maximize the usage of telemedicine in the future for the benefit of all citizens as everyone has the right to have availability of necessary healthcare services to improve the quality of life [12].

Telemedicine platform will be able to bring great revolution in the field of medicine and pharmacy with the utilization of technological advancements. It will facilitate to reach towards each individual in terms of healthcare in the large population and hetero geography of India. At all fronts India is taking initiatives in establishing and advancement in the telemedicine facilities with high-speed satellite, communication models, etc. There is still scope for upgrading the national policies, framework, laws, ethical framework, etc. to smooth implementation in healthcare services.

References

1. Mahar JH, Rosencrance JG, Rasmussen PA. Telemedicine: past, present, and future. Cleve Clin J Med. 2018;85(12):938–42.
2. Wurm EM, Hofmann-Wellenhof R, Wurm R, Soyer HP. Telemedicine and teledermatology: past, present and future. J Dtsch Dermatol Ges. 2008;6(2):106–12.
3. Sood S, Mbarika V, Jugoo S, Dookhy R, Doarn CR, Prakash N, Merrell RC. What is telemedicine? A collection of 104 peer-reviewed perspectives and theoretical underpinnings. Telemed e-Health. 2007;13(5):573–90.
4. Amadi-Obi A, Gilligan P, Owens N, O'Donnell C. Telemedicine in pre-hospital care: a review of telemedicine applications in the pre-hospital environment. Int J Emerg Med. 2014;7(1):1–1.
5. Nicogossian AE, Pober DF, Roy SA. Evolution of telemedicine in the space program and earth applications. Telemed J E Health. 2001;7(1):1–5.
6. Xiao Y, Takahashi D, Liu J, Deng H, Zhang J. Wireless telemedicine and m-health: technologies, applications and research issues. Int J Sensor Netw. 2011;10(4):202–36.
7. Takahashi T. The present and future of telemedicine in Japan. Int J Med Inform. 2001;61(2–3):131–7.
8. Mishra SK, Kapoor L, Singh IP. Telemedicine in India: current scenario and the future. Telemed e-Health. 2009;15(6):568–75.
9. Ohinmaa A, Hailey D, Roine R. Elements for assessment of telemedicine applications. Int J Technol Assess Health Care. 2001;17(2):190.
10. Bratton RL, Cody C. Telemedicine applications in primary care: a geriatric patient pilot project. Mayo Clin Proc. 2000;75(4):365–8.
11. Angaran DM. Telemedicine and telepharmacy: current status and future implications. Am J Health Syst Pharm. 1999;56(14):1405–26.

12. Whitten PS, Mair F. Telemedicine and patient satisfaction: current status and future directions. Telemed J E Health. 2000;6(4):417–23.
13. Bashshur R, Doarn CR, Frenk JM, Kvedar JC, Woolliscroft JO. Telemedicine and the COVID-19 pandemic, lessons for the future. Telemed J E Health. 2020;26(5):571–3.
14. Hailey D, Roine R, Ohinmaa A. Systematic review of evidence for the benefits of telemedicine. J Telemed Telecare. 2002;8(Suppl. 1):1–7.
15. Available at https://www.isro.gov.in/applications/tele-medicine
16. Available at: https://www.rcctvm.gov.in/telemedicine.php
17. Available at: https://mea.gov.in/Uploads/PublicationDocs/176_india-and-afghanistan-a-development-partnership.pdf
18. Bashshur RL, Shannon GW, Smith BR, et al. The empirical foundations of telemedicine interventions for chronic disease management. Telemed J E Health. 2014;20(9):769–800.
19. Cryer L, Shannon SB, Van Amsterdam M, Leff B. Costs for 'hospital at home' patients were 19 percent lower, with equal or better outcomes compared to similar inpatients. Health Aff (Millwood). 2012;31:1237–43.
20. Leff B, Burton L, Mader SL, et al. Hospital at home: feasibility and outcomes of a program to provide hospital-level care at home for acutely ill older patients. Ann Intern Med. 2005;143(11):798–808.
21. Leff B, Soones T, De Cherrie L. The hospital at home program for older adults. JAMA Intern Med. 2016;176(11):1724–5.
22. Wechsler LR, Demaerschalk BM, Schwamm LH, et al. American Heart Association Stroke Council; Council on Epidemiology and Prevention; Council on Quality of Care and Outcomes Research Telemedicine quality and outcomes in stroke: a scientific statement for healthcare professionals from the American Heart Association/ American Stroke Association. Stroke. 2017;48(1):e3–e25.
23. Wilcox ME, Wiener-Kronish JP. Telemedicine in the intensive care unit: effect of a remote intensivist on outcomes. JAMA Intern Med. 2014;174(7):1167–9.
24. Perednia D, Allen A. Telemedicine technology and clinical applications. JAMA. 1995;273:483–8.
25. Strode S, Gustke S, Allen A. Technical and clinical progress in telemedicine. JAMA. 1999;281:1066–8.
26. Gustke SS. Telemedicine in developing health care networks. New Med. 1997;1:61–6.
27. Rudd G. Physician extender models reduce costs of telemedicine services. Telemed Telehealth Netw. 1998;19:21.
28. Kane B, Sands D. Guidelines for the clinical use of electronic mail with patients. J Am Med Inform Assoc. 1998;5:104–11.
29. Flahault A, Dias-Ferrao V, Chaberty P, et al. FluNet as a tool for global monitoring of influenza on the Web. JAMA. 1998;280:1330–2.
30. McMaster T, Wright T, Mori K, Stelmach W, To H. Current and future use of telemedicine in surgical clinics during and beyond COVID-19: a narrative review. Ann Med Surg. 2021;102378

Secure and Privacy Issues in Telemedicine: Issues, Solutions, and Standards

21

Shaweta Sachdeva, Aleem Ali, and Shahnawaz Khan

21.1 Introduction

As we all know, protection and privacy are top priorities of healthcare practices when it comes to online access to electronic health records (EHR). EHR is increasingly replacing paper in healthcare organizations and is becoming more common. Patients, as well as healthcare organizations and practitioners, will benefit from this online access to medical records and transactions related to diagnosis. However, it poses significant privacy concerns about medical data; for example, no patient wants to reveal health details that might embarrass him or jeopardize his professional career. Patients can view their entire medical history at any time using internet-based EHR programs. As a result, protection and privacy are important considerations. Financial rewards, obstacles, rules and regulations, the state of technology used, and organizational influences are all important factors for EHR adaptation.

In a healthcare information system, there are three correlated records:

- A patient's personal health record is defined as a record that is kept only by the patient. It contains a comprehensive medical history review compiled from a variety of sources, including EMR and electronic health record (EHR).
- Healthcare practitioners develop, use, and maintain an electronic medical record (EMR) to track, control, and to control healthcare system as shown in Fig. 21.1.

S. Sachdeva (✉) · A. Ali
Department of CSE, Glocal University Saharanpur, Saharanpur, Uttar Pradesh, India
e-mail: aleem@theglocaluniversity.in

S. Khan
Faculty of Engineering, Design and Information & Communications Technology, Bahrain Polytechnic, Isa Town, Bahrain
e-mail: shahnawaz.rs.cse@itbhu.ac.in

© The Author(s), under exclusive license to Springer Nature Switzerland AG 2022
T. Choudhury et al. (eds.), *Telemedicine: The Computer Transformation of Healthcare*, TELe-Health, https://doi.org/10.1007/978-3-030-99457-0_21

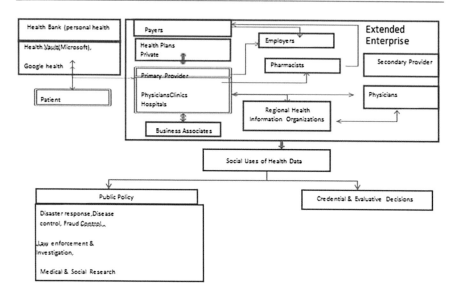

Fig. 21.1 Graphical representation of the flow of information in the telemedicine system

- An electronic health record (EHR) is a segment of an electronic medical record (EMR) that is produced and held by the patient and managed by each CDO. The electronic health record incorporates patient feedback and can be used by various healthcare distribution agencies within a community.

For successful healthcare delivery, privacy is an essential between patient–doctor relationships. Patients should exchange details with their doctors to ensure an accurate diagnosis and treatment plan, especially to prevent drug interactions.

Medical records include information such as a patient's identity, medical diagnosis history, medical images, prescription history, eating patterns, genetic information, psychological histories, job history, and a physician's subjective observations of personality and mental state, among other things.

A standard knowledge flow in the healthcare system is depicted in Fig. 21.1. Aside from diagnosis and care, patient health records could be used for a variety of purposes. To justify reimbursement of physician services, a patient's medical records are also shared with amount payer agencies such as insurance companies, Medicare, or Medicaid. Records may be used by healthcare providers to monitor their operations, measure service quality, and identify opportunities for quality enhancement. Providers can also exchange health information via a regional network .

21.2   Associated Work

Sinha [1] proposed the numerous technological problems and their drawbacks in India have been addressed in an eye-opening aspect of telemedicine in Punjab. It is essential to enforce a set of standards. They have spoken about telemedicine in terms of neurosurgical emergencies, and they suggest that the requirements for effective application of this growing technology be refined on a regular basis.

Mishra [2] proposed the current state of telemedicine in India. Many efforts are being made by the public and private sectors to enhance the quality of medical services, according to the study of Design and Implementation platform of Telemedicine Network in a Sub Himalayan State of India. Different digital medical repositories have also been added to provide additional support.

Mohandas [3] identified a telemedicine healthcare system that can be used for patient monitoring in an emergency and suggested an Improved Three Pattern Huffman Compression Algorithm for Medical Images in Telemedicine. The proposed telemedicine system included a portable and non-portable telemedicine component. The use of TCP/IP greatly increases the system's operability.

Yang Xiao [4] discusses the use and future aspects of telemedicine technology with examples. In his paper, he discussed wireless telemedicine systems and mobile health technologies, implementations, and research issues. There was also a brief discussion about the LINCOS initiative. There was an extensive debate on various technical problems such as compression and artificial intelligence. Medical monitors, home monitoring devices, and electrical medical records (EMRs), which are thought to be the future of telemedicine, were also discussed.

Pal [5] presented a comprehensive review of the existing state of telemedicine in a developing country such as India in a report. Since the majority of India's population lives in rural areas, the authors discuss the importance of telemedicine in different countries. They also present case studies and discuss some of the critical reasons for telemedicine to be applied more actively.

21.3   Main Components of Telemedicine

21.3.1 Collaboration Software

Smartphones, laptops, and tablets are examples of devices that enable the hospital to communicate patients with providers.

21.3.2 Medical Peripherals

Stethoscopes, ultrasound devices, and optical stethoscopes are examples of peripheral diagnostic instruments used in telemedicine. When peripheral devices are combined with communication tools and workflow agenda, caregivers can provide high-definition audio, video, images, and data from various locations, allowing them to provide

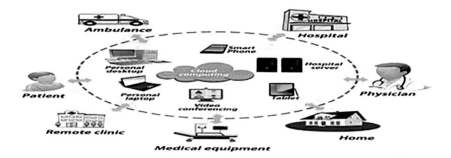

Fig. 21.2 Cloud-based services used in telemedicine

better treatment and diagnosis [6]. To help patients, multiple service lines with the same equipment, ease of use, and flexibility of peripherals are essential.

21.3.3 Workflow

It refers to the ability to provide thorough documentation across a wide range of subspecialties and modalities. This means, in addition to the requirement of various telemedicine hardware (such as medical peripherals), hospitals also need various software to handle the whole process of linking patients with doctors and integrating telemedicine with existing IT systems like EHR. A telemedicine program can also provide clinicians with the number of tools they need, such as safe messaging, store and forward functionality, EHR integration, and billing process.

21.3.4 Cloud-Based Services

Traditionally, telemedicine services have been run on enterprise systems, which can cost thousands of dollars to run only one telemedicine system. This is not a problem for large organizations because they have extensive telemedicine services [7]. However, as telemedicine becomes more widely used in nursing homes and small clinics, the cost of telemedicine may become prohibitively expensive for smaller organizations as shown in Fig. 21.2. A cloud-based service will save an organization thousands of dollars, directly affecting their bottom line.

21.4   Telemedicine Advantages and Disadvantages

Our aim is to compile a list of these factors in one location and to elaborate on a few of them. The main advantages of telemedicine can be summarized as follows:

- Better access to healthcare.
- Having access to quality treatment.
- Improved inter-career contact.

- Continuing education that is both easier and better.
- Improved information accessibility.
- More efficient use of resources.
- Minimal costs.

The following are the results of our survey of telemedicine recorded limitations:

- Relationships between patients and their caregivers are often strained.
- Relationships between healthcare professionals are strained.
- Technology that is impersonal.
- Organizational disruption.
- Additional training needs.
- Protocol development is a difficult task.
- Uncertainty about the accuracy of health data.
- Low usage rates.

21.5 Opportunities in Telemedicine

Telemedicine has exploded in popularity in India's healthcare industry. What factors have influenced rural healthcare practices? Owing to a variety of logistical issues, people living in rural areas do not have access to adequate medical care [8]. They will get healthcare delivered to their homes using this technology. Apart from these some other benefits are as follows:

- Telemedicine is less expensive. Such amenities are accessible to everyone.
- It is often used when there are not as many options available.
- It aids in the provision of services in rural and remote areas of the country.
- It facilitates the exchange of information among health professionals.
- It aids in the training of healthcare practitioners.
- It aids in the rescue of people during wars, floods, earthquakes, and other natural disasters.
- It also helps in the collaboration of healthcare professionals.

21.6 Challenges in Telemedicine

The following are some of the obstacles to telemedicine effective implementation in the Indian health sector:

- Health professional's attitudes: Health professionals are unsure about the telemedicine system and are unfamiliar with it.
- Patients' apprehension: Patients are concerned about the effective results of the telemedicine system.
- Financial unavailability: The high costs of equipment and connectivity make telemedicine impractical.

- Lack of basic amenities: Almost half of India's population lives in poverty. Transportation, power, telecommunications, clean drinking water, primary healthcare, and other basic infrastructure services have all vanished. When an individual has nothing to improve, no technological innovation can help.
- Language diversity and literacy rate: Only 65.38% of India's population is literate, with only 2% fluent in English.
- Technical limitations: The telemedicine method, which is aided by a variety of software and hardware, is still in its infancy. Advanced biological sensors and more bandwidth support are needed for proper diagnosis and data pacing.

21.7 Security and Privacy Issues

Because of the risks associated with EHR, it is important to ensure patient privacy. When accessing or transacting EHR, every healthcare institution should be aware of the following security concerns:

21.7.1 User Authentication

When a user wants to access a health record, only those who have been approved or registered are allowed to do so.Several solutions based on smart cards have been suggested [9, 10]. Biometric-based system is one of the best ways used for ensuring the authorized person to access the records.

21.7.2 Confidentiality and Integrity

This refers to the quality and consistency of medical records, as well as the integrity and consistency of physical device and network systems. Patient data may be altered or clinical infrastructure may be destroyed as a result of EHR device hacking events.

21.7.3 Access Control

Access control is one of the critical security issues for sharing in computing environments because medical records are stored in internal databases and shared through heterogeneous file systems. Since responsibilities and privileges are assigned differently depending on the system and organization, users' rights to use such resources must be controlled by granting or denying access to resources. If the remote link is not safe, an unidentified user can easily gain access to the network [11]. Role-based access, passwords, and audit trails should all be available via electronic systems. Genetic research raises significant privacy concerns. Individuals are concerned about job loss and life insurance. As a result, refusing to use successful genetic testing is harmful.

21.7.4 Data Ownership

When delegating access to a patient's record, it is also necessary to remember data ownership. Who will own which data, and how will control over data be delegated? Data ownership obligations and duties should also be done transparently.

21.7.5 Data Protection Policies

Since the healthcare diagnostic system involves many organizations that cross organizational and functional boundaries, appropriate and consistent data protection is needed. All organizations must have specific policies and way of limiting the use of physical media and portable devices to prevent fraudulent or loss of medical records. EHR systems demand continuing functionality concept creation to preserve security, by adding different levels of security, and block access to specific notes, lab results, monitoring process, and sensitive entries for information that is to be released.

21.7.6 User Profiles

Patient, doctor, healthcare company, trusted third party, pharmacist, and other organizations are all active in the healthcare system. Patient identification systems in hospitals differ widely and are incompatible, by making it more difficult to identify patients individually within a facility or through the organizations. Interoperability requires the existence of a mechanism for distinguishing patients through institutions. There is currently no industry-wide record-to-record matching requirement.

21.7.7 Misuse of Health Record of Patients

Many EHR-related websites, especially those that offer free storage space, are unconcerned about privacy issues. They may sell the information to other businesses or put ads on the same page as the patient's information. Protection of health records can be difficult in a multi-specialty environment. Since the care of these patients can span various medical specialties and document forms, organizations must be able to segregate all documents relevant to substance abuse treatment [12–14].

21.8 Security and Privacy Threats

Figure 21.3 defines how attacks can be divided into four different groups based on the type of disruption of normal information flow as shown in Fig. 21.3.

(a) Interruption: This is an assault on information availability (A). Information becomes inaccessible or destroyed.

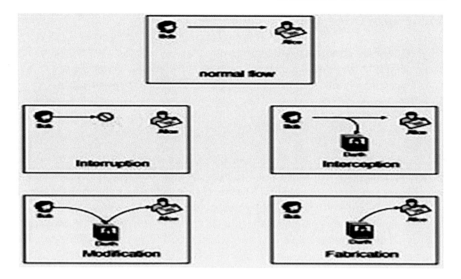

Fig. 21.3 Categories of security threats in telemedicine

(b) Interception: This is a breach of knowledge confidentiality(C). Data is accessed by an unauthorized third party.
(c) Modification: This is an assault on the information's credibility (I). The information is not only accessed but often interferes with by an unauthorized third party.
(d) Fabrication is an attempt to deceive the public about the accuracy of facts. The information interferes with by an unauthorized third party who inserts a fake message.

Depending on the type of attack, telemedicine network attacks can be divided into two categories:

21.8.1 Active Attacks

There are three types of active attacks, each of which involves the alteration, disruption, or fabrication of patient information:

21.8.1.1 Masquerade
This has the potential to compromise information's confidentiality (C) and honesty (I). In this scenario, a person tries to deceive a system by misrepresenting itself and posing as someone else.

21.8.1.2 Modification of Messages
This has an effect on the information's credibility (I). This happens when a portion of a valid message is changed, or when messages are withheld and then replicated to create an unauthorized effect.

21.8.1.3   Denial of Service

The availability of information is harmed by a denial of service attack. An intruder uses this attack to make a memory resource or computing too busy to handle legitimate requests, denying legitimate communication facility usage or management [15].

21.8.2 Passive Attacks

Knowledge is intercepted but not altered in these attacks. These attacks are carried out by watching the devices while performing relevant functions for gathering the data. These tasks include eavesdropping, sniffing, and traffic analysis. Passive attacks cause information or data files to be disclosed to an attacker without the user's permission or awareness. Such attacks are broadly grouped into two categories:

21.8.2.1   Release of Message Content

A telephone call, an e-mail address, or a patient data transfer can all be easily accessed without affecting the message.

21.8.2.2   Traffic Analysis

All network incoming and outgoing traffic is processed, but not changed, by an unauthorized third party in order to obtain knowledge necessary to comprehend the essence of communication.

21.9   Security and Privacy Solutions

21.9.1 Enabled by Smart Card E-prescribing Systems That Protect Your Privacy

Smart cards are extremely important. The smart cards are designed to be portable storage devices for up-to-date personal medical records and insurance documents, allowing doctors to access data quickly and accurately during the diagnosis process [16]. Hospitals, general practitioners (GPs), and corporate partners such as insurance providers, billing firms, and pharmacists are all interested in providing healthcare. This approach focuses on a smart card-based portable personal information repository to streamline the drug-prescribing process by allowing doctors to skip many bureaucratic measures [17–19].

Smart cards can be used not only as a storage unit, but also to perform intelligent tasks such as digital signature signing, which allows users to sign electronic pads, and patient authorization. Delegated signing is a smart card task extension that includes the delegation of prescription signing capability among users.

It is for a designated individual who signs the prescription on behalf of the patient and collects the drug using his own smart card [20]. It has the capability of being borne by anyone other than the user. Furthermore, it does not add to the system's complexity. This system allows patients and physicians to communicate with each other while limiting data disclosure [21, 22].

The following are some of the benefits of this smart card-enabled solution:

1. Patients' authenticity is automatically assured by keeping cards.
2. It eliminates the need for numerous prescriptions from various doctors.
3. It can be used to keep track of public health campaigns.

21.10 Conclusion

Telemedicine, the most difficult aspect of e-governance, provides rural patients with affordable and reliable healthcare. However, telemedicine programs continue to face privacy and security concerns, owing to the widespread use of emerging communication technologies. In order to preserve patient safety, dignity, and confidentiality, medical records contain highly classified information that should not be made available to unauthorized individuals. At the same time, registered users should be able to access patient information anytime they need it for legitimate purposes. Information security resources such as confidentiality, honesty, and availability (C-I-A) are threatened by attacks such as interruption, surveillance, alteration, and fabrication. Depending on whether they alter, fabricate, or intercept information, these attacks may be classified as active or passive. Despite the use of various preventive, deterrent, and control measures, a security or privacy threat may exploit a small vulnerability to inflict massive harm. As a result, the risk of privacy and security violations on a telemedicine network should be evaluated so that effective mitigation steps can be taken to mitigate potential damages.

References

1. Sinha VD, et al. Telemedicine in neurosurgical emergency: Indian perspective. Asian J Neurosurg. 2012;7(2):75–7. https://doi.org/10.4103/1793-5482.98648.
2. Mishra SK. Telemedicine in India: current scenario and the future. Telemed e-Health. 2009;15(6):568–75. https://doi.org/10.1089/tmj.2009.0059.
3. Mohan D, et al. An improved three pattern Huffman compression algorithm for medical images in telemedicine. In: Information processing and management, communications in computer and information science, vol. 70. Berlin, Heidelberg: Springer; 2010. p. 263–8. https://doi.org/10.1007/978-3-642-12214-9_43.
4. Xiao Y, et al. Wireless telemedicine and m-health: technologies, applications and research issues. Int J Sensor Netw. 2011;10(4):202–36. https://doi.org/10.1504/ijsnet.2011.042770.
5. Pal A, et al. Telemedicine diffusion in a developing country: the case of India. IEEE Trans Inform Technol Biomed. 2004:59–65. https://doi.org/10.1109/TITB.2004.842410.
6. Mandl KD, et al. Public standards and patients control: how to keep electronic medical records accessible but private. Brit Med J. 2001;322(7281):283–7.
7. T. Ermakova et al. Security and privacy system requirements for adopting cloud computing in healthcare data sharing scenarios security and privacy system requirements for adopting cloud computing in healthcare data sharing scenarios, August, 2013.

8. Knut H, et al. Proposal for a security management in cloud computing for health care. Scientific World J. 2014;146970., 7 pages https://doi.org/10.1155/2014/146970.

9. Rao BT, et al. A study on data storage security issues in cloud computing. Procedia Comput Sci. 2016;92:128–35.

10. Alowolodu OD, et al. Elliptic curve cryptography for securing cloud computing applications. Int J Comput Appl. 2013;66(23)

11. Mell P, et al. The NIST definition of cloud computing recommendations of the National Institute of Standards and Technology. Nist Spec Publ. 2011;145:7.

12. Wang C, et al. Toward secure and dependable storage services in cloud computing. IEEE Trans Serv Comput. 2012:220–32.

13. Al-Nayadi, et al. An authorization policy management framework for dynamic medical data sharing. Int Conf Intell Pervas Comput. 2007:313–8.

14. Angst et al. An empirical examination of the importance of defining the PHR for research and for practice, Robert H. Smith School Research Paper No. RHS-06-011 Available at SSRN: http://ssrn.com/abstract=904611, 2006.

15. Applebaum, et al. Privacy in psychiatric treatment: threats and response. Am J Psychiatry. 2002;159:1809–18.

16. Ball, et al. Patient privacy in electronic prescription transfer. IEEE Security Privacy. 2003:77–80.

17. Baumer, et al. Privacy of medical records: IT implications of HIPAA. ACM Comput Soc. 2000;30(4):40–7.

18. Becker, et al. Detecting medicine abuse. J Health Econ. 2005;2005(24):189–201.

19. Aleem Ali, Neeta Singh, M/M/1/n+Flush/n model to enhance the QoS for Cluster Heads in MANETs. Published in International Journal of Advanced Computer Science and Applications (IJACSA) , U.K. 2018. ESCI, Scopus.

20. Parveen N, Ali A, Ali A. IOT Based automatic vehicle accident alert system. In: 2020 IEEE 5th International Conference on Computing Communication and Automation (ICCCA), Oct. 2020, Greater Noida. p. 330–3. https://doi.org/10.1109/ICCCA49541.2020.9250904. (Scopus Indexed).

21. Sachdeva S, Ali A. A hybrid approach using digital Forensics for attack detection in a cloud network environment. Int J Future Gener Commun Netw. 2021;14(1):1536–46.

22. Kaur R, Ali A. A novel blockchain model for securing IoT based data transmission. Int J Grid Distrib Comput. 2021;14(1):1045–55.

Perception of Parents About Children's Nutritional Counseling Through Telemedicine

22

Swapan Banerjee, Tanupriya Choudhury, Digvijay Pandey, Hilda Emmanuel-Akerele, Tayana Silva de Carvalho, and Manish Taywade

22.1 Introduction

Health and wellness are the top priorities for any nation, and diet is essential. It works in both scenarios during good health and disease. Simultaneously, counseling is an integral part of the health care world in all the medical fields. We all are aware that child health care is more important because children are the future of any nation. Children are one of the vulnerable sections of so many infectious and non-communicable diseases, for which a country runs various immunization programs and other area-wise awareness programs. Therefore, children's health and wellness have been considered for significant research and policy implementation by most countries [1]. Caring for the child means the role of the mother who comes first as friend, philosopher, guide, and a complete caregiver since birth. Some studies

S. Banerjee (✉)
Department of Nutrition, Seacom Skills University, Kendradangal, Birbhum, West Bengal, India

T. Choudhury (✉)
School of Computer Science, University of Petroleum and Energy Studies (UPES), Dehradun, Uttarakhand, India

D. Pandey
Department of Technical Education, IET, Dr. A.P.J. Abdul Kalam Ajad Technical University, Lucknow, Uttar Pradesh, India

H. Emmanuel-Akerele
Department of Biological Sciences, Anchor University, Ipaja, Lagos, Nigeria

T. S. de Carvalho
Heart and Diabetes Center NRW, Bad Oeynhausen, Germany

M. Taywade
Department of Community Medicine & Family Medicine, All India Institute of Medical Sciences, Bhubaneswar, Odisha, India

T. Choudhury et al. (eds.), *Telemedicine: The Computer Transformation of Healthcare*, TELe-Health, https://doi.org/10.1007/978-3-030-99457-0_22

showed that if a mother gets proper awareness, there is a positive impact on the child's health from childhood till adulthood [2]. However, parents are mainly responsible for planning for the diet and nutrition of the child. In the metro and major cities of most advanced countries, father and mother both are working at offices or fields, although, during the COVID pandemic, they are getting closer to their children due to work from home system.

22.1.1 Child Malnutrition

Malnutrition can be undernutrition or overnutrition. Undernutrition is due to food insecurity, mostly in rural areas, whereas overnutrition leads to obesity. Malnutrition showed tremendous momentum as a dual burden during the last few years, including COVID-19 phases. Infectious diseases usually lead to vitamin A deficiency, micronutrients, and macronutrients due to poor absorption and increased excretion. Poor diet ultimately leads to an increased possibility of infection. Micronutrients are essential to maintain the immunological mechanism response to any microbial infections, and COVID is one of the burning examples [3]. Before COVID pandemic, malnutrition in India has already a considerable burden. National Family Health Survey-5 (NFHS-5), 2019–2020 clearly shows that malnutrition has increased compared to the NFHS-4, reported in 2015–2016. The children are the country's future, and if malnutrition is not declining, they miss the opportunity to contribute to its development in subsequent years. Undoubtedly, the situation due to COVID-19 will accelerate the burden of malnutrition in the coming days [4].

Figure 22.1 shows that the United Nations Children's Fund (UNICEF) reports the global prevalence of weight status of children under 5 years who are much more vulnerable. In the rural sections, children predominantly suffer from undernutrition from mild to severe, leading to anemia, tuberculosis, and other nutrition-related disorders. However, overweight status is equally visible considering the growing cases of obesity, starting from children to older adults.

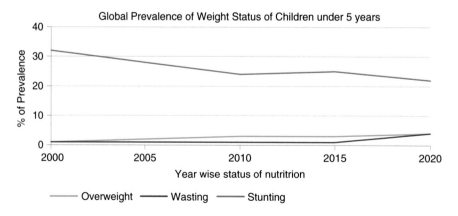

Fig. 22.1 Global status of infant and young child nutrition [5] (Source https://data.unicef.org)

In Fig. 22.2 we have shown the girls' population under tremendous focus by all the world's best public health agencies, regulatory bodies, and respective countries ministry of women and child care. The girls' population under 5–19 years are significantly vulnerable to obesity.

As like Figs. 22.2 and 22.3 also emphasized the nutritional status of the boys in the global population under the age of 5–19 years. This section falls under child cum adolescents who are the future of any nation. Nutrition is equally essential for the urban population of boys and girls suffering from overweight, obesity, and other lifestyle diseases. Type-1 diabetes or juvenile diabetes has been considered one of the significant autoimmune disorders globally.

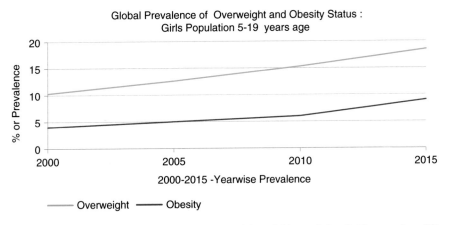

Fig. 22.2 Global status of child and adolescent nutrition: girls' population 5–19 years of age [6] (Source: http://ncdrisc.org)

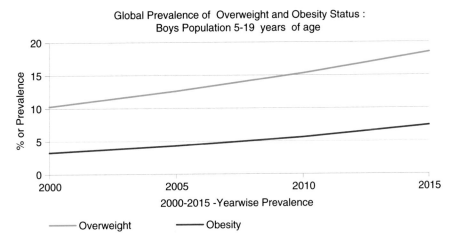

Fig. 22.3 Global status of child and adolescent nutrition: boys' population 5–19 years of age [6] (Source: http://ncdrisc.org)

22.1.2 Children Nutrition and SARS CoV-2 Infections

Children were not directly affected by SARS CoV-2 in 2020, although in 2021, they are getting affected comparatively. Children below 12 years are at the risk of contacting the COVID-19. However, the infection was mild to moderate; only 5–6% has landed up so far with the severe case. Children with chronic diseases, like diabetes, asthma, rheumatic arthritis, etc., are more prone to compromised immune systems. One cross-sectional study reported reducing intake of fruits and vegetables by 41.4% and exacerbating food insecurity in the last few years [7]. A study from Italy showed the parents' perception of food security. The study showed an alarming rise in food insecurity before the COVID pandemic (8.3%) and after (16.2%). Almost 27% of parents reported their children eating more, 31.8% of respondents said children gained weight within the lockdown phases [8].

COVID-19 pandemic has influenced the physical, mental, and social domains of life. The diet and nutrition component is one of them, significantly impacting human health. The COVID-19 and dietary pattern are both associated with the risk of COVID infections [9]. Undernutrition and overnutrition are associated with a high prevalence of anemia and other lifestyle diseases. Therefore, it is vital to have a balanced diet to reduce the potential risk of contracting with the COVID-19. Data shows that the deterioration of dietary practices has a significant impact on the public health system in India. The infectious (e.g., tuberculosis) and noncommunicable diseases (e.g., diabetes, hypertension) are increasing the burden of diseases with COVID-19 since 2020 [10–12].

22.1.3 Urban and Rural Differences

The dietary diversity in the idea has its issues and may contribute to the variation in the COVID-19 cases. Nutritional patterns and behavior in the COVID-19 pandemic have changed a lot. Overeating and meal frequency has increased in most urban families. Therefore, to disseminate the knowledge on healthy dietary and eating processes, many initiatives have been pointed out as a "call for action." [13]

22.1.4 Opportunities and Challenges of Telemedicine and Nutritional Awareness During COVID-19 Outbreak

Nutrition and diet counseling should be encouraged during the COVID-19 pandemic by dietary recommendations and counseling regarding the intake of fruits, vegetables, and whole-grain food items. Diet should be rich in fruits and vegetables containing fat-soluble (A, C, D, E) A and water-soluble B complex. Fruits and vegetables are also good sources of fibers, water, and antioxidants that play an essential role in controlling noncommunicable diseases like hypertension, diabetes, and improper weight. In addition, micronutrients like zinc, selenium, iron, copper,

Fig. 22.4 Challenges around the corner of the world

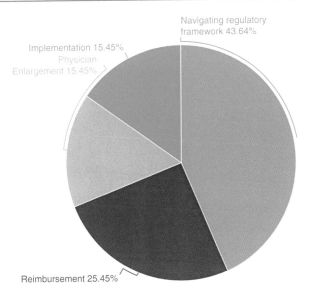

folate, omega 3 fatty acids, etc., are essential to balance the diet. Thus, a healthy diet can prevent COVID-19 indirectly and also reduce the risk associated with COVID-19 deficiency [14, 15].

Figure 22.4 shows the significant challenges in telemedicine all over the world and the distribution of challenges by following different factors as mentioned below serially:

- Navigating country by a country regulatory framework
- Reimbursement process and its issues
- Physician enlargement and implementation of plans

Similarly, Fig. 22.5 depicts an overview of telemedicine's utilization on various core and demanding departments' growing practices at global level medical institutions and services centers, including trade settings. It indicates that telemedicine is preferred in metro cities compared to non-metro towns. The top two chosen segments are radiology, followed by psychiatry and primary care based on global data. One study showed significant improvements in diet and clinical outcomes of chronic kidney disease (CKD) patients using telehealth intervention. The study explored the food group consumption, vegetable serving, dietary fiber intake, and body weight [16]. The telehealth system has already been operating in rural settings for the diabetic prevention program.

Further, quarantine has restricted the movement to visit health facilities during this COVID period; hence, proper dietary counseling over teleconsultation and a healthy diet will help. To maintain the nutritional status, diet is critical in any infections. The importance of dietary advice helps to reduce undernutrition over nutrition and boosts immunity for all illnesses, including COVID-19 disease [17, 18].

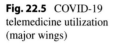

Fig. 22.5 COVID-19
telemedicine utilization
(major wings)

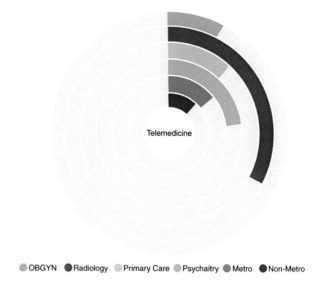

Telemedicine

● OBGYN   ● Radiology   ● Primary Care   ● Psychaitry   ● Metro   ● Non-Metro

22.2 Methodology

Study Design: A qualitative study with a convenience sampling method was used. The study was conducted through focus group discussion by a reliable, popular virtual platform using video-meeting mode. Three different dates were selected from April 2021 to May 2021 within a span of 45 days from 3 pm to 4.30 pm each day. The group meetings were subsequently accomplished three days in the same week with one practicing dietitian (moderator). One doctor (as an advisor) from a reputed national medical institute and hospital was also in the research team apart from other contributors. A pre-tested semi-structured questionnaires format was prepared and duly filled by each respondent well in advance and considered for the discussion during the FGD [19, 20].

Selection of Samples: In this study, 24 interested parents, either father or mother of the class-1 to class-7 students from the age group 6 years to 12 years, participated in the FGD. Hence, we selected as convenience sampling all the working parents who are usually busy in the job or their business. In addition, the email consent was also taken from each parent for participation about children's diet and nutrition by filling online questionnaires [19].

Geographical Area: All the 24 parents were from Kolkata city as permanent residents.

Tools and Techniques: The study followed the mixed-method research often used in public health research: (i) FGD through pre-tested semi-structured question- naires, (ii) BMI calculation through height and weight measurements of the chil- dren that received from the parents 7 days before to start of first FGD, (iii) collection and screening of current medical reports including laboratories tests as available but mandatorily all records collected for juvenile diabetes data, (iv) anthropometric measurements from every parent, (v) assessments of children's dietary habits and basic nutrition knowledge of parents, and (vi) dichotomous questions to fill in the questionnaire [20, 21].

Data Collection: Data was collected through the questionnaires duly filled by every parent and subsequently discussed in the FGD in the presence of the moderator. The FGD was conducted fortnightly by using a similar virtual platform. The discussions were based on nutrition and its application to children's health. Three themes were considered: parent awareness on nutrition, parent attitude towards telemedicine, and perception of underweight, overweight, diabetes, and routine diet counseling for their child. In addition, a few attributes and related factors were focused on content analysis also [21].

Statistical Methods: Mixed methods by using NVIVO-10 for statistical and content analysis.

Consent from Participants: We got written consent from each parent as per our prescribed format following all ethical norms of FGD and collection of other and their uses [22].

22.3 Results

22.3.1 Frequency and Percentage Analysis

In the study, we found that 24 parents participated actively in the focussed groups for their children studying classes 1–7, under the age group 6–12. Table 22.1 showed that a minimum of 4.2% of class 6 students' parents to a maximum of 20.8% of class 3 level parents was assessed by their perceptions with the presence of a moderator on each FGD [21, 23].

A total of 3 group meetings were subsequently conducted weekly, repeated fortnightly. Hence calculation of 9 FGD was performed within 45 days for three focus groups at a median of 8 participants [19]. This study intended to understand the parents' perception of their child's health and diet. Therefore, we considered all convenience sampling regarding parents and their children. The inclusion criteria were children with undernutrition or overnutrition, also called obesity.

Table 22.1 Participants children's frequency

Age	Class	Frequency	Percent%
6	1	4	16.7
7	2	4	16.7
8	3	5	20.8
9	4	3	12.5
10	5	4	16.7
11	6	1	4.2
12	7	3	12.5
$N = 24$	1–7	100	100

We also added very few parents of juvenile diabetes (type-1 diabetes mellitus) children, an autoimmune disorder common in children and adolescents worldwide. Therefore, our study analyzed the status as per health and nutrition is concerned. Table 22.2 showed that 20.8% were mild underweight and obese children whereas 8.3% of each in the category of mild to moderate underweight and juvenile diabetes cases among the children of participated parents.

22.3.2 Analysis of 8 Attributes Cum Themes Applied in Questionnaires and FGD

Tables 22.3 and 22.4 identified and analyzed the participants' perceptions through their dichotomous answers and percentages based on our pre-tested semi-structured questionnaires. The easy, nonsensible, and adjustable questions were provided in the questionnaires filled by the parents without hesitation well in advance before

Table 22.2 Health and nutrition frequency of children

Health issues	Frequency	Percentage
Mild underweight	5	20.8
Moderate underweight	2	8.3
Severe underweight	2	8.3
Overweight	4	16.7
Pre-obesity	6	25
Obesity	5	20.8
Juvenile diabetes (yes)	2	8.3
Juvenile Diabetes (No)	22	91.7

Table 22.3 Analysis of attributes and content of participants received from questionnaires and FGD

Questions	Attributes in the questionnaires	Yes	%	No	%	May be	%	SD = Standard deviation*
1	Teleconsultation awareness of nutrition and diet	7	29.2	17	70.8	NA	0	0.464
2	Following any diet by a dietician	3	12.5	21	87.5	NA	0	0.187
3	How many teleconsultations availed so far on diet	3	12.5	21	87.5	NA	0	0.676
4	Interested in routinely diet counseling	16	66.7	2	8.3	6	25	0.881
5	Interested in teleconsultation for diet	13	54.2	3	12.5	8	33.3	0.932
6	Getting awareness, now you are confident about teleconsultation	22	91.7	2	8.3	NA	0	0.282

their second FGD meet. A total of eight closed-ended questions were prepared [24]. We got the replies from the parent about their pre-existing perception and reasons towards their child's nutrition status where we mentioned the question "Perception of child's nutrition status." We got the replies also 20.8% less eating and 37.5% due to overeating, 12.5% genetic, and 29.2% lack of awareness.

We revealed that 91.7% (SD = 0.282) of participants were hopeful and interested in starting a diet consultation through teleconsultation during a COVID pandemic or while unable to visit clinics or hospitals. Similarly, 66.7% of parents (SD = 0.881) showed their interest in routinely diet counseling anyways for their children's better health and nutrition.

22.3.3 Focus Group Discussions Analysis

As per the video recording of each FGD, we transcripted word by word, following the protocol of FGD analysis: underlined, capitalized, and bold as applicable. The process quickly helped to track the discussions on precise questions. We did not follow punctuation but focused on the highlighted words while parents talked. In our web meetings, we just discussed in more uncomplicated, easy, and accurate ways.

The above tables (Tables 22.5–22.12) are in the results section concerned about mean analysis. The analysis has been done to determine the mean and standard deviation (SD) irrespective of all eight attributes. Attributes are named A1 to A8 as per eight tables that show the standardization of dependent variables regarding each attribute under the FGD themes. Before starting this research, the themes we considered were parent awareness on nutrition, parent attitude towards telemedicine, perception of underweight, overweight, diabetes, and routine diet counseling.

Additionally, we enlisted the dependent variables list: 1. participants, 2. sex of children, 3. the age group of children, 4. classes they are studying, 5. weight status: underweight (mild, moderate, severe); overweight (overweight, pre-obesity, obesity), and 6. type-1 diabetes (juvenile DM). Same way, all attributes are in the list of independent variables.

22.4 Discussion

In our research paper, we partially applied mixed-method (qualitative cum quantitative) to analyze all collection of data and information [20]. However, our study is primarily qualitative as it tried to understand and assess the perception and gross attitude of all participants who were parents of classes 1-to 7. From Tables 22.5–22.12, we showed the mean and SD analysis in the above, irrespective of every attribute and participants' demographic cum health details [24]. We planned and prepared eight different attributes to get responses from the respective parents. First-round (at first video conference), moderator interacted with the parents about their current health and troubles due to COVID lockdown and post lockdown phases

Table 22.4 Analysis of attributes and content of participants received from the questionnaires and FGD

Questions	Attributes in the questionnaires	Busy	%	Physical visit	%	Financial	%	After pandemic	%	SD*
7	If not teleconsulted then reason	4	16.7	9	37.5	2	8.3	9	37.5	1.167
Questions	**Attributes in the questionnaires**	**Less eating**	**%**	**Overeating**	**%**	**Genetical**	**%**	**Lack of awareness**	**%**	**SD***
8	Perception of child's nutrition status	5	20.8	9	37.5	3	12.5	7	29.2	0.1.574

Table 22.5 Mean and SD analysis: attribute no.1 vs. participants' demographic and health details

A1. Teleconsultation awareness of nutrition and diet		Participants	Boy or girl	Age group	Children classes	Weight status	Juvenile diabetes
Yes	Mean	13.14	1.43	7.86	2.86	3.29	1.86
	N	7	7	7	7	7	7
	SD	6.793	0.535	2.116	2.116	2.215	0.378
No	Mean	12.24	1.41	8.88	3.88	4.00	1.94
	N	17	17	17	17	17	17
	Std. deviation	7.370	0.507	1.867	1.867	1.732	0.243
Total	Mean	12.50	1.42	8.58	3.58	3.79	1.92
	N	24	24	24	24	24	24
	SD	7.071	0.504	1.954	1.954	1.865	0.282

Table 22.6 Mean and SD. Analysis: attribute no.2 vs. participants' demographic and health details

A2. Following any diet by the dietician		Participants	Boy or girl	Age group	Children classes	Weight status	Juvenile diabetes
Yes	Mean	12.33	1.33	10.00	5.00	2.67	2.00
	N	3	3	3	3	3	3
	SD	4.509	0.577	3.464	3.464	2.082	0.000
No	Mean	12.52	1.43	8.38	3.38	3.95	1.90
	N	21	21	21	21	21	21
	SD	7.447	0.507	1.687	1.687	1.830	0.301
Total	Mean	12.50	1.42	8.58	3.58	3.79	1.92
	N	24	24	24	24	24	24
	SD	7.071	0.504	1.954	1.954	1.865	0.282

Table 22.7 Mean and SD. Analysis: attribute no.3 vs. participants' demographic and health details

A3. How many teleconsultations availed so far on diet		Participants	Boy or girl	Age group	Children classes	Weight status	Juvenile diabetes
One	Mean	12.33	1.33	10.00	5.00	2.67	2.00
	N	3	3	3	3	3	3
	SD	4.509	0.577	3.464	3.464	2.082	0.000
No yet	Mean	12.52	1.43	8.38	3.38	3.95	1.90
	N	21	21	21	21	21	21
	Std. deviation	7.447	0.507	1.687	1.687	1.830	0.301
Total	Mean	12.50	1.42	8.58	3.58	3.79	1.92
	N	24	24	24	24	24	24
	SD	7.071	0.504	1.954	1.954	1.865	0.282

Table 22.8 Mean and SD. Analysis: attribute no.4 vs. participants' demographic and health details

A4. If not, then reason		Participants	Boy or girl	Age group	Children classes	Weight status	Juvenile diabetes
Busy	Mean	15.00	1.75	8.75	3.75	4.00	1.75
	N	4	4	4	4	4	4
	SD	9.592	0.500	2.754	2.754	2.160	0.500
Physical visit prefer	Mean	10.56	1.33	8.44	3.44	4.22	2.00
	N	9	9	9	9	9	9
	SD	6.307	0.500	1.740	1.740	1.922	0.000
Financial issues	Mean	17.50	2.00	6.50	1.50	3.50	1.50
	N	2	2	2	2	2	2
	SD	2.121	0.000	0.707	0.707	3.536	0.707
After pandemic is over	Mean	12.22	1.22	9.11	4.11	3.33	2.00
	N	9	9	9	9	9	9
	SD	7.429	0.441	1.900	1.900	1.581	0.000
Total	Mean	12.50	1.42	8.58	3.58	3.79	1.92
	N	24	24	24	24	24	24
	SD	7.071	0.504	1.954	1.954	1.865	0.282

Table 22.9 Mean and SD. Analysis: attribute no.5 vs. participants' demographic and health details

A5. Your perception of child's nutrition status		Participants	Boy or girl	Age group	Children classes	Weight status	Juvenile diabetes
Less eating	Mean	8.20	1.20	8.20	3.20	1.40	1.80
	N	5	5	5	5	5	5
	Std. deviation	5.357	0.447	2.280	2.280	0.894	0.447
Overeating	Mean	12.50	1.50	8.17	3.17	5.00	2.00
	N	6	6	6	6	6	6
	Std. deviation	6.348	0.548	1.602	1.602	0.894	0.000
High calorie foods	Mean	16.33	1.33	9.33	4.33	6.00	1.67
	N	3	3	3	3	3	3
	Std. deviation	5.686	0.577	0.577	0.577	0.000	0.577
Genetical	Mean	13.67	1.67	9.00	4.00	3.67	2.00
	N	3	3	3	3	3	3
	Std. deviation	10.017	0.577	3.000	3.000	2.309	0.000
Lack of awareness	Mean	13.43	1.43	8.71	3.71	3.57	2.00
	N	7	7	7	7	7	7
	Std. deviation	8.384	0.535	2.289	2.289	1.272	0.000
Total	Mean	12.50	1.42	8.58	3.58	3.79	1.92
	N	24	24	24	24	24	24
	Std. deviation	7.071	0.504	1.954	1.954	1.865	0.282

Table 22.10 Mean and SD. Analysis: attribute no.6 vs. participants' demographic and health details

A6. Interested in routinely diet counseling		Participants	Boy or girl	Age group	Children classes	Weight status	Juvenile diabetes
Yes	Mean	11.38	1.44	8.81	3.81	3.38	1.87
	N	16	16	16	16	16	16
	Std. deviation	7.302	0.512	1.834	1.834	1.857	0.342
No	Mean	11.50	1.50	6.00	1.00	5.50	2.00
	N	2	2	2	2	2	2
	Std. deviation	10.607	0.707	0.000	0.000	0.707	0.000
May be	Mean	15.83	1.33	8.83	3.83	4.33	2.00
	N	6	6	6	6	6	6
	Std. deviation	5.456	0.516	2.137	2.137	1.862	0.000
Total	Mean	12.50	1.42	8.58	3.58	3.79	1.92
	N	24	24	24	24	24	24
	Std. deviation	7.071	0.504	1.954	1.954	1.865	0.282

Table 22.11 Mean and SD. Analysis: attribute no.7 vs. participants' demographic and health details

A7. Interested in teleconsultation for diet		Participants	Boy or girl	Age group	Children classes	Weight status	Juvenile diabetes
Yes	Mean	12.54	1.38	8.85	3.85	3.85	1.92
	N	13	13	13	13	13	13
	Std. deviation	7.827	0.506	1.819	1.819	1.625	0.277
No	Mean	14.67	1.33	9.33	4.33	2.33	2.00
	N	3	3	3	3	3	3
	Std. deviation	8.145	0.577	2.309	2.309	2.309	0.000
May be	Mean	11.62	1.50	7.88	2.88	4.25	1.87
	N	8	8	8	8	8	8
	Std. deviation	6.116	0.535	2.100	2.100	2.053	0.354
Total	Mean	12.50	1.42	8.58	3.58	3.79	1.92
	N	24	24	24	24	24	24
	Std. deviation	7.071	0.504	1.954	1.954	1.865	0.282

Table 22.12 Mean and SD. Analysis: attribute no.8 vs. participants' demographic and health details

A8. Getting awareness, now you are confident about teleconsultation		Participants	Boy or girl	Age group	Children classes	Weight status	Juvenile diabetes
Yes	Mean	12.73	1.41	8.41	3.41	3.86	1.91
	N	22	22	22	22	22	22
	Std. deviation	7.192	0.503	1.943	1.943	1.910	0.294
No	Mean	10.00	1.50	10.50	5.50	3.00	2.00
	N	2	2	2	2	2	2
	Std. deviation	7.071	0.707	0.707	0.707	1.414	0.000
Total	Mean	12.50	1.42	8.58	3.58	3.79	1.92
	N	24	24	24	24	24	24
	Std. deviation	7.071	0.504	1.954	1.954	1.865	0.282

in 2020. The participants got familiar with the experienced moderator, one of our authors. After that, the questionnaires were sent by emails to fill, followed by the FGD. The process of filling questionnaires was also discussed in the first FGD [24].

22.4.1 FGD Process and Data Transcription

Similarly, all three video conferences were conducted in the same week as three groups of 8 participants in each. We received all the filled questionnaires within the next 7 days from every participant and intimated the next FGD date accordingly. In the second round, everyone participated seriously, and the moderator directed the induction of the whole online FGD. Moderator (one author) first recorded, and subsequently, we as a team transcribed all the words one by one as participants communicated. Four questions were mainly highlighted as most suitable on this round that is: (first FGD round)

A1. "Teleconsultation awareness of nutrition and diet."
A2. "Following any diet by the dietician."
A5. "Your perception of child's nutrition status."
A3. "How many teleconsultations availed so far on a diet."

We transcripted and edited out all content at our convenience, following the technical aspects of non-verbatim transcription. This method significantly extends the readability and clarity of transcripts. The transcription we prepared clearly and unambiguously, cleaning up the words or sounds related to "thinking noises" that were "you know," "I think," "um," "okay," "uh," "er," "like," "ah," "I mean," etc. [25, 26].

Remain three questions were as most pertinent questions on the second round FGD.

A4. "If not teleconsultation, then reason."
A6. "Interested in routinely diet counseling."
A7. "Interested in teleconsultation for diet."

In the third cum last round FGD, we finally interacted and discussed the necessity of a balanced diet through good food that can provide the best nutrition to the child of the respective parent. In this last round of FGD, we concluded only one question, as mentioned below. Most importantly, the moderator and other authors tried to provide the essential awareness and nutritional knowledge on child nutrition that was easy to understand.

The final question:

A8. "Getting awareness, now you are confident about teleconsultation."

In this series of FGD, we can conclude that almost every parent was motivated and positive-minded after getting awareness of a home-based easy, low-cost diet. However, they finally realized that an experienced and skilled dietitian could help diet consultation through teleconsultation during the pandemic. Physical consultation also was encouraged if no such pandemic or time crisis of parents or need for a physical visit. Ultimately, diet consultation is required for every child that should not be stopped or must be started without further delay [27, 28].

22.4.2 Nutritional Guidelines for Parents

Children are most beloved by their parents always. The children's health is more concerned not only by their parents but also by all family members. Fathers are busy with their jobs or business, whereas mothers manage the home and kitchen. Mothers are more knowledgeable about food, ingredients, and the entire cooking process [29, 30]. In urban areas, most parents are working outside of their homes, and there is a growing trend that working parents are busy with their work in a day. Despite work pressure, some of them are interested in spending some time with their children [31].

Moreover, there is a gap in childcare that is total care of a child's nutrition, health, education, and psychosocial well-being. During the COVID pandemic since March 2020, various media such as print, broadcast, social, and other digital media are the knowledge sharing tools from where everyone is getting multiple information about COVID-19 and related health issues [31, 32]. In addition, social media are partly used for discussion and mass awareness of various important social, health, and other problems among friends, families, educational, and business groups [27, 33].

Our research work tried to share the need for awareness of essential nutrition following the information provided in recommended dietary guidelines (RDA). We discussed for the children nutrition under 6–12 years of age that there is 1360–2220 kcal per day. In a day, 16–33 g protein, 550–650 mg calcium, 125–250 mg magnesium, iron 11–28 mg, 4.5–8.5 mg zinc, and 90–100 mcg iodine are minimum required for the Indian children population. In addition, a child needs 35–50 mg vitamin C, 510–790 mcg of vitamin A, and 600 IU of vitamin D [34, 35]. Moreover, protein, minerals, and vitamins must not be deficient in children. In a nutshell, nutrition not only boosts immunity but protects the entire human body through healthy foods. However, at the end of the awareness sessions, 22 parents self-evaluated and subsequently accepted their responsibility for the child's diet and exercises. Despite their busy lifestyles and other factors, they agreed upon easy and affordable access through telemedicine by their smartphone despite their active lifestyles and other factors [27, 28].

22.5 Conclusion

Many people depend on teleconsultation, a part of telemedicine, sitting at home during the COVID-19 pandemic. In this crisis phase, the diet has become a critical factor for all children's proper health. Large numbers of parents living in urban areas are busy with their online work or scaring about COVID infection, resulting in less attention to their children's nutrition. Essential awareness of children's nutrition and telemedicine can change their perception about the non-consultation of diet during the pandemic. Diet is an integral part of telemedicine offered by all the private and public settings at an affordable cost. Therefore, parents need to develop a positive mindset towards periodical diet consultation for various health issues, mainly weight management, diabetes, and other lifestyle disorders, by the easily accessible teleconsultation process during and post COVID pandemic.

References

1. Fairbrother H, Curtis P, Goyder E. Making health information meaningful: children's health literacy practices. SSM—Popul Heal. 2016;2:476–84. https://doi.org/10.1016/j.ssmph.2016.06.005.
2. Al-Ayed IH. Mothers' knowledge of child health matters: are we doing enough? J Family Commun Med. 2010;17:22–8. https://doi.org/10.4103/1319-1683.68785.
3. Covid-19 lockdown means 115 million Indian children risk malnutrition. https://www.new-scientist.com/article/2251523-covid-19-lockdown-means-115-million-indian-children-risk-malnutrition/. Accessed on 25th May 2021.
4. Fact Sheets. KEY INDICATORS. National Family and Health Survey (NFHS-5).2019–2020. http://rchiips.org/NFHS/factsheet_NFHS-5.shtml. Accessed on 25th May 2021.
5. Child and Adolescent Nutrition Status. UNICEF/WHO/World Bank Joint Child Malnutrition Estimates: Stunting, Wasting and Overweight (July 2020, New York). Available at: https://data.unicef.org/resources/dataset/malnutrition-data. Accessed on 10th June 2021.
6. NCD Risk Factor Collaboration 2017. Available at: http://ncdrisc.org/data-downloads.html. Accessed on 15th June 2021.
7. Sharma SV, Chuang RJ, Rushing M, Naylor B, Ranjit N, Pomeroy M, Markham C. Social determinants of health-related needs during COVID-19 among low-income households with children. Prev Chronic Dis. 2020;17:E119. https://doi.org/10.5888/pcd17.200322.
8. Dondi A, Candela E, Morigi F, Lenzi J, Pierantoni L, Lanari M. Parents' perception of food insecurity and of its effects on their children in Italy six months after the COVID-19 pandemic outbreak. Nutrients. 2020;13:121. https://doi.org/10.3390/nu13010121.
9. Bousquet J, et al. Is diet partly responsible for differences in COVID-19 death rates between and within countries? Clin Transl Allergy. 2020;10:16.
10. Das A, Das M, Ghosh S. Impact of nutritional status and anemia on COVID-19- is it a public health concern? Evidence from national family health survey-4 (2015–2016). Public Health India. 2020;185:93. Accessed on 21st May 2021
11. Jayawardena R, Misra A. Balanced diet is a major casualty in COVID-19. Diab Metab Syndr Clin Res Rev. 2020;14:1085–6.
12. Mishra Diabetes (India). National Diabetes Obesity and Cholesterol Foundation (NDOC), and Diabetes Expert Group, India Strict glycemic Control is needed in times of COVID 19 epidemic in India: a call for action for all nutritionists and physicians. Diab Metab Syndrome: Clin Res Rev. 2020;14:1747–50.
13. Maggini S, Pierre A, Calder PC. Immune function and micronutrient requirements change over the life course. Nutrients. 2018;10:1531. https://doi.org/10.3390/nu10101531.
14. Wang B, Li R, Lu Z, Huang Y. Does comorbidity increase the risk of patients with COVID-19: evidence from meta-analysis. Aging (Albany NY). 2020;12:6049–57.
15. De Faria Coelho-Ravagnani C, Corgosinho FC, Sanches F, Prado C, Laviano A, Mota JF. Dietary recommendations during the COVID-19 pandemic. Nutr Rev. 2021;79:382–93. https://doi.org/10.1093/nutrit/nuaa067.
16. Campo SS, Samouda H, La Frano MR, Bohn T. Strengthening the immune system and reducing inflammation and oxidative stress through diet and nutrition: considerations during the COVID-19 crisis. Nutrients. 2020;12:1562. https://doi.org/10.3390/nu12061562.

17. Vadheim LM, Patch K, Brokaw SM, Carpenedo D, Butcher MK, Helgerson SD, Harwell TS. Telehealth delivery of the diabetes prevention program to rural communities. Transl Behav Med. 2017;7:286–91. https://doi.org/10.1007/s13142-017-0496-y.

18. Mattioli AV, Sciomer S, Cocchi C, Maffei S, Gallina S. Quarantine during COVID-19 outbreak: changes in diet and physical activity increase the risk of cardiovascular disease. Nutr Metab Cardiovasc Dis. 2020;2020(30):1409–17. https://doi.org/10.1016/j.numecd.2020.05.020.

19. Suen LJ, Huang HM, Lee HH. A comparison of convenience sampling and purposive sampling. Hu Li Za Zhi. 2014;61:105–11. https://doi.org/10.6224/JN.61.3.105.

20. Halcomb LJ, Davidson PM. Is verbatim transcription of interview data always necessary? Appl Nurs Res. 2006;19:38–42. https://doi.org/10.1016/j.apnr.2005.06.001.

21. Tausch AP, Menold N. Methodological aspects of focus groups in health research: results of qualitative interviews with focus group moderators. Glob Qual Nurs Res. 2016;3 https://doi.org/10.1177/2333393616630466.

22. Sim J, Waterfield J. Focus group methodology: some ethical challenges. Qual Quant. 2019;53:3003–22. https://doi.org/10.1007/s11135-019-00914-5.

23. Burrows D, Kendall S. Focus groups: What are they, and how can they be used in nursing and health care research? Soc Sci Health. 1997;3:244–53.

24. Garrison MB, Pierce SH, Monroe PA, Sasser DD, Shaffer AC, Blalock LB. Focus group discussions: three examples from family and consumer science research. Fam Consum Sci Res J. 2009;27:428–50. https://doi.org/10.1177/1077727X99274004.

25. Krueger RA, Casey MA. Chapter 4: Participants in a focus group. In: Focus Groups A practical guide for applied research. Sage Publications, Inc.., Published online; 2000. p. 63–83.

26. Ochieng NT, Wilson K, Derrick CJ, Mukherjee N. The use of focus group discussion methodology: Insights from two decades of application in conservation. Methods Ecol Evol. 2018;9:20–32. https://doi.org/10.1111/2041-210X.12860.

27. Banerjee S. The Essence of Indian Indigenous Knowledge in the perspective of Ayurveda, Nutrition, and Yoga. Res Rev Biotechnol Biosci. 2020;7:20–7.

28. Vasiloglou MF, Fletcher J, Poulia KA. Challenges and perspectives in nutritional counselling and nursing: a narrative review. J Clin Med. 2019;8:1489. https://doi.org/10.3390/jcm8091489.

29. Bhandari R, Thakur S, Singhal P, Chauhan D, Jayam C, Jain T. Parental awareness, knowledge, and attitude toward conscious sedation in North Indian children population: a questionnaire-based study. Indian J Dent Res. 2018;29:693–7.

30. Daifallah A, Jabr R, Al-Tawil F, et al. An assessment of parents' knowledge and awareness regarding paracetamol use in children: a cross-sectional study from Palestine. BMC Public Health. 2021;21:380. https://doi.org/10.1186/s12889-021-10432-5.

31. Kagan J. The role of parents in children's psychological development. Pediatrics. 1999;104:164–7.

32. Soenens B, Deci E, Vansteenkiste M. How parents contribute to children's psychological health: the critical role of psychological need support. In: Development of self-determination through the life-course. Dordrecht: Springer; 2017. https://doi.org/10.1007/978-94-024-1042-6_13.

33. Banerjee S, Srivastava S, Giri AK. Possible nutritional approach to cope up COVID-19 in Indian perspective. Adv Res J Med Clin Sci. 2020;06:207–19.

34. Nutrients Requirement for Indians. Recommended dietary allowances and estimated average requirements—2020. ICMR-National Institute of Nutrition. India. Available at https://www.nin.res.in. Accessed on 20th June 2021.

35. Longvah T, Ananthan R, Bhaskarachary K, Venkaiah K, Indian Food Composition Tables 2017. National Institute of Nutrition (ICMR). Department of Health Research, MoHFW, Government of India. Accessed on 20th June 2021.

Telemedicine: A Future of Healthcare Sector in India

23

Upagya Rai, Anurag Upadhyay, and Richa Singh

23.1 Introduction

This chapter on telemedicine is written at a time when countries and the entire world are battling a pandemic COVID-19. This pandemic COVID-19 has brought back the spotlight on the healthcare sector in a big way; countries with better healthcare facilities have also had their share of struggles and developing countries with huge populations like India have realized how unequipped and unprepared their healthcare sector is for a situation like this. Today the healthcare sector is an area that concerns everyone, and particularly for a developing country like INDIA. Before this pandemic telemedicine has not had the due it deserved. Only a few countries had regulations put in place as regards telemedicine practices and teleconsultation. It was mostly looked at with skepticism in comparison to in-person visits to the healthcare facilities which were more reassuring and conforming whereas telemedicine lacked these properties [1]. 2020 COVID-19 forced the global healthcare providers and regulatory bodies to look for alternatives cater to the needs of rising concerns across the globe and telemedicine came to rescue be it sharing crucial information related to the virus that was spreading across the continents or catering to the needs of patients in remote villages with bare minimum or no healthcare facilities it was telemedicine that made it possible without risking the lives as it does not require the healthcare provider to reach the individual physically it was all virtual. COVID-19 forced the world to look at telemedicine as an alternative to the healthcare system [2].

U. Rai (✉)
IILM University, Gurugram, Haryana, India

A. Upadhyay
Udai Pratap College, Varanasi, Uttar Pradesh, India

R. Singh
Vasanta College for Women, B.H.U., Varanasi, Uttar Pradesh, India

© The Author(s), under exclusive license to Springer Nature
Switzerland AG 2022
T. Choudhury et al. (eds.), *Telemedicine: The Computer Transformation of Healthcare*, TELe-Health, https://doi.org/10.1007/978-3-030-99457-0_23

23.2 Telehealth and Telemedicine

The World Health Organization says, "Surveillance, health promotion, and public health function" are the components that come together to make what we understand as term telehealth. It comprises a broad variety of technology that involves healthcare resources, services, delivery infrastructure, and the healthcare system as a whole. Telemedicine and telemedicine are used interchangeably, but telehealth is different from telemedicine in terms of scope; telehealth has a broader scope than telemedicine. Telehealth involves both clinical and nonclinical services that are remote and not accessible such as providing training to medical professionals and facilitating the studies of individuals so that they can complete their degrees and courses; if there is a condition due to which they cannot be physically present. Telemedicine and telehealth can be distinguished with the previous being limited to benefit conveyance by doctors as it were, and the last-mentioned meaning administrations gave by well-being experts in common, counting medical attendants, drug specialists, and others. Be that as it may, telemedicine and telehealth have been utilized correspondingly. Telehealth is a broader umbrella, and telemedicine is one of the crucial components under that umbrella (Chironhealth.com) [3].

23.2.1 Telemedicine

As explained by the World Health Organization 2010 [4], telemedicine, which is "healing for a distance," came into being in the 1970s. After it struggled to find a single definition for telemedicine World Health Organization endorse a broader description *"The delivery of health care services, where distance is a critical factor, by all health care professionals using information and communication technologies for the exchange of valid information for the diagnosis, treatment and prevention of disease and injuries, research and evaluation, and for the continuing education of health care providers, all in the interests of advancing the health of individuals and their communities."*

Sood et al. [5] reported that definitions of telemedicine is an ever-evolving field of science, incorporating and adapting to technological advances that change the perspective about the healthcare system in our society. It uses Information Communication Technology (ICT) to make healthcare and information about healthcare accessible to all. According to Sood et al. [5], started to define telemedicine. Domain that involves practice of medicine without the physician-patent confrontation with the help of new technology like audio-visual communication system, evolved over the years the essence of that evolution can bee seen in its changing definitions over the years as presented by Sood et. al., in his paper after reviewing 104 perspectives of different researchers. In 1975, Bashshur RL, Reardon TG, and Shannon GW gave an elaborate definition, according to which telemedicine may be a framework of care composed of six components: (1) geographic partition between supplier and beneficiary of data, (2) utilization of data innovation as a substitute for individual or face-to-face interaction, (3) staffing to perform essential capacities (counting doctors, colleagues, and professionals), (4) an organizational structure reasonable for framework or organize advancement and usage, (5) clinical conventions for treating and triaging patients, and (6) regulating guidelines of behavior in terms of doctor and chairman respect for the quality of care, secrecy, and the like. According to Bashshur [6], telemedicine is a framework to hone the pharmaceutical depending on the utility of broadcast communications innovation in the absence of normal face-to-face interaction between client and healthcare provider. According to Denton [7] "Telemedicine is patient-ware". Preston in [6] suggests that temedicine is a delivery of a healthcare system by physician to patients who are distant using telecommunication and other technological tools as reported by Sood et al. [5].

Sood et al. [5] peer-reviewed available works of literature on telemedicine give us a glimpse into the growing popularity of this topic as the year progressed. In the year 1994, two major definitions of telemedicine were given by Hostetler [9]. Over the years, telemedicine evolved as advances took place; as a result, the definition of telemedicine also evolved and the number of researches done in the area increased exponentially; Table 23.1 gives an account of year-wise names of researchers who worked on the topic of telemedicine and contributed to the existing definition and understanding.

Sood et al. [5] revealed that apart from researchers, various institutions, commissions, and observatories also gave definitions of telemedicine based on their understanding. Few of them are described in the given paragraph so that we can develop an understanding about vast majority of domains that were interested in telemedicine and how it served its purpose to all the stake holders. *European Health Telematics Observatory* defines "Telemedicine is the investigation, monitoring and management of patients and the education of patients and staff using systems which allow ready access to expert advice and patient information no matter where the

Table 23.1 List of contributors to the definition of telemedicine from 1995 to 2006

Year	Contributors of definitions of telemedicine
1995	Perednia and Brown; Merrell; Klein and Manning; Grigsby et.al.; Au et.al.; Tangalos; Chimiak
1996	Petersen, Baune, and Huggins; Wyatt; Villaire; Goldberg; Ried
1997	Kunihiko, Bongsik, and Grace; Kunihiko, Bongsik, and Grace; Baquet; Coiera; Mulliner; LaMay and Craig; Krol; Bashshur, Sanders, and Shannon; Yellowlees
1998	Wootton; Taylor; Schlachta; Morabito; Taylor; Strauss; Jerant, Schlachta, and Ted; Grigsby and Sanders; Buckner; Coiera; Wright
1999	Beolchi et.al.; Rajani and Perry; Craig; Paul et.al.; Bangert, Doktor, and Warren; Garshnek and Burkle; Garshnek and Hassell; Jen-Hwa
2000	Whitten; Gupta and Kant; Currell et.al.; Nagendran et.al.; Bangert et. al.; Garshnek and Hassell
2001	Chun et.al.; Roine, Ohinmaa, and Hailey; Tyler; Bareiss; Miller et.al.; Miller; Maheu, Whitten, and Allen; Patterson et.al.; Wootton
2002	Linkous; Liqiong; Gonzalez
2003	Reichlin et.al.; Demiris; Lymberis and Olsson
2004	Kim; Jones, Banwell, and Shakespeare PG; Spooner and Gotlieb; Menachemi, Burke, and Ayers
2005	Rafiq and Merrell; Pal et.al.; Stain et.al.; Spivack; Miscione; Sood, Bhatia; Smith et al.
2006	Dena and Barbara, Stuart S; Hung and Zhang

patient or relevant information is located." European Commission DG XIII suggests that telemedicine is a quick way to access the distributed and distant medical expertise employing telecommunication and information technology, irrespective of the patient's location or the location of relevant information. Institute of Medicine, National Academy, Press23 explains that telemedicine saying that it is "The use of audio, video, and other telecommunications and electronic information processing technologies to provide health services or assist healthcare personnel at distant sites." Institute of Medicine, National Academies, United States of America (USA) defined "Telemedicine is the use of electronic information and communications technologies to provide and support healthcare when distance separates the participants." National Telecommunications and Information Administration "Employing the rising data and innovations using modern techniques, to pass caregiver and data where it is determined to be, instead of shifting the understanding to centralized places that provides well-being of administrations as well as data. Telemedicine is advancing towards "teleconsultation," In this case doctor counsels the patients after considering the pros and cons, and develops an understanding with the help of a high-tech videoconferencing, followed with a personal interview to empower the online data access." House of Representatives Standing Committee on Family and Community Affairs, Australia, defined "Telemedicine is the practice of medicine and delivery of healthcare between two distant locations by the use of interactive videoconferencing facilities." Report of the International Consultation (WHO) said telemedicine is "The delivery of healthcare services, where distance is a critical factor, by all healthcare professionals using information and communication technologies for the exchange of valid information for the diagnosis, treatment, and prevention of disease and injuries, research, and evaluation, and for the continuing education of healthcare providers, all in the interests of advancing the health of individuals and their communities." Working Group on telemedicine reporting to congress (US) explained telemedicine as a "Situations where the physician and patient are geographically separated and rely on electronic devices in the delivery of healthcare." Information for Health, NSH (UK), defined telemedicine as "Any healthcare-related activity (including diagnosis, advice, treatment, and monitoring) that normally involves a professional and a patient (or one professional) and another who is separated in space (and possibly also in time) and is facilitated through the use of information and communications technologies." Finnish National Research and Development Centre for Welfare and Health reported that "Telemedicine refers to telematics which is as automatic system used for distribution of information that is located in remote places, these systems can be used in healthcare, enable diagnosis or seeking medical help from a faraway place." Association of Telehealth Service Providers defines that "Telemedicine uses electronic communication and information technologies to deliver medical facilities when remoteness isolate the healthcare providers from their patients. It can also be used for imparting educational information to the medical fraternity as well as streamlining the administrative functioning and make it more efficient to support healthcare via videoconferencing." Telemedicine for the Medicare Population is explained as "Telemedicine is the use of telecommunications technology for medical diagnostic, monitoring, and therapeutic purposes when distance separates the users. Modern computer and communications technology can record and rapidly circulate textual, audio, and video information. This quick and easy access might have advocated the use of technology to improve healthcare facilities in rural areas, homes, and in remote an obscure place that lacks proper medical facility or availability of medical personnel." American Telemedicine Association said that "Telemedicine is a tool used to exchange medical information from one place to another via electronic communications to boost patients' health condition." According to Swiss Telemedicine Association, "Telemedicine is an apply telecommunication and information technology in the healthcare apparatus to get the better outcome of a physical disconnection between patient and practicing physician, also between physicians separated by distance." Telemedicine Glossary ITS and European Commission say that telemedicine is "Using the remote medical expertise made available at the place it is needed. Consisting of two domains: First is home care – this works as the care and medical help is provided where it is required using sensors, hubs, middleware. Second is reference centers and cooperative working – this works as a network of medical expertise linked together." Telemedicine Information Exchange, define telemedicine "as the employing of electronic communication to pass on medical data between two physically distant places. Telemedicine refers primarily to clinical or supportive medical practice delivered across distances via telecommunication technology, performed by licensed or otherwise legally authorized individuals." Telemedicine and E-health Information Service, UK, defines "Telemedicine could be a better approach of conveying healthcare permitting an alteration from a centralized benefit to one which is patient-centered resource-efficient and where choices are made at a neighborhood level near to the persistent. The term telemedicine is utilized when alluding to a few applications of data and communication innovation (ICT) to pharmaceutical. A few of these, like teleradiology or 3D reenactment computer programs, are progressed data administration strategies, and although amazingly profitable in contributing to moved forward healthcare, are not telemedicine. We save the term telemedicine for "remote, telematic healthcare," which includes patients more closely in their healthcare process" [5].

Sood et al. [5] have also categorized the definitions in terms of benefits of telemedicine they particularly focusing on; a total of 25 definitions have indicated that telemedicine is a way to "improve access", other 19 of them indicate that telemedicine could be a way to improve adequacy, quality, conveyance, the effectiveness of healthcare administrations, 9 definitions emphasize that telemedicine ensures equality of distribution of healthcare services and remaining 2 focus that telemedicine also helps in lowering the cost of treatment if employed as a medium of treatment. Separated from their accentuation being distinctive these definitions highlight that telemedicine is an open and continually advancing range; it joins unused progressions in innovation and reacts and adjusts to the changing healthcare needs and social settings of social orders. Telemedicine is moving forward and trying to make a clinical supply better, overcoming geological obstruction, connecting the medical professionals and patients who are located in different physical locations to give a better well-being by utilizing the power and magic of information, communication and technology.

23.2.2 Types of Telemedicine

Telemedicine can be classified into three types but with the numerous definitions by now you might know that it is not limited to only three types but these three are major classifications for technical purposes [10].

Interactive Medicine—Exchange between patient and healthcare provider is happening in real-time and also there is compliance to HIPAA.

Store and Forward—Healthcare providers have the permission to share the patients' health-related information with other healthcare providers at other locations away from the patient.

Remote Patient Monitoring—Both the patient and the healthcare providers are at different locations and the caregiver uses mobile medical devices to gather the information related to the patient's health and monitor their health.

23.2.3 History of Telemedicine

Telecommunication technology gave birth to the concept of telemedicine; advances in telecommunication like telegraph, radio, and telephone made it became possible to send information over distance in the form of electromagnetic signals. In the nineteenth century, these communication channels started to gain acceptance as a viable mode of communication. The twentieth century showed a shift in imagining these technologies to have the potential of being applied in the medicine and healthcare sector. In 1952, Science and Invention magazine featured an imaginary invention called "teledactyl" by Dr. Hugo Gernsback. He imagined that the tool described will use the long and tall fingers of a robot and radio and will present the doctor with a video of the patient, then they will use this video feed to examine the patients who are far away. This is the concept that eventually led to the formation of telemedicine that we know of today, i.e., remote consultancies between doctor and patient using video as a tool [11]. In the 1950s educational medical fraternity experimented with the idea of telemedicine; during this process, they shared radiologic images via telephone. In Canada, a Teleradiology system, i.e., a practice of a radiologist interpreting medical images while not physically present in the location, was practiced in the same years the 1950s. In 1959, healthcare professionals at the University of Nebraska used a two-way shared television to transmit neurological examination data to students and by 1964 they had a telemedicine link established with another campus that was 112 miles away. With telemedicine gaining its ground in the beginning, it was mostly used to get access to the rural population. But very soon medical staff and governments started to see the greater potential and a tool to reach even urban populations that have healthcare shortages, patient's health records, medical emergencies, sharing medical consultations without much delay. In the 1960s, telemedicine attracted investment for research and innovation by the US government, NASA, Public Health Department, Department of Defense, and Health and Human Science Department. Space Technology Applied to Rural Papago Advanced Health Care (STARPAHC) in partnership with NASA and Indian Health Services is worth mentioning as it also propelled research in medical engineering and other developments in telemedicine and researches at organizations, medical centers, and universities [12]. Since its inception, the field of telemedicine is evolving every day and advances in technology have worked as a catalyst and transformed telemedicine into an intricate integrated service used in hospitals, homes, private physician offices, and healthcare facilities. Table 23.2 inspired by the extensive work done by Teresa Iafolla [13, 14] gives a glimpse into the history of telemedicine starting from 1924-2016.

Table 23.2 History of telemedicine

History of Telemedicine 1924–2016
1876—Alexander Graham Bell invented the telephone; launched the beginning of an era of telecommunication
1924—Dr. Hugo Gernsback conceptualizes the term 'teledactyle," equipment with robotic claws and a protruded video feed that examines the patient from a distance. It was a fantasy at that time
1950s—Individuals in the medical profession started conducting experiments with close circuit television
1959–1964—Very first interactive video link was created by Nebraska Institute and Norfolk State Hospital
1960s—NASA engages with telemedicine and explores ways to provide healthcare to astronauts in space and improve telecommunication technology
1964—AT & T releases the Picturephone. Designed to transmit interactive video using telephone lines
1967—The first telehealth system was created that connects paraprofessionals to physicians-patients encounters
1970s—Late 1960s and 1970s was a golden age of telemedicine research and expansion in the USA
1972–1975—Space Technology Applied to Rural Papago Advanced Health Care (STARPAHC). NASA partnered with Indian Health Services to deliver remote healthcare to the Papago Indian Reservation in Arizona
1974—NASA tests how to utilize video for telemedicine. Partnered with SCI Systems to study the minimum video requirements to do a remote medical diagnosis
1989—First International telemedicine Project. Launched Space Bridge to offer medical support to Soviet Republic of Armenia after an earthquake
June 25, 1989—The first time a patient was successfully defibrillated by telephone
1989—World Wide Web invention expands the capabilities of telemedicine and changes the world we know
1993—The American Telemedicine Association (ATA) a nonprofit organization is created
1999—Medicare gets in the Telemedicine Game
2000s—Video chat and skype take off, making virtual video chat a reality and an everyday technology for many
2009—American Recovery and Reinvestment Act (ARRA) help stimulate the telemedicine sector. It includes health IT and telemedicine to stimulate business in the industry
2010s—The decade brings rapid expansion in telemedicine as the U.S looks for ways to cut down the cost and provide convenient care for patients
2014—eVIsit Launches! eVIsit team creates a safe space that allows healthcare providers and patients to video chat at anytime, anywhere
2015—Healthcare is now mobile. Pew Research Center reports that in 2015. 2/3 of America is now accessing healthcare information and resources using smartphones and using these resources for research
2020—It is anticipated that telemedicine is a $34 billion industry and plays a key part in modern healthcare delivery

Sourced from: Blog Post by Teresa Iafolla [13, 14]

23.3   Telehealth Regulations

Like any other medical practice, telemedicine is also governed by certain regulations and laws; they are referred to as telemedicine regulations. Telemedicine is growing rapidly as one of the prominent options that make healthcare accessible to many and also reduces the hassle of physically traveling for the consultation. It also makes healthcare accessible to patients who are in remote areas and does not have the means, ways, or reach a decent healthcare facility. With all these points that make a very good argument in favor of telemedicine, it also brings in certain concern among organizations that want to implement telemedicine. Reimbursement of the healthcare provider is a major concern as it varies from one state to another state. In many states in the USA, although there is parity in the payment for services provided under telemedicine, only a selected few will be reimbursed. Patient consent is another point that needs to be looked into in telemedicine regulation. Regulation regarding medical licensing that allows practitioners to provide their services across states also creates concerns and hurdles in the smooth functioning of telemedicine. Telemedicine is a fast-growing field and policymakers and regulators are finding it very difficult to cope with the advances in this field [15].

23.3.1 Benefits of Telemedicine

Advances in telemedicine are beneficial to everyone equally across the continuum. It is changing the way we have understood healthcare all this while. Patients, doctors, and service-providing organizations are gaining benefit from the technological advances happening in the healthcare system. Prominent benefits of telemedicine are increase in revenue, medical professionals can attend to more patients as a result more revenue, the care provider can reach places that are far as a result accommodate more patients. Another benefit is being cost-effective, with telemedicine in existence a practitioner does not need a physical clinic to practice medicine, he/she can run its virtual clinic managing the record of the patients online which is far cost-effective in comparison to maintaining an office space or paper records, convenience; telemedicine is convenient to both the patient and the healthcare provider as it cuts down the travel time, waiting time, convenience cost, etc., getting a second opinion on a critical illness or a second opinion of a reputed expert is now easy due to telemedicine as this can be done using a secure software platform and without physically travelling to that destination, improved healthcare quality it has been reported as another important benefit of telemedicine as with telemedicine the readmission of patients is significantly reduced compared to physical visits because doctors are able to do frequent follow-ups. telemedicine is also beneficial for health care providers as with telemedicine in place a doctor can tap into new technological advances much easily and at lesser cost, they can add different updated modules to the existing software making it more effective, last but not the least patients just love telemedicine especially those who are familiar to the technology and its advances they just love the flexibility, privacy and freedom that they receive with telemedicine [16].

23.3.2 Shortcomings of Telemedicine

There are several benefits of telemedicine but also some shortcomings, downsides telemedicine has when it comes to policymakers, providers, and payers. A gray area that was difficult to keep up as telemedicine is a fast-growing enterprise that brings challenges of technological and practical nature. Disadvantages related to telemedicine are lack of clarity on policies related to telemedicine, fast-paced technology advances and for policymakers it is difficult to modify and change the policies at such a fast pace, Physicians and patients are finding it difficult to cope with this new virtual interaction between the two, another very crucial shortcoming of telemedicne is that there is always a possibility of technological error while detecting a symptom or making a diagnosis. Telemedicine can also be seen as an expensive option in the beginning as it requires setting up new equipment and training the staff that was traditionally trained to handle patients in person. With all these concerns it would be a good idea to consult an expert before a physician decides to shift from physical mode to telemedicine mode as these experts do make things look easier and much more adaptable [17].

23.3.3 Researches on Telemedicine

Grigsby et al. [18] concluded on the effectiveness of telemedicine. The researches on telemedicine initially focused on the way to transmit the data, which involved a gamet of technologies as reported by Perednia and Allen [19] and by Perednia and Grigsby [20]. Minsky [21] research indicated that prominent ways to transfer data were through audio (telephone or radio), images, or in the form of video.

Satava [22] and Kelly [23] talk about the use of Robotics and virtual reality as a medium of data transfer respectively being tested in experiments and other applications. Evidence related to the transmission of data in the form of images in radiology can be traced back to 1972, as reported by Andrus and Bird [24]. Pieces of evidence suggest that diagnostic services like teleradiology, telepathology, and telecardiology can be used to study the application of telemedicine [25–27]. Literature review in telemedicine leads to a realization that the changes in the technology used in the area of healthcare are changing faster when compared to the concerns they cater to. Replication and cross-validation is another major concern that comes to the forefront when we are talking about researches done in the area of telemedicine [28]. Bashshur et al. [29], Park and Bashshur [30], Bashshur and Lovett [31] and Bashshur [32] provide valuable information on telemedicine and its evolution that concerns the researchers and policymakers of today. The viability of technologies that can be used for telemedicine ranges from fax-radio-telephone to printed images-video conferences and consultations. This journey has been long as reported by various researches done in the area of telemedicine [33–41]. Telemedicine has also been tested in space, dessert, and warfare [42, 43], respectively. Others traditional settings for which telemedicine has been tested are homes, care facilities, clinics and hospitals [44, 45]. Researches done have also tested telemedicine for its effectiveness in various domains of healthcare and have found that overall telemedicine is an effective way to provide healthcare facilities to the patients by a registered healthcare practitioner [46]; another research by Houtchens et al. [47] suggests that telemedicine is an effective way to manage patients. The review indicates that telemedicine has come a long way since its conception and is going to play a crucial role in shaping the future of healthcare.

23.3.4 Application of Telemedicine

Telemedicine has made it possible for patients to connect to the physicians who they were not able to see before due to various issues like distance, access, waiting time, work timings, etc.; they can see them now almost without any effort; thus, it is very important to understand the most valuable places where telemedicine can be applied. Obtained data suggest that 75% of the money that is spent on healthcare in the US is dedicated to diseases like cancer, diabetes, and heart conditions. This has led to the focus of physicians and other healthcare providers to create a system where they can monitor the reading of the patients from the hospital and can intervene if required in time. Telemedicine is becoming high-tech, and these medical devices are making it possible for family members to participate and collaborate with the healthcare system. Now conditions like heart rate, blood pressure, and glucose level can be measured at home with the help of a device that is easy to handle and read which was not possible before the advances of telemedicine took place. Another application of telemedicine is using technology to manage the medication of older adults; with the help of technology it becomes easier for the caretaker of the healthcare provider to make sure that the patient has taken the medicine as a result of better recovery and less consultation and visits to the doctor. With telemedicine giving a facility to have the information in digital form, it is easier to share it with another expert from another far-off location. X-rays, blood reports, and other important information can be shared in real-time, and life can be saved. The application of telemedicine can also be seen in places like the emergency room of the hospitals; they are mostly crowded and stressful environments to be in. With telemedicine, we can easily avoid those expensive visits. Telemedicine can also be applied to gather 2nd opinions from the comfort of one's house which is a very convenient way of getting information by just sending once a report online or an image of the report. Telemedicine consultation as an application is not limited to services like medical reports sharing, telemedicine as a service is all has the capability and competence to revolutionize the neonatal intensive care unit (NICU) and intensive care unit (ICU) as well, where the time is of crucial essence. Progress in tele-neonatal intensive care can be of crucial importance as an expert opinion can be obtained in fairly less time, and also without transporting infant from one location to another physically. With the help of a secure video feed experts sitting at a faraway place can guide the physician who is handling the case in person [48]. The same facility can be employed when it comes to ICU or during a surgical procedure where due to time or any other constraint a physician cannot be physically present. Telemedicine can also be applied for follow-ups in almost all cases which make the whole process of healing and recovery smoother and free of hassle like travel and wait. Telemedicine application during disaster relief is another important facet that needs to be focused on and is worth the mention. In times of a disaster usually seen is a crunch of physicians and other healthcare experts; during these times telemedicine can be applied as an effective alternative and also help reduce the crunch of healthcare professionals. It is usually seen that the emergency division of the hospitals reaches its capacity limit very quickly; as a result, the patients are directed to other hospitals only once they reach and find out that there is no space available. Technology can help get this information about the capacity of emergency rooms in real-time; as a result, time, energy, and resources all can be directed towards helping the patient who needs immediate care and attention. Telemedicine is also applicable when we talk about clinics that are in remote areas of the country especially applicable for a country like India; having access to a healthcare provider at a click can do wonders in case of not so complex cases and this can also help people to continue with the symptoms and make it sever where they could have got treatment at a very early stage. Another fascinating application of telemedicine is how gradually your mobile device is changing into a diagnostic tool that can measure your heart rate, blood pressure, oxygen saturation, etc., and can reveal a lot about your health or at least alert you that you need to see a practitioner. Advances in technology have increased the application and scope of telemedicine; it had made possible that just by downloading an app on your mobile you can have access to 24×7 access to healthcare; it also made possible that in scenarios where the situation is critical one can get help in much lesser time than it used to happen before; it also allowed us to transfer data obtained from various test to across the world. Telemedicine application seems to be limitless [49].

Telemedicine is beneficial for primary healthcare, but several specialties can use telemedicine to break time barriers and expand their reach. Mental health is one such area where telemedicine can contribute immensely. Mental health professionals can take sessions from anywhere in the world; they can streamline their practice by using software that helps in organizing the flow of the patients, documentation, and effective time management. Radiology is another area that can leverage the benefits of telemedicine; instead of bringing the sick child to the clinic, pediatrics can use telemedicine as a tool to make sure the visits are minimized to absolute important ones and rest can be done remotely from the comfort of the home. A report published by WHO in 2010 [4] titled "TELEMEDICINE Opportunities and developments" was WHO's second global survey on eHealth. The survey concluded that telemedicine services are far less advanced in upper-middle-lower income countries and services are less established on all the parameters than the countries that are high income. Under the preview of WHO only 30% of the countries who responded to the survey have reported that they have agencies in place for the development and promotion of telemedicine and only 20% stated that they have developed and implemented a national telemedicine policy in their countries. WHO also recognizes the most prominent barrier is the perception that implementing telemedicine infrastructure is very expensive. Few telemedicine setups are expensive but a lot of it is possible by using the existing infrastructure like internet and computer or mobile device. WHO is making recommendations to its member states to invest in cost-effective and multipurpose telemedicine solutions that are feasible and can be applied using locally available ICT infrastructure; there should be an attempt to provide funds to these initiatives under the aegis of integrated health service delivery strategy and member states should work in collaboration with the regional, national, and global government and non-government agencies. WHO also recommends the member states that there should be a discussion among the stakeholder as to how healthcare can be improved using telemedicine and what training should be given to the professionals to make them familiar with the telemedicine solutions.

23.4 Technologies for Telemedicine

According to a blog post by Netscribe [50], the combination of technology and telemedicine gained a high speed during the pandemic. Since the pandemic, it is reported that 60–90% of practicing clinicians are now using some form of technology to reach their clients (American Medical Association). Innovation in the area of technology and medicine is unprecedented and will help optimize the field even after the global pandemic. The advances in technology help healthcare providers to the services more effective, efficient, and transparent; they also ease the overburdened system and reduce the cost and time. In the domain of telemedicine, technology plays a crucial role. Glimpse into the technological advancements shaping the future of telemedicine. Artificial Intelligence (AI) is revolutionizing telemedicine by innovations like care-assistive apps that are operated by AI and don't require human assistance. Predictive algorithms are equipped in translating prescriptions into Electronic Health Records (EHRs) and generating medical reports, thus reducing the burden on healthcare professionals (HCPs). The scope of Artificial Intelligence is expanding in the areas such as teleradiology, telepsychiatry, teledermatology, and telepathology. Another popular way to implement AI in healthcare is chatbots; they help educate the person about symptoms, collect information on behalf of healthcare practitioners, schedules appointments, etc. Augmented and Virtual Reality is the second advancement in the field of technology shaping the future of telemedicine. These tools are equipped to provide real-time data making the virtual diagnosis more efficient and accurate. Augmented and Virtual Reality can be used as a tool in Health tracking, managing, and streamlining the workflow in the hospitals, better collaboration among healthcare providers, diagnosis, and sharing of 3D images for better clarity during virtual consultations. Tele-robots, advances in this area of technology, and their use in healthcare are gaining strength; these robots are now being used for diagnosis, monitoring patients in real-time, inpatient wards, and also in ICUs. Tele-robots are also being tested for postoperative consultation. Internet of Things (IoT) and nanotechnology focus on the interaction between technology and human; nanotechnology-based IoT uses the physiological and health data obtained via apps and other devices to make advances in this area. One such example is Smart pills and bandages; these bandages and pills unlike ordinary bandages and pills also record body temperature, collect a sample of affected tissue for further analysis, and take a picture. Another path breaking innovation in the area of telemedicine is 3D Printing. 3D printing is revolutionizing the aspects of healthcare at the level of bone creation, creation of lung tissues, cartilage, surgery as well as diagnosis. 3D printing can be done using scan reports present at remote places. It would be heartwarming to imagine the prospects of 3D printing when it comes to prosthetics. As these advances are evolving, it is seen that technology and medicine together are here to make the world a better place [51].

23.5 Telemedicine in India

In a country like India, it is no less than a Utopia if every individual has access to a specialist and gets a medical consultation. India's current situation of healthcare is negligible or absent in villages at present whereas, even in suburban and urban areas does not have healthcare facilities available uniformly to all its citizens. Attempts to have specialists practice in villages or suburban areas by giving those incentives have failed. But it is interesting to observe that computer literacy is developing at a very fast pace in a country like India.

Looking at its reach and scope, healthcare providers are now looking at the term "e" as the new avatar that can reach these villages and suburban areas without them physically being present there. It is far easier to set up a telecommunication healthcare infrastructure in remote areas than to set up and deploy hundreds of healthcare specialists in these places. As Ganapathy [52, 53] reported, in India, it was 1997 when Information and Communication Technology (ICT) was used as a tool to provide secondary and tertiary medical expertise in rural and suburban India. A pilot project was launched in a village called Aragonda with a population of 5000 called as Aragonda Project. March 2000 was the year when first 2000 Very Small Aperture Terminal (VSAT) was established. Apollo Telemedicine Networking Foundation (ATNF) is the oldest and largest multispecialty network with 115 centers and 9 overseas centers, providing 57,000 teleconsultations to patients that are 120–4500 miles away ranging from sexual medicine to neurosurgery. 85% of these consultations were reviewed about the existing consultation or report. From 2000 to 2001 a proof-of-concept study that Apollo did was used by the Indian Space Research Organization (ISRO) in making telemedicine a major thrust area. Apollo being a pioneer in this area also played a significant role in establishing a VSAT enabled hospital on wheels. In India telemedicine programs are actively supported by the Department of Information Technology (DIT), Indian Space Research Organization (ISRO), NEC telemedicine program for North-Eastern states, Apollo Hospitals, Asia Heart Foundation, State Governments, and also by certain private organizations. With a long-term objective, the Department of Information Technology who is working as a facilitator is taking prominent leads into potent application and amalgamation of Information Technology in all the important sectors like its development of technology related to telemedicine, initiating telemedicine schemes that are related to specialties such as tropical diseases and oncology, standardization of the processes involved with telemedicine, and building an infrastructure that supports good quality telemedicine services in the healthcare sector. All India Institute of Medical Sciences (AIIMS), New Delhi, Postgraduate Institute of Medical Education and Research (PGIMER) Chandigarh, and Sanjay Gandhi Post Graduate Institute of Medical Sciences (SGPGIMS) Lucknow these three prominent institutes of the country are now connected using telemedicine software developed by Center for Development of Advanced Computing C-DAC, these telemedicine software provide, facilities like telecardiology, teleradiology, telepathology, etc. An expansion plan using these telemedicine techologies includes connecting other medical institutes in Rohtak, Shimla, and Cuttack [54].

Telemedicine network is growing at a much faster pace in India [55]. 2001 was the year when telemedicine as a system was encorporated in School of Tropical Medicine (STM) Kolkata and two state run hospitals, the first in Siliguri District hospital situated in Siliguri West Bengal this hospital inaugurated its first telecoronary care unit and the second telemedicine center was in Bankura Sammilani Hospital, Bankura on 21 July 2001. Others who implemented the telemedicine project were Webel ECS at two Referral Centers, namely Nil Ratan Sircar Medical College and Hospital in Kolkata and Burdwan Medical College and Hospital in Burdwan. Four nodal centers also got roped in for telemedicine practices so that it reaches the remote areas where healthcare facilities were either scarce or absent: Nodal Centers of Midnapore (W) District Hospital, Behrampur District Hospital, Suri District Hospital, and Purulia District Hospital. In association with ISRO telemedicine network is now expanded and it connects 45 remote and rural hospitals as well as 15 super-specialty hospitals. With ISROs effort telemedicine is now reaching areas like offshore islands of Andaman and Nicobar and Lakshadweep regions of Jammu and Kashmir hilly areas like Kargil and Leh, medical college hospitals in remote areas of Orissa, and rural hospitals of mainland states. Narayana Hrudayalaya (NH) Bangalore, Rabindranath Tagore International Institute of Cardiac Sciences (RTIICS) Calcutta, Hewlett Packard and Indian Space Research Organization (ISRO), and also the state governments of all the seven North-Eastern states of India all are sponsoring a non-profitable project of telemedicine. RTIICS and NH will be the hub that will work as a link between these institutes, and specialists from the institution will offer their services free of cost to propagate telemedicine practices in hospitals that do not have coronary care units. Karnataka has already reported a success story as far as telemedicine is concerned with over 10,000 teleconsultations as a part of their pilot project in their next phase; they plan to bring multispecialty facilities to the rural and remote population of Karnataka. These efforts will work as a launching pad for the "HEALTHSAT" to be launched in the future to facilitate the process of telemedicine [55].

23.6 Telemedicine's Perception in India

The process of getting cure or healing is a combination of treatment and the perception about the treatment in the mind of the patient. In this profession, many say that the strong will to get a cure and the trust that the medicines are working in the mind of the patient can do wonders. All this is achieved to a large extent by the human interaction that a patient has with its doctor or healthcare provider. The perception that is formed during these interactions is a combination of several components like human touch (open your mouth, take a deep breath, show me your eyes, checking the pulse rate), consolatory statements like "don't worry you will be fine very soon" (chinta mat kariye aap jaldi theek ho jayenge), patient listening to the problems of patients, in-person follow-up sessions and thought that if something goes wrong I can visit the hospital and be in safe hands. These build a perception of being safe and trustable as far as the treatment process is concerned. Telemedicine in India is still trying to gain trust; individuals seeking healthcare facilities are fully aware that telemedicine is new age technology; it is fast and has a vast reach but there is something that is missing. In India telemedicine is still at a stage where it is finding it difficult to find firm ground. According to research done by Pew research center using data that was published by the World Bank, it was estimated that 134 million people have a purchasing power parity of 2$ or less than that due to pandemic induced recession. With the absence of basic facilities as drinking water, electricity, and primary healthcare, it is difficult to have the focus shifted to advances in telemedicine and encourage people to believe that it is a better alternative. Another hindrance that telemedicine witnesses in India are the rate of diversity in language making it difficult to implement telemedicine as a tool to reach the remote parts of the country; as a result, patients in these areas are not able to develop trust towards a tool which does not speak or understand their language. To change this perception software must be made available that translates the information into patients' regional language. Process must be in place to remove various concerns related to telemedicine and the Healthcare fraternity will have to work towards making patients familiar with the processes and functioning of telemedicine, also what benefits telemedicine brings to them especially to those who are in the remote part of the country. telemedicine as a domain also need to work towards gaining the trust of patients. This process is a long drawn process as both the patients and the doctors are not yet fully convinced that telemedicine can be a substitute to human presence or assurance of physical human touch. Apart from these perceptions building exercises telemedicine needs to work on improving its biological sensors, making cost effective equipment, supported by policy and guidelines that streamlines the process and ensures quality control.

23.7 Humanization of Telemedicine

Keeping the technology human is the most difficult or one of the most difficult things to do. A media report by CNN brought back the spotlight on this matter when a doctor appeared on a live stream and informed a 78-year-old patient that "all the treatment options are exhausted"; this incident was a realization that technology with all its benefits cannot be a substitute to human warmth and compassion and what could be lost if we replace doctors with technology [56]. There is going to be a learning curve to this shift of human touch to technology and healthcare providers need to be aware of this. The power of the human touch has been well documented in various researches done in the area of healthcare. A book titled "In the Hands of Doctors: Touch and Trust in Medical Care" by historian Paul Stepansky expresses that before the nineteenth century the profession of medicine and healthcare was all about touching and patients welcomed their touch, as physicians were integral part of the community. In research published in the International Journal of Complementary & Alternative Medicine, North East Australian rainforest shamans used touch to heal both mental and physical disorders for thousands of years [12]. Nadi Pariksha is a way of diagnosis, uses to read the pulse of the patient, the recording of pulse reveals information about physical and mental conditions [57]. Aboriginals used touch as a key way to learn the secrets of the body and the root cause of the problem. Modern-day research also corroborates and establish the authenticity of these time-tested methods like Nadi Pariksha, These researches also emphasis that fact that if a doctor or medical professional shows compassion towards the patients it reduces the pain, improves the rate of survival, and boosts the immune system. Patient satisfaction and compliance are seen to be better if the doctor shows empathy towards the patient. Researchers have found that human touch can reduce the elevated cortisol level in the patient as a result of stress. Evidences like these gives strength to the fact that touch can human touch play a pivotal role in the process of recovery and healing of the patient. Human touch is an established powerful tool in the process of comforting, diagnosing, and treating patients; human touch is something that every individual craves at a very primal level. Patients are always worried about the intervention of Artificial Intelligence (AI) and other technological advances and intervention as reported by Harvard Business Review report; patients feel that their medical concerns are unique and can be addressed by a machine or algorithm. Various steps can be taken by the healthcare providers to make sure that the intervention of technology does not give an impression that it is replacing human interaction; they need to find a perfect balance and keep a close eye on the nuances that are required to maintain this balance. Patients' experience must not be 100% digital; healthcare providers are sensitive to the emotional needs of their patients, and life-altering news must be delivered by the practitioner who is a living being who can understand and feel the needs of other human beings. Abraham Verghese who is a physician, author, and professor at Stanford University expresses that practices like physical examination are reassuring and restorative and they are at the heart of patient and physician relationships; when a physician is resorting to shortcuts like ordering tests rather than doing a physical examination of the patient and talking to them they are losing on a ritual that is transformational and transcendent and is a core of the relation between the two. Healthcare practitioners must always keep their eye on the goal, i.e., their patients, and keep patients' problems at the center rather than getting distracted by solutions technology can provide. Physicians and the technicians should always be mindful that technology offers tools to make things better but there is always a possibility of errors like misdiagnosis, symptoms that are overlooked or not looked at all as there was no physical examination done by the doctor and there was too much reliance on the lab test results, little or no rapport formation between the patient and the doctor leading to unintended consequences. Human touch is powerful; it is a basic unit to all human experiences; a touch shapes the connection between two individuals; it is a gateway to emotion, trust, and healing. However, one cannot deny the importance of devices like EMR's, devices that track blood pressure, blood sugar, oxygen level, etc. Technology helps the caregiver have a larger reach and make the administrative work more efficient. Healthcare professionals must find a common ground that allows them to blend the advances of technology and the power of the human touch.

23.8   Future of Telemedicine in India

Implementation and innovation of telemedicine in India is a complex task due to factors like demographic differences, differences in landscape, accessibility to technology, and technology literacy. The future of telemedicine is bright; the telemedicine market is growing at a fast pace and is impacting the growth, revenue, market share, and sale of the international economy. Indian government wants to utilize this opportunity to reach the rural areas and bridge the gap formed due to distance and lack of healthcare infrastructure. Rural areas present several problems to both the service provider and the individual seeking those services; telemedicine can work as a bridge between the two and make healthcare facilities accessible to every individual with a basic device like mobile and an internet connection. The year 2018 and 2019 witnessed a significant increase in the telemedicine industry; the inclusion of Artificial Intelligence to identify prospective medical conditions like Asthma attack, heart attack, diabetes, or blood pressure with the help of connected devices that one can wear around the wrist or carry in their pockets was revolutionizing the healthcare at a very fast pace. Facility to reach a doctor over the phone for basic consultation and over-the-counter medicine was able to save many lives and was the first unofficial encounter with telemedicine. The data published in a magazine named Data Labs by Mandal [58] reported that telemedicine is expected to be 5.5 $US Billions by 2025 in India. Telemedicine in India was governed by a statutory body before the pandemic; it was March 25, 2020, due to COVID-19 pandemic government of India has come with guidelines for telemedicine solutions. Any medical professional who is enrolled in the Indian medical register can practice telemedicine in their state and also inter-state as there was no specific regulation. Initially, telemedicine was governed by IT Act 2000; this lacked clarity on several aspects like privacy, security, and the confidentiality of data. In 2003, these guidelines were revised by the IT ministry based on certain recommendations to make the practice of telemedicine in India more conducive. March 2020 saw a major shift in the policy and guidelines of telemedicine; due to COVID-19 pandemic, restrictions of movement impacted the healthcare system and its reach to every individual, and telemedicine played an important role in these testing times. Telemedicine guidelines in collaboration with the Medical Council of India (MCI) and NITI Aayog came up with the Telemedicine Practice Guideline, Professional Conduct, Etiquette, and Ethics Regulation 2020 [15] to enable all the registered medical practitioners to provide healthcare using telemedicine. Telemedicine guideline was an extensive document that includes the definition of telemedicine, how it is different from telehealth, and who all come under the purview of the term registered medical practitioner. The telemedicine guideline document also included details about the scope of telemedicine and also cautions the practitioners that they must refrain from using digital devices and facilities to conduct any type of surgical procedures remotely and refrain from providing consultation outside of the jurisdiction of India. As for tools to be used for telemedicine consultation, the guidelines say the RMP can use any tool that works for them; it can be telephone, video, LAN, WAN, Internet devices, mobile phones, Chat platforms, and messengers like WhatsApp and Facebook messenger to name the popular ones, mobile apps, skype, email, fax, irrespective of the tools; the telemedicine practice and its core principle to make healthcare available to the remote part of the country is paramount. Application of telemedicine can be classified into four categories in India: mode of communication (video—skype, facetime, Audio—Phone, Apps, Text-based—smartphone apps like Practo, General messaging—text, chat, WhatsApp, Facebook messenger, google hangout, zoom); Timing of the information transmitted (real-time video/audio/text interaction or asynchronous exchange of relevant information); Purpose of the consultation (first consult with any RMP for diagnosis/treatment/health education/counseling or follow-up consult with the same RMP); and Interaction between the individuals involved (Patient to RMP, Caregiver to RMP, RMP to RMP, Health worker to RMP).

MCI and NITI Aayog 2020 [15] Guidelines prepared also gave directions related to the use of technology and that can qualify as a potential mode of communication for telemedicine consultation. Video, Sound, and Content (chat, informing, mail, fax, etc.) each have their particular qualities and shortcomings. Rules moreover emphasized that the hone of telemedicine in India ought to depend on the proficient judgment of the enrolled restorative professional. Enrolled restorative experts ought to have the specialist to choose whether a technology-based meeting is adequate sufficient or an in-person visit and audit is required. 2020 guidelines that are established for telemedicine consultation help facilitate the process by abiding to the following given points; the first one is context it means that registered medical practitioners should base their decision of telemedicine consultation on the context that they are presented with, the second guidelne is identification of registered medical practitioners and patients must be known to each other, they cannot be anonymous. The third guideline is the mode of communication the practitioner can use multiple modes of telecommunication based on the convenience, weakness, and strength of these mode communications. The fourth guideline to be followed during telemedicine consultation is that every practitioner must abide by is the consent of the patient before they start the telemedicine practice. The practitioner must obtain explicit patient consent which must be recorded and kept for future purposes. The fifth point is the type of consultation; this is to give clarity on the first time consulting the practitioner or this is a follow-up or had an in-person consultation before moving to teleconsultation. The sixth one is the evaluation of a patient's condition and whether that can be managed by the practitioner via telemedicine or not; based on that judgment the practitioner can go ahead with providing counseling, medical education related to the condition or medicine. The seventh one is patient management; this part involves components like medical ethics that need to be taken care of while engaging in teleconsultation, the importance of data privacy of the patient, and the confidentiality clauses that need to be kept in place as there is more likely that teleconsultation is prone to these lapses. Telemedicine process in Indian now also have to follow a framework, and this framework provides a guideline for teleconsultation between patient to a registered medical practitioner, consultation between caregiver to registered medical practitioners, consultation between health worker to registered medical practitioners, registered medical practitioners to registered medical practitioners and also during emergencies.

Practo, doconline, 1mg, Portea medical providing telemedicine consultation service providers as well as agregators also have to follow certain guidelines if they are operating in India, They must abide to the guidelines suggested by ICMR and NITI Aayog. These platforms must ensure that the patient is consulting a registered practitioner only. These practitioners can be registered with either the national medical council or respective state medical council and comply with them. Platforms also must provide name, qualifications, registered mobile number, and contact details of all the practitioners listed on their platform; any non-compliance must be reported to BoG or to MCI to take appropriate action; they must do their due diligence before listing the practitioner on the platforms; platforms based on artificial intelligence/machine learning must not be used to counsel the patients or prescribe medicines to a patient; only a registered practitioner is entitled to provide counseling or provide medicine only after directly communicating with the patient; technologies like artificial intelligence, internet of things, etc. can assist the registered practitioner but the final prescription or counseling must be delivered by the registered practitioner only. Mechanism to ensure that there is a place to record the grievances of the customer should be there. Any violation of the abovementioned regulation the platform can be blacklisted. The medical council of India and the board of governors can modify the drug list used for telemedicine purposes; these bodies can also give directives and make changes to the existing directives. Telemedicine guidelines must be amended at regular intervals and necessary directions or clarification must be provided from time to time keeping the larger interest of people in mind and approval must be obtained by the Central Government, Ministry of Health and Family Welfare, Government of India [15].

23.9 Conclusion

No creative ability is required to comprehend that telemedicine has the potential to form each little check by gathering clinical information from numerous patients at the same time and thus bridging the distance and increasing the accessibility to healthcare. Teleconsultation has supported the need of all across the globe at the time of pandemic, when it was impossible and scary to move out of our homes due to the lockdown that was imposed as a method to prevent the spread of the virus. The Healthcare system and professionals were overburdened and overwhelmed by the number of patients who required medical facilities. Around such times telemedicine and teleconsultation has relieved the healthcare provider of their huge burden and made it possible for them to reach the person who is in the remote village and has no means to reach or consult a doctor, it was then the telemedicine gave hope and relief to many. With all its concern and shortcomings telemedicine still holds a key to the future of the healthcare system.

References

1. Mahapatra R.. Mass poverty is back in India. 2021, April 07. Down to earth. https://www.downtoearth.org.in/blog/governance/mass-poverty-is-back-in-india-76348
2. TMF: The Medical Futurist. COVID-19 and the rise of Telemedicine. 2020, March 31. https://medicalfuturist.com/covid-19-was-needed-for-telemedicine-to-finally-go-mainstream
3. Chiron a Medical Company. What is telemedicine? 2019, November 4. https://chironhealth.com/telemedicine/what-is-telemedicine/
4. World Health Organization. Telemedicine opportunities and developments in member states Report on the second global survey on eHealth Global Observatory for eHealth series—Volume 2, 2010
5. Sood S, Mbarika V, Jugoo S, Dookhy R, Doarn CR, Prakash N, Merrell RC. What is telemedicine? A collection of 104 peer-reviewed perspectives and theoretical underpinnings. Telemed J E Health. 2007;13(5):573–90. https://doi.org/10.1089/tmj.2006.0073.
6. Bashshur RL. Telemedicine and health policy. Proceedings from the Tenth Annual Telecommunications Policy Research Conference: Telemedicine and health policy, 1993.
7. Denton I. Telemedicine: a new paradigm. Healthc Inform. 1993;10(11):44–6, 48, 50. PMID: 10130474.
8. Preston J. The Telemedicine Handbook: Improving Health Care with Interactive Video. Austin, TX: Telemedical Interactive Consultative Services, 1993.
9. Hostetler S. Modern medicine (using telemedicine). LAN Magazine 1994;9:125–132.
10. Gray GR. What is telemedicine, and how does it work? GoodPx. 2020, October 12. https://www.goodrx.com/blog/what-is-telemedicine/
11. eVisit. What is Telemedicine? 2018, May 5. https://evisit.com/resources/what-is-telemedicine/
12. Olsen R. At the height of digital wellness, are we missing the human touch? Mid City News. 2021, Jan 14; https://medcitynews.com/2021/01/at-the-height-of-digital-wellness-are-we-missing-the-human-touch/
13. See V. What is telemedicine? 2021, January 9. https://vsee.com/what-is-telemedicine/
14. Iafolla T. History of Telemedicine Infographic. 2019, June 4. eVisit. https://blog.evisit.com/virtual-care-blog/history-telemedicine-infographic
15. Board of Governors In supersession of the Medical Council of India. Telemedicine Practice Guidelines Enabling Registered Medical Practitioners to Provide Healthcare Using Telemedicine, 2020. https://www.mohfw.gov.in/pdf/Telemedicine.pdf
16. See V. Telemedicine benefits. 2021, January 9. VSee. https://vsee.com/telemedicine-benefits
17. Wu B. What are the benefits and advantages of telemedicine? 2016, December 19. Healthline. https://www.healthline.com/health/telemedicine-benefits-and-advantages
18. Grigsby J, Kaehny MM, Sandberg EJ, Schlenker RE, Shaughnessy PW. Effects and effectiveness of telemedicine. Health Care Financing Rev. 1995;17(1):115–31.
19. Perednia DA, Allen A. Telemedicine technology and clinical applications. J Am Med Assoc. 1995;273:483–8.
20. Perednia DA, Grigsby J. Telephones, telemedicine, and a rational reimbursement policy. 1995. Under review.

21. Minsky M. Toward a remotely-manned energy and production economy. Cambridge, MA: Massachusetts Institute of Technology Artificial Intelligence Laboratory; 1979. A.I. Memo No. 544

22. Satava RM. Robotics, telepresence and virtual reality: a critical analysis of the future of surgery. Minimally Invasive Ther. 1992;1:357–63.

23. Kelly PJ. Quantitative virtual reality surgical simulation, minimally invasive stereotactic neurosurgery and frameless stereotactic technologies. In: Paper presented at medicine meets virtual reality II: Interactive technology and healthcare conference; San Diego, January 1994.

24. Andrus WS, Bird KT. Teleradiology: evolution through bias to reality. Chest. 1972;62:655–7.

25. Gitlin JN. Teleradiology. Radiol Clin N Am. 1986;24:55–68.

26. Batnitzky S, Rosenthal SJ, Siegel EL, et al. Teleradiology: an assessment. Radiology. 1990;177:11–7.

27. Ho BKT, Taira RK, Steckel RJ, Kangarloo H. Technical considerations in planning a distributed teleradiology system. Telemed J. 1995;1:53–65.

28. Grigsby J, Kaehny MM, Schlenker RE, et al. Telemedicine: literature review and analytic framework. Denver: Center for Health Policy Research; 1993.

29. Bashshur RL, Armstrong PA, Youssef ZI. Telemedicine: explorations in the use of telecommunications in health care. Springfield, IL: Charles C. Thomas; 1975.

30. Park B, Bashshur R. Some implications of telemedicine. J Commun. 1975;25:161–6.

31. Bashshur R, Lovett J. Assessment of telemedicine: results of the initial experience. Aviation Space Environ Med. 1977;48:65–70.

32. Bashshur R. A proposed model for evaluating telemedicine. In: Parker L, Olgren C, editors. Teleconferencing and interactive medicine. Madison, WI: University of Wisconsin; 1980.

33. Sanders JH, Samsor L. Telecommunications in health care delivery. In: Proceedings of the First Symposium on Research Applied to National Needs (RANN); National Science Foundation; 1973.

34. Sanders JH. Increasing productivity through telecommunications. In: Proceedings of the NSF symposium on research applied to national needs (RANN-2); November 1976.

35. Bertera EM, Bertera RL. The cost-effectiveness of telephone vs. clinic counseling for hypertensive patients: a pilot study. Am J Public Health. 1981;71:626–9.

36. House M, Keough E, Hillman D, et al. Into Africa: the telemedicine links between Canada, Kenya and Uganda. Can Med Assoc J. 1987;136:398–400.

37. Wasson J, Gaudette C, Whaley F, et al. Telephone care as a substitute for routine clinic follow-up. J Am Med Assoc. 1992;267:1788–93.

38. Smego RA, Khakoo RA, Burnside CA, Lewis MJ. The benefits of telephone-access medical consultation. J Rural Health. 1993;9:240–5.

39. Rinde E, Nordrum I, Nymo BJ. Telemedicine in Rural Norway. World Health Forum. 1993;14:71–7.

40. Bertrand CA, Benda RL, Mercando AD, et al. Effectiveness of the fax electrocardiogram. Am J Cardiol. 1994;74:294–5.

41. Turner J, Brick J, Brick JE. MDTV telemedicine project: technical considerations in videoconferencing for medical applications. Telemed J. 1995;1:67–71.

42. Pool SL, Stonsifer JC, Belasco N. Application of telemedicine systems in future manned space flight. In: Paper presented at Second Telemedicine Workshop; Tucson, AZ, December 1975.

43. Cawthon MA, Goeringer F, Telepak RJ, et al. Preliminary assessment of computed tomography and satellite teleradiology from operation desert storm. Invest Radiol. 1991;26:854–7.

44. Finkelstein SM, Lindgren B, Prasad B, et al. Reliability and validity of spirometry measurements in a paperless home monitoring diary program for lung transplantation. Heart Lung. 1993;22:523–33.

45. Sparks KE, Shaw DK, Eddy D, et al. Alternatives for cardiac rehabilitation patients unable to return to a hospital-based program. Heart Lung. 1993;22:298–303.

46. Grigsby J, Barton PL, Kaehny MM, et al. Telemedicine policy: reimbursement, quality assurance, and utilization review. Denver: Center for Health Policy Research; 1994a.

47. Houtchens BA, Clemmer TP, Holloway HC, et al. Telemedicine and international disaster response: medical consultation to Armenia and Russia via a telemedicine spacebridge. Prehospital Disaster Med. 1993;8:57–66.
48. See V. Intermountain NICU gets makeover with VSee simple telemedicine. 2013, May 15. https://vsee.com/blog/intermountain-nicu-uses-vsee-telehealth/
49. Grigsby B, Brown N. ATSP 1999 Report on US Telemedicine Activity. 2000. Association of Telehealth Service Providers. https://people.eou.edu/bgrigsby/files/2013/02/TMReport99.pdf
50. https://www.netscribes.com/technology-in-telemedicine/, 2020
51. Tulu B, Chatterjee S, Laxminarayan S. A taxonomy of telemedicine efforts with respect to applications, infrastructure, delivery tools, type of setting and purpose. In: Proceedings of the 38th IEEE Hawaii International Conference on System Sciences (HICSS'05), January 2005, 2005.
52. Saxena G, Singh JP. E-medicine in India: hurdles and future prospects. In: [paper presentation] International seminar organized at The International Institute of Professional Studies, 2003. Devi Ahilya University
53. Ganapathy K, Ravindra A. Telemedicine in India: the Apollo story. Telemed J E Health. 2009;15(6):576–85. https://doi.org/10.1089/tmj.2009.0066.
54. Dasgupta A, Deb S. Telemedicine: a New Horizon in Public Health in India. Indian J Community Med. 2008;33(1):3–8. https://doi.org/10.4103/0970-0218.39234.
55. Bedi BS. Telemedicine in India: Initiatives and perspective, eHealth. 2003, Oct 17. Addressing the Digital Divide.
56. Finnegan J., Landi H. As telehealth tech explodes in use, can medicine preserve the human touch? Fierce Healthcare. 2019, March 19. https://www.fiercehealthcare.com/tech/replacing-doctors-technology-feature
57. Art of Living. (2021). NadiPariksha- precision in diagnosis to heal you. https://www.artofliving.org/in-en/ayurveda/therapies/pulse-diagnosis
58. Mandal S.. Why telemedicine is the next big opportunity in Indian Healthtech.Inc42. 2020, April 16. https://inc42.com/datalab/telemedicine-market-opportunity-in-indian-healthtech/